A Clinician's Guide to Aphasia

A Clinician's Guide to Aphasia

Editor: Adlan Brooks

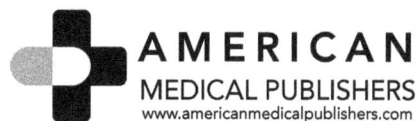

AMERICAN
MEDICAL PUBLISHERS
www.americanmedicalpublishers.com

AMERICAN
MEDICAL PUBLISHERS
www.americanmedicalpublishers.com

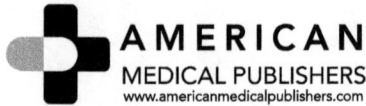

Cataloging-in-Publication Data

A clinician's guide to aphasia / edited by Adlan Brooks.
   p. cm.
Includes bibliographical references and index.
ISBN 978-1-63927-574-8
1. Aphasia. 2. Aphasia--Diagnosis. 3. Aphasia--Treatment. 4. Brain--Diseases.
5. Language disorders. 6. Speech disorders. I. Brooks, Adlan.
RC425 .C55 2023
616.855 2--dc23

American Medical Publishers,
41 Flatbush Avenue,
1st Floor, New York,
NY 11217, USA

ISBN 978-1-63927-574-8 (Hardback)

Contents

Preface

It is often said that books are a boon to mankind. They document every progress and pass on the knowledge from one generation to the other. They play a crucial role in our lives. Thus I was both excited and nervous while editing this book. I was pleased by the thought of being able to make a mark but I was also nervous to do it right because the future of students depends upon it. Hence, I took a few months to research further into the discipline, revise my knowledge and also explore some more aspects. Post this process, I begun with the editing of this book.

Aphasia is a communication disorder that results from damage caused to those portions of the brain which are responsible for language. The disorder may develop slowly and occur suddenly following a stroke or head injury, as the result of a progressive neurological disease. Aphasia impairs the expressions, reading, writing and ability of a person to understand language. Broadly, there are two types of aphasia, namely, fluent and non-fluent aphasia. However, there are several sub-types of aphasia within these broad categories. The most common type of fluent aphasia named Wernicke's aphasia, results from damage to the temporal lobe of the brain. The most significant type of non-fluent aphasia is Broca's aphasia. People suffering from this disorder experience damage in the frontal lobe of the brain. This damage results in right-sided weakness or paralysis of the arm and leg. Treatment of aphasia primarily involves use of therapy which lays emphasis on restoring a person's communication abilities and making patients learn alternate ways of communication, such as gestures, pictures or electronic devices. This book contains some path-breaking studies on aphasia. It explores all the important studies on this disorder in the present day scenario. This book is a resource guide for experts as well as students.

I thank my publisher with all my heart for considering me worthy of this unparalleled opportunity and for showing unwavering faith in my skills. I would also like to thank the editorial team who worked closely with me at every step and contributed immensely towards the successful completion of this book. Last but not the least, I wish to thank my friends and colleagues for their support.

Editor

Agraphia in bulbar-onset amyotrophic lateral sclerosis: Not merely a consequence of dementia or aphasia

Hiroo Ichikawa*, Nobuyoshi Takahashi, Soutaro Hieda, Hideki Ohno and Mitsuru Kawamura
Department of Neurology, Showa University School of Medicine, Shinagawa-ku, Tokyo, Japan

Abstract. The clinical significance and characteristics of writing errors in bulbar-onset amyotrophic lateral sclerosis (ALS) are not clear. We retrospectively investigated writing samples in 19 patients with bulbar-onset ALS without preceding extra-motor symptoms. Co-development of dementia and/or aphasia was also explored and single photon emission computed tomography (SPECT) images of the brain were reviewed. As a result, a high prevalence of writing errors (15 of the 19 patients) was found. Of note were isolated writing errors with neither dementia nor aphasia verified in 2 patients whose dysarthria was mild enough to evaluate spoken language. The remaining 13 patients also showed agraphia, but either dysarthria was too severe to evaluate aphasia or frontotemporal dementia (FTD)-like features co-existed. Of these patients, one who initially lacked dementia subsequently developed FTD-like features. The frequent writing errors were omission or substitution of kana letters and syntactic errors. SPECT images showed bilateral or left-side dominant hypoperfusion in the frontotemporal lobes as a consistent feature. These results show that patients with bulbar-onset ALS frequently exhibit agraphic writing errors and that these are not merely consequences of dementia or aphasia. However, these writing errors may indicate the involvement of frontotemporal language-related areas beyond the primary motor cortex.

Keywords: Amyotrophic lateral sclerosis, writing error, agraphia, syntactic error, frontotemporal dementia

1. Introduction

Motor neuron disease (MND) and/or amyotrophic lateral sclerosis (ALS) has been documented to accompany varying degrees of cognitive impairment more often than previously considered [1,2,23,26,31, 33,40]. Of the cognitive changes in MND and/or ALS (MND/ALS), the most consistent feature has been reported to be executive dysfunction represented by impaired verbal fluency, based on detailed neuropsychological assessments [1,2,23,26,31,33,40]. Besides, impaired confrontation naming has been repeatedly reported with speculation of underlying language dysfunction in MND/ALS [1,2,40], although the af-

fected processes are not completely clear. However, detailed neuropsychological assessments can only be applied for less severely affected patients with MND/ALS. Meanwhile, full-blown dementia associated with MND/ALS, in other word ALS/MND with dementia (ALS/MND-D), is now understood to show typically the feature of frontotemporal dementia (FTD) [28,36], and aphasic syndrome associated with MND/ALS has also been reported as rare cases [4–7,10,17,22,29,38]. In general, dementia is usually recognized to precede motor symptoms, but the opposite observation has also been documented [18, 31]. It is of note that full-blown dementia or aphasic syndrome has been reported most frequently in combination with bulbar-onset MND/ALS [4–7,10,17,22, 23,29,31,33,38], suggesting a strong linkage between such extra-motor and bulbar symptoms.

Bulbar-onset ALS presents with dysarthria which causes early deterioration of spoken language leading

*Corresponding author: Hiroo Ichikawa, Department of Neurology, Showa University School of Medicine, 1-5-8 Hatanodai, Shinagawa-ku, Tokyo 142-8666, Japan.
E-mail: h_ichikawa0527@yahoo.co.jp.

to mutism and make subsequent evaluation of language functions difficult. However, in contrast to limb-onset ALS, the motor functions of the hand are relatively well preserved in bulbar-onset ALS, which enables evaluation of writing as one aspect of language. Nonetheless, the characteristics of writing problems in bulbar-onset ALS have not been analyzed in detail, and we consider that investigation of writing errors may provide further insights into language functions in patients with bulbar-onset ALS. Recently, we reported a high prevalence of writing errors, suggesting involvement of language dysfunction, in patients with ALS/MND-D, most of whom showed the features of bulbar-onset ALS [18]. This observation raised a further question whether writing errors were resultant or partial features of dementia and/or aphasia (dementia/aphasia), or could appear independently of dementia/aphasia in patients with bulbar-onset ALS. In the present study, we investigated the prevalence, onset time, and characteristics of writing errors in patients with bulbar-onset ALS without preceding extra-motor symptoms including dementia/aphasia. We also studied co-development of dementia/aphasia as motor symptoms progress, to clarify the association between writing errors and these conditions. Additionally, we reviewed single photon emission computed tomography (SPECT) images of the brain to assess the potential lesions and pathomechanisms that may underlie writing errors.

2. Methods

2.1. Patient selection

We reviewed the medical records of Japanese patients with MND/ALS who were admitted to our department from May, 1990 to November, 2007, and found 87 patients who fulfilled the clinical and electrophysiological criteria for clinically definite ALS according to the Revised Criteria for the Diagnosis of Amyotrophic Lateral Sclerosis of the World Federation of Neurology Research Group on Motor Neuron Disease: El Escorial revised [41]. Of these 87 ALS patients, bulbar-onset ALS was diagnosed in 27 patients, two of whom were excluded since they had preceding dementia. In the remaining 25 patients, writing samples were searched from medical records, interview forms, diaries, and letters to doctors, as well as from confrontation writing tests. Finally, we employed 19 patients from whom writing samples were obtained. At the time when these samples were written, the patients had the ability to write legible letters with their own hand and could ambulate free from artificial respiratory ventilation

2.2. Evaluation of writing errors

The presence of critical writing errors and the onset-time and characteristics of the writing errors were evaluated in the samples (spontaneous writing and dictation of words and sentences) obtained from 19 patients. To describe these results, we explain the Japanese writing system, which consists of two types of letters: kana (phonogram) and kanji (morphogram). A kana letter represents a spoken syllable, with a strict one-to-one correspondence of sound-to-script. Kana words consist of one or more kana and always have only one phonetic pronunciation; therefore, kana words correspond to regular words in European languages. In contrast, kanji is not used in spoken language. Each kanji letter conveys a particular meaning, but has several different pronunciations. Kanji words consist of more than two kanji letters and usually have one pronunciation attached to the meaning; therefore, Kanji words are comparable with irregular words in European languages. There are 2,000 kanji letters in common use, and these are learned during compulsory education in Japan from age 6 to 15 years old. Today, normal Japanese adults are able to write, read and comprehend these basic kanji letters as well as all kana letters. Generally, a Japanese sentence is written by mixing kana and kanji letters: kanji is usually used for writing most nouns and roots of verbs, adverbs and adjectives, and kana letters are mainly used to write inflectional endings, conjunctions and postpositions (prepositions) that integrate syntax.

The 25 patients in the study had education ranging from 9 to 16 years, and in the premorbid state the patients had ability to write, read and comprehend Japanese letters as well as normal adults. This information about writing ability was confirmed through interviews with their family. The presence of writing errors was defined as three or more repeated mistakes in basic kana or kanji letters, which can be written correctly by students at the end of their first six years of education. To assess the types of mistakes, we evaluated writing errors for both kana and kanji letters in words based on the classification of Sakurai et al. [31]: non-response, partial response, and morphologic, phonologic and semantic paragraphia. Syntactic problems involving mistakes with suffixes or postpositions were also investigated.

2.3. Evaluation of dementia and aphasia

Co-development of dementia and aphasia was evaluated in patients for whom writing errors were found to assess the association of these conditions with the writing errors and to investigate the pathomechanism. Since all the subjects had bulbar-onset ALS, all suffered from dysarthria as an initial symptom followed by dysphagia and atrophy with fasciculation of the tongue. These clinical characteristics sometimes made it difficult to evaluate dementia and aphasia, although the severity differed among the patients. Dementia was diagnosed based on daily activities, and particularly behavioral changes, with reference to the clinical diagnostic criteria for FTD [28,36], and the International Classification of Diseases-10 [42]. To avoid overlooking the possible development of FTD, we focused on behavioral changes including reduced volition, disinhibition, attention deficits, and restlessness. We also performed several neuropsychological tests, including the Mini-Mental State Examination (MMSE), the Hasegawa Dementia Scale-Revised (HDS-R) test, and the Adult Intelligent Scale-Revised (WAIS-R) test for measurement of general cognitive function. The HDS-R is a simple test that is similar to the MMSE and is thought to correlate well with the MMSE [16]. The HDS-R is commonly used to diagnose dementia in Japan, with a score under 20 points (the highest possible score is 20 points) usually considered to indicate dementia. We also used the Frontal Assessment Battery (FAB) as a measurement of frontal lobe dysfunction. Since these neuropsychological tests were not conducted systematically and the timing of the tests was diverse across patients, all examinations were not necessarily performed for all patients. In addition, the tests were executed through writing for some patients whose spoken language was incomprehensible due to severe dysarthria. Aphasia was evaluated if dysarthria was mild enough to allow evaluation of spoken language through spontaneous speech, naming, repetition and auditory comprehension. However, for most patients evaluation of speech was difficult due to the reasons discussed above.

2.4. Evaluation of SPECT images

SPECT images were acquired with ^{99m}Tc-ethylcystinate dimmer (ECD), ^{99m}Tc- hexamethyl propyleneamine oxide (HMPAO), or N-isopropyl-p-[^{123}I] iodoamphetamine (IMP). The images were assessed visually to evaluate the lesions that were potentially associated with the writing errors.

3. Result

3.1. Prevalence of writing errors and its relationship with dementia or aphasia

Writing errors were observed in 15 of 19 patients. We were unable to exclude the possibility that the other 4 patients had writing errors because the number of writing samples was relatively small for these patients. The following investigations were performed only in the 15 patients with confirmed writing errors. A summary of the clinical backgrounds of these patients is shown in Table 1. Of theses patients, 2 were autopsied and the diagnoses of ALS were confirmed neuropathologically (a precise investigation of extra-motor brain pathology is now in progress). The onset age of ALS with bulbar symptoms ranged from 43 to 80 years old (mean: 69.3 ± 8.8 years old). All patients were right-handed. The interval from onset of ALS to the time when the writing errors were first encountered varied from 3 to 40 months (mean: 18.6 ± 13.3 months). In the 4 patients without confirmed writing errors, the interval from onset of ALS to the time when the samples were written was considerably shorter at 3 to 10 months (mean: 7.3 ± 3.1 months).

At the time when the writing errors were encountered, dysarthria was too severe to evaluate speech or the speech was completely aphonic in 10 patients (patients 3–6, 8–12 and 15), thereby rendering a detailed evaluation of spoken language impossible. Prior to the time when the samples were written, aphasia had not been noted by family members, doctors, or other medical staff. In the other 5 patients (patients 1, 2, 7, 13 and 14) speech was mildly dysarthric, but sufficiently comprehensible to allow confirmation of absence of aphasia at the time of evaluation.

Only 2 patients had been diagnosed with dementia by testing with the MMSE or HDS-R at the time when the samples were written. However, 9 patients (patients 7–15) showed varying degrees of behavioral changes that suggested development of FTD. The other 6 patients (patients 1–6) showed neither behavioral changes nor decline in neuropsychological tests, indicating the absence of dementia. Of these patients, one patient (patient 6) subsequently developed behavioral changes, and therefore FTD-like behavioral changes have been observed in 10 of 15 patients during the clinical courses to date. In the other 5 patients, the observation period may have been too short to evaluate dementia or the development of dementia is unclear.

Table 1
Summary of background of 15 patients with writing errors

Patient	Age/Gender	Handedness	Duration from the onset of ALS to writing errors (months)	Aphasia	FTD-like Behavioral change	Neuropsychological tests
1	80 F	Right	15	−	−	MMSE 27; FAB 16
2	68 M	Right	9	−	−	MMSE 30; FAB 16; WAIS-R 92
3	71 M	Right	36	N.A.	−	HDS-R 27
4	68 M	Right	23	N.A.	−	HDS-R 27
5	64 M	Right	6	N.A.	−	HDS-R 30
6	67 M	Right	9	N.A.	−[1]	HDS-R 29
7	71 M	Right	4	−	+	MMSE 23; FAB 12
8*	73 F	Right	16	N.A.	+	HDS-R 26
9*	43 F	Right	40	N.A.	+	HDS-R 19
10	65 M	Right	37	N.A.	+	FAB 15
11	71 F	Right	23	N.A.	+	N.A.[2]
12	80 M	Right	18	N.A.	+	N.A.[2]
13	74 F	Right	4	−	+	HDS-R 24
14	75 F	Right	3	−	+	MMSE 12; FAB 12
15	69 F	Right	36	N.A.	+	HDS-R 26; FAB 11
Mean age, 69.3 ± 8.7			18.6 ± 13.3	Absent in 6	Absent in 6 Absent in 6	

Abbreviations: M, male; F, female; ALS, amyotrophic lateral sclerosis; FTD, frontotemporal dementia; MMSE, Mini-Mental State Examination; Fab, Frontal assessment Battery; WAIS-R, Wechsler Adult Intelligence Scale-Revised; HDS-R, Hasegawa's Dementia Scale-Revised; N.A. not available. Mean ± SD is shown for mean age, and duration at the bottom. N.A. in the aphasia indicates that spoken language was too severely dysarthric to evaluate or completely aphonic at the time when writing errors were encountered (patients 3–6, 8–12, and 15). N.A. in neuropsychological tests indicates that tests were tried but unable to be accomplished. *Autopsied cases. [1]Behavioral change developed 6 months after.

Table 2
Characteristics of writing errors in 15 patients

Types of writing errors	Patients															Total number of patients
	1	2	3	4	5	6	7	8	9	10	11	12	13	14	15	
Kana																
Nonresponse																0
Partial response	+	+	+			+	+	+		+	+	+		+	+	11
Phonologic error	+	+		+	+	+	+				+			+		8
Morphologic error	+						+			+				+		4
Semantic error																0
Syntactic error						+		+		+	+			+	+	6
Kanji																
Nonresponse																0
Partial response			+						+					+		3
Phonologic error	+								+			+				3
Morphologic error	+								+			+				3
Semantic error																0

It is of note that the two patients (patients 1 and 2) whose dysarthria was mild enough to allow evaluation of spoken language showed isolated writing errors without dementia/aphasia. The errors observed in writing did not appear in spoken language and their reading was perfect. In addition, the patients were very polite, well oriented and well aware of their illness, with excellent scores in neuropsychological tests and a Digit Span Forward score of 7, suggesting lack of dementia and attention deficit. These characteristics suggest a feature of "pure agraphia". Subsequent development of aphasia and dementia remains unclear over the short period after encountering the writing errors.

3.2. Characteristics of writing errors

Representative samples of different types of writing errors are shown in Fig. 1 and the characteristics of writing errors observed in 15 patients are summarized in Table 2. As shown in Fig. 1, the observed writing errors were partial response and phonologic and morphologic errors in both kana and kanji. In addition to

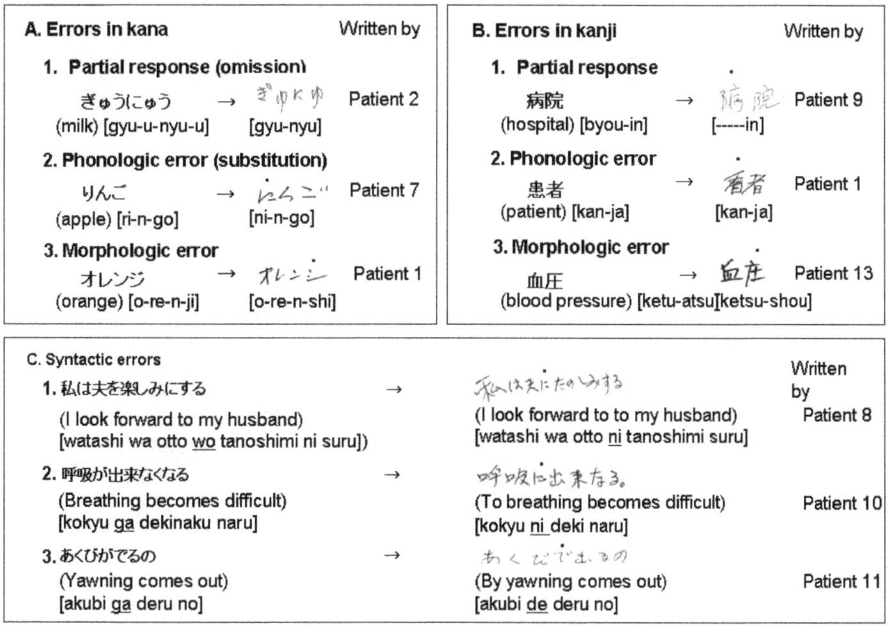

Fig. 1. Samples of writing errors observed in the study. Samples of writing errors in kana (A) and kanji (B) are shown in the upper half of the figure. For each type of error the correct text is typed on the left of the arrow and the samples written by the patients themselves are on the right with the wrong letters indicated by dots for all errors except omission. The corresponding English and the pronunciation for correct and incorrect text are shown below each word in the parentheses and blankets, respectively. Writing errors in kana, included partial responses, with omission of one or more kanas that constitute a kana word (A-1); phonologic errors, in which one or more kanas that constitute a kana word is substituted for other kanas (A-2); and morphologic errors, with omission or addition of a component of kana (A-3). Writing errors in kanji included partial responses, in which part of the kanji components were correct but the written kanji does not really exist (B-1); phonologic errors, with substitution of another kanji that has the same value as the correct component but a different meaning (B-2); and morphologic error, with substitution of another kanji that has visual resemblance to the correct component (B-3). Samples of syntactic errors are shown in the lower half of the figure (C). Mistakes with postpositions (prepositions) are indicated by dots in each sentence written by patients and the corresponding pronunciation is underlined. Mistakes included misuse of a postposition that modifies an indirect object instead of a postposition that modifies a direct object (C-1); misuse of a postposition that modifies an indirect object instead of a postposition that modifies a subject (C-2); and misuse of a postposition that modifies an adverb instead of a postposition that modifies a subject (C-3).

these errors, some patients showed misuse of kana letters mainly for postpositions, thereby suggesting syntactic errors. The most frequent type of writing errors was the partial response (omission) of kana letters observed in 11 patients, followed by phonologic errors (substitution) of kana in 8 patients, and syntactic errors in 6 patients (Table 2). Non-response and semantic errors were not observed and there were no apraxic or spatial features of writing errors in any patients.

3.3. Characteristics of SPECT images

The characteristics of SPECT images acquired from 14 patients exhibited feature of reduced uptake in the bilateral frontal lobes beyond the primary motor cortex (Table 3). Reduced uptake was also observed frequently in the temporal lobes and occasionally in the parietal lobe. Uptake in the occipital lobes was preserved in all patients. Reduced uptake was predominant on the left-side in 8 patients and symmetrical in 6 patients; none of the patients showed right-sided predominance of reduced uptake.

4. DISCUSSION

Cases of ALS presenting with progressive aphasia have been reported as a rare condition and most cases are preceded by aphasic syndrome followed by motor symptoms with predominant bulbar features, namely bulbar-onset ALS [4–7,10,17,22,29,38]. Some writing errors have been mentioned as a part of aphasia [5,6, 10,17,38], but less attention has been paid to writing problems. Our study is the first in which writing errors were investigated in a number of patients with bulbar-onset ALS, and we found a high prevalence of writing errors in these patients. This prevalence may not be generally applicable to patients with ALS due to the study design, but our observation suggests that writing errors are common feature in patients with bulbar-onset ALS. Writing errors were first encountered from 3 to 40 (mean 18.6 ± 13.3) months after the onset of bulbar symptoms, although these errors might have existed prior to the evaluation of writing. At the time when writing errors were encountered, co-development

Table 3
Summary of SPECT analysis

Patient	Area of reduced uptake								Dominant side of reduced uptake
	Right				Left				
	F	T	P	O	F	T	P	O	
1	+	+			+	+	+		Left
2	+	+			+	+			Symmetric
3	+	+			+	+	+		Left
4	+	+			+	+	+		Left
5	+	+	+		+	+	+		Left
6	+	+			+	+			Symmetric
7	+	+			+	+	+		Left
8	+	+	+		+	+	+		Left
9	+	+			+	+			Symmetric
10	+				+				Symmetric
11	+	+	+		+	+	+		Left
12	+	+			+	+	+		Left
13	+	+	+		+	+	+		Symmetric
14	+	+			+	+			Symmetric
Total	14	13	4	0	14	13	9	0	

Abbreviations. F = frontal; T = temporal; P = parietal; O = occipital.

of FTD-like behavioral changes were observed in 10 of 15 patients, but features of dementia were not present in the other 5 patients, one of whom subsequently developed behavioral changes suggesting FTD. Thus, development of dementia after the onset of ALS symptoms was frequent in this study, similarly to a report indicating the possible underestimation of developing dementia in bulbar-onset ALS [31], and writing errors might precede overt dementia. It was of note that two patients (patients 1 and 2) showed isolated writing errors without either aphasia or dementia, indicating features of "pure agraphia". These findings suggest that writing errors can develop independently from or precede clinical manifestation of dementia/aphasia in some patients. Interestingly, Luzzi et al. [25] documented a patient with slowly progressive isolated pure dysgraphia who initially presented with only omission of letters and then developed apraxia of speech after 7 years. The authors speculated that the disease was frontotemporal lobar degeneration without dementia [25]. Some cases with peripheral progressive agraphia have also recently been reported in the context of corticobasal degeneration [12–14], although they had features of apraxic agraphia, in contrast to our ALS patients. Fukui et al. [12] stressed that progressive agraphia can be a harbinger of degenerative dementia, and we believe that the different types of agraphia documented in our study may be an early sign for development of dementia/aphasia in ALS.

Writing errors in ALS, in Western countries, first documented by Ferguson and Boller in 1977 [9]. They reported 2 cases of bulbar-onset ALS, one of whom was neuropathologically confirmed to have ALS, presenting with syntactic writing errors in sentences and spelling errors of words [9]. Although their speech was almost abolished and detailed neuropsychological evaluations were not performed, the features of writing errors were described as "pure agraphia" [9]. However, subsequent descriptions of writing errors in ALS patients did not appear until the late 1990 s [4–6,10,22,29], with a major focus on aphasia. These reports documented progressive aphasia combined with MND/ALS, and provided descriptions of spelling errors or paragraphia [6, 10,29], and syntactic errors [4]. Similarly to our observations, recent Japanese case reports have described the omission of kana, paragraphia, and syntactic errors [17,19,20], and all the patients in these reports appear to have features of bulbar-onset ALS. Among these reports, Kanzaki et al. [20] reported a patient with bulbar-onset ALS, who presented omission of kana but lacked overt dementia, subsequently developed apparent dementia, although his speech was incomprehensible and evaluation of aphasia was difficult. Our study is the first to indicate that partial response (omission) of kana is the most frequent and common writing errors in ALS patients with bulbar-onset, with or without dementia/aphasia.

The SPECT images acquired in the study did not reveal a detailed topographical correlation with each type of writing error, but involvement of the left frontotemporal lobe was a consistent feature in SPECT images. This suggests that dysfunction of this region may be associated with the pathomechanism underlying the writing errors. Considering the anatomical relationship, involvement of the frontal regions located adjacent to the primary motor cortex corresponding to the orolingual area may be important. Historically, the writing center is considered to be located at the foot of the middle frontal gyrus, the so-called Exner area [3,8,37]. Recently, functional magnetic resonance imaging (fMRI) studies have also suggested that the left middle frontal region is crucial to writing, along with other regions such as the intraparietal sulcus, cingulate gyrus, supplementary motor cortex, and posterior inferior temporal cortex [21,27,34]. An interesting study of direct cortical stimulation under awake surgery conducted in patients with a brain tumor showed that writing-specific interference was localized in the posterior part of the dominant middle frontal gyrus and that stimulation of this region elicited writing errors such as letter omission and paragraphia [24]. With regard to syntactic errors, Bak et al. [4] reported that patients with MND presented with impaired syntactic comprehension and selective impairment of verb processing and showed selective pathological changes in Brodmann areas 44 (Broca's area) and 45. Several neuropsychological studies and recent neuroimaging studies have also suggested that Broca's area plays an important role in the processing of syntax [11,35,39]. Other than the frontal lobe, it has also been documented that the posterior inferior temporal cortex is important in spelling [30]. Taken together, these findings suggest that writing errors are closely associated with the language-related frontotemporal lobe.

We recognize several limitations of the study, including the nature of the non-systematic retrospective study, the evaluation of writing errors without well-organized writing tests, the lack of a comparable investigation of limb-onset ALS patients, and analyses of SPECT images only visually and without control data for patients without writing errors. However, a systematic study with various neuropsychological tests is not practical clinically, since at the time of the first visit to neurologists spoken language is already poor and writing is the only way to communicate with many of patients with bulbar-onset ALS. Conversely, it is often difficult to evaluate writing in limb-onset ALS patients due to progressive hand disabilities. Regarding to the SPECT images, most of our patients without writing errors have not undergone SPECT, and therefore we were unable to investigate differences in imaging features between patients with and without writing errors.

Within these limitations, we consider that our results are consistent with previously documented evidence and that our observations provide further information for clinical practice and clinicopathological studies. Regarding to word retrieval impairment, recent studies using fMRI and ^{11}C-flumazenil positron emission tomography have shown that poor performance on confrontation naming correlates with localized dysfunction in the prefrontal region, including the middle or inferior frontal gyrus extending to Broca's area [1,2]. These results indicate that language dysfunction is present in ALS patients, in addition to executive dysfunction, and suggest that this condition occurs due to selective involvement of extra-motor regions, rather than diffuse brain dysfunction [1,2]. These studies were conducted exclusively for patients with limb-onset ALS or without severe bulbar involvement [1,2], but the results are somewhat supportive of our conclusions, and *visa versa*. Respiratory dysfunction has also been argued to influence cognitive functions, but limb-onset ALS patients with respiratory failure do not necessarily develop dementia or aphasia. This does not explain the enigma of the close relationship between dementia/aphasic syndrome and bulbar-onset ALS, and we believe that writing errors are attributable to the primary pathological involvement of selected brain regions, as seen in a report of MND/ALS with aphasia [4], and are not due to secondary brain damage caused by respiratory dysfunction.

In conclusion, our results suggest that writing errors are the common clinical feature of bulbar-onset ALS and are not merely consequences of dementia/aphasia. Such writing errors may develop independently from or precede clinical manifestation of dementia/aphasia, and may involve frontotemporal language-related areas beyond the primary motor cortex.

Acknowledgements

M.K. is supported by a grant from the Core Research for Evolutional Science and Technology (CREST, 17022035) and a Grant-in-Aid for Scientific Research on Priority Areas – System Study on Higher-order Brain Functions from the Ministry of Education, Culture, Sports, Science and Technology (MEXT, 18020027).

References

[1] S. Abrahams, L.H. Goldstein, A. Simmons, M. Brammer, S.C. Williams, V. Giampietro and P.N. Leigh, Word retrieval in amyotrophic lateral sclerosis: a functional magnetic resonance imaging study, *Brain* **127** (2004), 1507–1517.

[2]   S. Abrahams, P.N. Leigh and L.H. Goldstein, Cognitive change in ALS: a prospective study, *Neurology* **64** (2005), 1222–1226.

[3]   S.W. Anderson, A.R. Damasio and H. Damasio, Troubled letters but not numbers, Domain specific cognitive impairments following focal damage in frontal cortex, *Brain* **113** (1990), 749–766.

[4]   T.H. Bak, D.G. O'Donovan, J.H. Xuereb, S. Boniface and J.R. Hodges, Selective impairment of verb processing associated with pathological changes in Brodmann areas 44 and 45 in the motor neuron disease–dementia-aphasia syndrome, *Brain* **124** (2001), 103–120.

[5]   R.J. Caselli, A.J. Windebank, R.C. Petersen, T. Komori, J.E. Parisi, H. Okazaki, E. Kokmen, R. Iverson, R.P. Dinapoli, N.R. Graff-Radford and S.D. Stein, Rapidly progressive aphasic dementia and motor neuron disease, *Ann Neurol* **33** (1993), 200–207.

[6]   M. Catani, M. Piccirilli, M.C. Geloso, A. Cherubini, G. Finali, G. Pelliccioli, U. Senin and P. Mecocci, Rapidly progressive aphasic dementia with motor neuron disease: a distinctive clinical entity, *Dement Geriatr Cogn Disord* **17** (2004), 21–28.

[7]   M. Doran, J. Xuereb and J.R. Hodges, Rapidly progressive aphasia with bulbar motor neuron disease: a clinical and neuropathological study, *Behav Neurol* **8** (1991), 169–180.

[8]   S. Exner, Unterschungen über die Locarisation der Functionen in der Grosshimrinde des Menschen, W. Braumüller, Wien, 1881.

[9]   J.H. Ferguson and F. Boller, A different form of agraphia: syntactic writing errors in patients with motor speech and movement disorders, *Brain Lang* **4** (1977), 382–389.

[10] I. Ferror, C. Roig, A. Espino, G. Peiro and X. Matias Guiu. Dementia of frontal lobe type and motor neuron disease. A Golgi study of the frontal cortex, *J Neurology Neurosurg Psychiatry* **54** (1991), 932–934.

[11] C.J. Fiebach, M. Schlesewsky, G. Lohmann, D.Y. von Cramon and A.D. Friederici, Revisiting the role of Broca's area in sentence processing: syntactic integration versus syntactic working memory, *Hum Brain Mapp* **24** (2005), 79–91.

[12] T. Fukui and E. Lee, Progressive agraphia can be a harbinger of degenerative dementia, *Brain Lang* **104** (2008), 201–210.

[13] M. Grossman, D.J. Libon, X.S. Ding, B. Cloud, J. Jaggi, D. Morrison, J. Greenberg, A. Alavi and M. Reivich, Progressive peripheral agraphia, *Neurocase* **7** (2001), 339–349.

[14] K.M. Heilman, A. Coenen and B. Kluger, Progressive asymmetric apraxic agraphia, *Cogn Beghav Neurol* **21** (2008), 14–17.

[15] A.E. Hills, J.W. Robert, B.B. Peter and A. Caramazza, Neural regions essential for writing verbs, *Nature Neurosci* **6** (2002), 19–20.

[16] T. Hosokawa, Y. Yamada, A. Isagoda and R. Nakamura, Psychometric equivalence of the Hasegawa Dementia Scale-Revised with the Mini-Mental State Examination in stroke patients, *Percept Mot Skills* **79** (1994), 664–666.

[17] T. Hyodo, M. Ikeda, S. Ueno, K. Komori, K. Hokoishi, R Fukuhara and H. Tanabe, A case of motor neuron disease with progressive aphasia and dementia, *Brain Nerve* **54** (2002), 713–718.

[18] H. Ichikawa, S. Koyama, H. Ohno, K. Ishihara, K. Nagumo and M. Kawamura, Writing errors and anosognosia in amyotrophic lateral sclerosis with dementia, *Behav Neurol* **19** (2008), 107–116.

[19] A. Iroi, Y. Okuma, J. Fukae, K. Fujishima, K. Goto and Y. Mizuno, Amyotrophic lateral sclerosis presented with alexia

[20] of kanji and word meaning aphasia, *Brain Nerve* **54** (2002), 903–907.

M. Kanzaki, M. Sato, G. Ogawa, N. Miyamoto, K. Motoyoshi, K. Kamakura and K. Takeda, A case of dementia with motor neuron disease associated with agraphia the omission of kana letters, *Clin Neurol* **44** (2004), 673–676.

[21] K. Katanoda, Y. Yoshikawa and M. Sugishita, A functional MRI study on the neural substrates for writing, *Hum Brain Mapp* **13** (2001), 34–42.

[22] H.S. Kirshner, O. Tanridag, L. Thurman, W.O. Whetsell Jr., Progressive aphasia without dementia: two cases with focal spongiform degeneration, *Ann Neurol* **22** (1987), 527–532.

[23] C. Hoerth, J. Murphy, S. Langmore, J.H. Kramer, R.K. Olney and B. Miller, Are amyotrophic lateral sclerosis patients cognitively normal? *Neurology* **60** (2003), 1094–1097.

[24] V. Lubrano, F-E, Roux and J-F. Dēmonet, Writing-specific sites in frontal areas: a cortical stimulation study, *J Neurosurg* **101** (2004), 787–798.

[25] S. Luzzi and M. Piccirilli, Slowly progressive pure agraphia: A further variant of the focal cerebral degeneration, *Brain Lang* **87** (2003), 355–360.

[26] P.J. Massman, J. Sims, N. Cooke, L.J. Haverkamp, V. Appel and S.H. Appel, Prevalence and correlates of neuropsychological deficits in amyotrophic lateral sclerosis, *J Neurol Neurosurg Psychiatry* **61** (1996), 450–455.

[27] H. Matsuo, C. Kato, F. F. Ozawa, Y. Takehara, H. Isoda, S. Isogai, T. Moriya, H. Sakahara, T. Okada and T. Nakai, Ideographic characters call for extra processing to correspond with phonemes, *Neuroreport* **12** (2001), 2227–2230.

[28] D. Neary, J.S. Snowden, L. Gustafson, U. Passant, D. Stuss, S. Black, M. Freedman, A. Kertesz, P.H. Robert, M. Albert, K. Boone, B.L. Miller, J. Cummings and D.F. Benson, Frontotemporal lobar degeneration: a consensus on clinical diagnostic criteria, *Neurology* **51** (1998), 1546–1554.

[29] W. Rakowicz and J.R. Hodges, Dementia and aphasia in motor neuron disease: an under-recognised association? *J Neurol Neurosurg Psychiatry* **65** (1998), 881–889.

[30] Z.S. Rapcsak and P.M. Beeson, The role of left posterior inferior temporal cortex in spelling, *Neurology* **62** (2004), 2221–2229.

[31] F. Portet, C. Cadilhac, J. Touchon and W. Camu, Cognitive impairment in motor neuron disease with bulbar onset, *ALS* **1** (2001), 23–29.

[32] Y. Sakurai, K. Matsumura, T. Iwatsubo and T. Momose, Frontal pure agraphia for kanji or kana: Dissociation between morphology and phonology, *Neurology* **49** (1997), 946–952.

[33] M.J. Strong, G.M. Grace, J.B. Orange, H.A. Leeper, R.S. Menon and C. Aere, A prospective study of cognitive impairment in ALS, *Neurology* **53** (1999), 1665–1670.

[34] G. Sugihara, T. Kaminaga and M. Sugishita, Interindividual uniformity and variety of the "writing center": A functional MRI study, *Neuroimage* **32** (2006), 1837–1849.

[35] D. Swinney, E. Zurif and P. Prather, Neurological distribution of processing resources underlying language comprehension, *J Cogn Neurosci* **8** (1996), 174–184.

[36] The Lund and Manchester Groups, Clinical and neuropathological criteria for fronto-temporal dementia, *J Neurol Neurosurg Psychiatry* **57** (1994), 416–418.

[37] H. Tohgi, K. Saitoh, S. Takahashi, H. Takahashi, K Utsugisawa, H. Yonezawa, K Hatano and T. Sasaki, Agraphia and acalculia after a left prefrontal (F1, F2) infarction, *J Neurol Neurosurg Psychiatry* **58** (1995), 629–632.

[38] K. Tsuchiya, E. Ozawa, J. Fukushima, H. Yasui, H. Kondo, I. Nakano and K. Ikeda, Rapidly progressive aphasia and motor

neuron disease: a clinical, radiological, and pathological study of an autopsy case with circumscribed lobar atrophy, *Acta Neuropathol (Berl)* **99** (2000), 81–87.

[39] I. Wartenburger, H.R. Heekeren, F. Burchert, S. Heinemann, R. De Bleser and A. Villringer, Neural correlates of syntactic transformations, *Hum Brain Mapp* **22** (2004), 72–81.

[40] P. Wicks, M.R. Turner, S. Abrahams, A. Hammers, D.J. Brooks, P.N. Leigh and L.H. Goldstein, Neuronal loss associated with cognitive performance in amyotrophic lateral sclerosis: an (11C)-flumazenil PET study, *ALS* **9** (2008), 43–49.

[41] World Federation of Neurology Research Group on Motor Neuron Diseases, El Escorial revised: revised criteria for the diagnosis of amyotrophic lateral sclerosis, *ALS* **1** (2000), 293–299.

[42] World Health Organization, The ICD-10 Classification on Mental and Behavioral Disorders; Clinical Descriptions and Diagnostic Guidelines, World Health Organization, Geneva 1992.

2

Crossed aphasia and visuo-spatial neglect following a right thalamic stroke

Lieve De Witte[a], Jo Verhoeven[b,c], Sebastiaan Engelborghs[d,e,f,g], Peter P. De Deyn[d,e,f,g] and Peter Mariën[a,c,d,e,*]

[a]*Department of Linguistics, Vrije Universtiteit Brussel, Brussel, Belgium*
[b]*Department of Communication Sciences, City University, London, UK*
[c]*Institute of Behavioural Neuroscience, Antwerp, Belgium*
[d]*Department of Neurology and Memory Clinic, Middelheim General Hospital (ZNA), Antwerp, Belgium*
[e]*Laboratory of Neurochemistry and Behavior, Institute Born-Bunge Foundation, University of Antwerp, Antwerp, Belgium*
[f]*Department of Health Care Sciences, University College Antwerp, Antwerp, Belgium*
[g]*Department of Nursing Sciences, Faculty of Medicine, University of Antwerp, Antwerp, Belgium*

Abstract. Crossed aphasia in dextrals (CAD) following pure subcortical lesions is rare. This study describes a right-handed patient with an ischemic lesion in the right thalamus. In the post-acute phase of the stroke, a unique combination of 'crossed thalamic aphasia' was found with left visuo-spatial neglect and constructional apraxia. On the basis of the criteria used in Mariën et al. [67], this case-report is the first reliable representative of vascular CAD following an isolated lesion in the right thalamus. Furthermore, this paper presents a detailed analysis of linguistic and cognitive impairments of 'possible' and 'reliable' subcortical CAD-cases published since 1975. Out of 25 patients with a pure subcortical lesion, nine cases were considered as 'possibly reliable or reliable'. A review of these cases reveals that: 1) demographic data are consistent with the general findings for the entire group of vascular CAD, 2) the neurolinguistic findings do not support the data in the general CAD-population with regard to a) the high prevalence of transcortical aphasia and b) the tendency towards a copresence of an oral versus written language dissociation and a 'mirror-image' lesion-aphasia profile, 3) subcortical CAD is not a transient phenomenon, 4) the lesion-aphasia correlations are not congruent with the high incidence of anomalous cases in the general CAD-population, 5) neuropsychological impairments may accompany subcortical CAD.

Keywords: Crossed aphasia, subcortical to aphasia, thalamus, right hemisphere, visuospatial neglect, stroke

1. Introduction

At the end of the 19th century, the so-called Broca's doctrine assigned left hemisphere dominance for language to dextrals and right hemisphere dominance to sinistrals. As an exception to this dogma, Byrom Bramwell [5] introduced the term crossed aphasia (CA) to denote any aphasic syndrome resulting from a cerebral lesion 'ipsilateral' to the dominant hand. Bramwell considered this exceptional phenomenon as a transient condition in right-handers. However, during the following decades several studies documented persistent aphasia in dextrals due to a right hemisphere lesion [22–25,48,58]. When studies with left-handed aphasic patients in the 1950s [26,42] demonstrated that crossed

*Corresponding author: Prof Dr. P. Mariën, ZNA-Middelheim General Hospital, Department of Neurology, Lindendreef 1, 2020 Antwerp, Belgium. E-mail: peter.marien5@ telenet.be.

aphasia in left-handers is the rule and not the exception, crossed aphasia became the synonym for 'crossed aphasia in dextrals' (CAD).

Many hypotheses have been put forward to explain this exceptional anomalous lateralisation of language in the brain. The most frequent explanations of CAD in the earlier literature are hidden sinistrality [19,33,47, 84], absence of decussation of the pyramidal tract [48], familial left-handedness [6,21], bilateral hemispheric language representation [35,50,74] and undetected damage of the left hemisphere [22,24,38,69].

The view on crossed aphasia of the French neurologist Pierre Marie [65], who introduced the concept of subcortical aphasia at the beginning of the 20th century, was fundamental [64–66]. He argued against 'the over-emphasised role of the cortex in speech and language dysfunctions' by stating that lesions in the striato-capsular region, particularly of the lenticular nucleus, often cause aphasic symptoms in CAD-patients irrespective of the hemisphere involved. The findings of Ardin-Delteil et al. [58], Marinesco et al. [22] and Holmes and Sadoff [29] supported this hypothesis by attributing aphasia in their patients to a lesion of the lenticular nucleus. Marie speculated that the increased incidence of pure deep lesions in the group of crossed aphasics was due to a weaker functional lateralisation of the subcortical structures. Habib, Joanette, Ali-Cherif and Poncet [41] reintroduced this idea several decades later. Because of the lack of support for this hypothesis in population studies, Laiacona, Capitani, Stangalino and Lorenzi [42] compared the incidence of deep lesions in crossed and standard aphasia. Laiacona et al. largely based their analysis of crossed aphasic cases on the review of Joanette, Puel, Nespoulos and Rasid [87] and selected the group of standard aphasia patients from the Milan aphasia database of Anna Basso (post-doctoral dissertation of Laiacona, 1985) and the German survey of Willmes and Poeck [36]. Contrary to the hypothesis of Habib et al. [41], Laiacona et al. [42] concluded that the 'prevalence of deep lesions with or without cortical involvement was not higher in crossed aphasia than in standard aphasia (47.22% versus 48.23%)'.

In their review Mariën, Paghera, De Deyn and Vignolo [66] revisited 152 vascular CAD-cases reported in the literature between 1975 and 2003. In order to identify the cases suitable for reliable research, they developed a set of diagnostic criteria for 'vascular CAD' in adults. For the purpose of this paper we added all new cases published after 2003 til 2007 applying the same set of criteria.

The aim of this article is: 1) to report the neurolinguistic and neurocognitive findings in a right-handed patient who incurred CAD following a vascular lesion of the right thalamus and 2) to critically analyse CAD in adults following a pure subcortical lesion.

2. Case report

L.C. is a 70-year-old right-handed nurseryman with seven years of formal education. Medical antecedents consisted of diabetes mellitus type II and paroxysmal atrial fibrillation. He was admitted to the neurological department of our hospital after sudden onset of left-sided weakness, a mild left facial nerve paresis and language disturbances. On admission, clinical neurological examination revealed a co-operative patient with a left hemiparesis, a mild left facial nerve paresis of central origin, dysarthria as well as left visuo-spatial neglect. Examination of coordination by finger-to-nose and hiel-to-knee tests disclosed dysmetria of the left arm and leg that could be explained by muscular weakness. Comprehension was severely disturbed. The patient could not execute simple verbal commands. Speech was incomprehensible as it consisted of semantic jargon. A left homonymous hemianopsia was found on Goldmann perimetry. A CT-scan of the brain on admission did not reveal any structural abnormalities. Four days after admission repeat CT showed a right thalamic lesion. One month post-onset of neurological symptoms, magnetic resonance imaging of the brain (MRI) confirmed an infarction in the median region of the right thalamus. In addition some small hypointense lesions were found surrounding the anterior and posterior lateral ventricles (Fig. 1). A 99^{m}Tc –ethyl cysteinate (ECD) SPECT was performed 13 months poststroke using a Trionix (Ohio, USA) Triad three-detector gamma camera equipped with high resolution fan beam collimators. The projection data were reconstructed by a filtered backprojection using a Butterworth filter (with cut-off frequency of 0.7 cyc/cm and roll-off 5) resulting in trans-axial images with a pixel size of 3.56 mm. In comparison to normal database findings the quantified baseline ECD SPECT study showed a significantly decreased perfusion in the right fronto-temporo-parieto-occipital region and a severe hypoperfusion in the right thalamus (Fig. 2).

The strong right-handedness of the patient was confirmed by a laterality quotient of +100 on the Edinburgh Handedness Questionnaire [75]. After careful inquiry, no family history of left-handedness could be

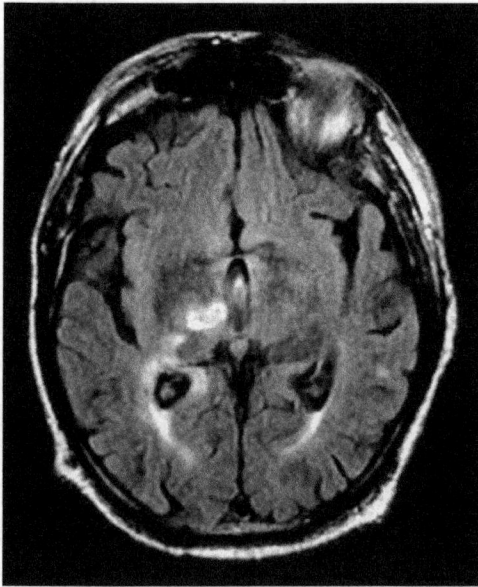

Fig. 1. Brain MRI axial FLAIR slices performed 1 month after stroke disclosing an infarction in the median region of the right thalamus as well as some small hyperintense lesions around the anterior and posterior lateral ventricles.

established. In addition, the patient had no history of brain injury or epileptic seizures and developmental milestones were entirely normal.

2.1. Neurocognitive examination

An in-depth neurolinguistic and neuropsychological assessment was carried out in the lesion phase (3 months post-onset) and the late phase (12 months and 18 months post-onset) of the stroke [18].

Formal language investigations consisted of standardised tests among which: the Aachen Aphasia Test (AAT) [62], the Token Test (TT) [15], the Boston Naming Test (BNT) [16,68] and a semantic verbal fluency task in which the patient had to name as many animals, clothes, vegetables and means of transport as possible within one minute (unpublished norms).

Cognitive functions were formally assessed by means of the Mini Mental State Examination (MMSE) [57], the Hierarchic Dementia Scale (HDS) [49], the Coloured Progressive Matrices (CPM) [28], the revised Wechsler Memory Scale (WMS-R) [12], the Rey Osterrieth Complex Figure Test (CFR) [71] and the Birmingham Object Recognition Battery (BORB) [51].

2.1.1. Neurolinguistic investigations

As shown in Table 1, AAT results for total *language comprehension* were severely defective in the lesion

phase in terms of both auditory and written comprehension. Subtest results additionally revealed a discrepancy between word and sentence comprehension. On these subtests, comprehension was strongly related to the degree of semantic and morphosyntactic complexity: results were worse on more complex instructions.

During the subsequent months, language comprehension gradually improved but still remained defective when tested 12 months poststroke.

One month post-onset *oral language* investigations showed fluent speech characterized by paragrammatic semantic jargon in which prolonged pauses indicated word-finding difficulties. On the AAT confrontation naming tests, a defective global score of 62/120 was found. The patient obtained a normal result for the naming of colours. Naming of simple nouns and compound nouns were severely deficient. Most errors were of the semantic type (8/13 errors): semantic paraphasias (e.g. vlam [flame] for kaars [candle]), semantic neologisms (e.g. 'oliemuts' [oil cap] for muts [cap] and onomatopoeias (e.g. 'tikketikketik' for 'schrijfmachine' [typewriter]).

Twelve months post-onset, a remission of paragrammatic semantic jargon was observed in spontaneous speech. In addition, a normal result was found on the AAT naming subtest 'simple nouns'. Naming of compound nouns improved but had not normalised. Defective test scores on the BNT at 12 months and 18 months poststroke confirmed the persistence of word-finding difficulties the late phase. At 12 months post-onset, the BNT error profile was dominated by semantic paraphasias (8/35 errors) (e.g. stoel [chair] = bank [bench]; kantoor [office] = huis [house]; muis [mouse] = bever [beaver]), semantic neologisms (5/35) (e.g. 'meetboog' [measure bow] = gradenboog [protractor]; 'ijshuis' [ice cottage] = iglo[o]) and circumlocutions (8/35) (e.g. het woont in het water en heeft veel poten [it lives in the water and has many legs] = inktvis [octopus]). In a semantic word fluency task the patient only produced 21 correct items. On the AAT-sentence construction subtest, he obtained a deficient score of 10/30. As demonstrated by the AAT results, repetition was normal.

Test performance at 18 months poststroke showed a decline of semantic errors (21/35 = 60%; 9/26 = 34,61%). However re-examination of the BNT and the semantic word fluency task still revealed pathological scores. A normal score on the sentence construction subtest was found.

Scores on the AAT-subtests of *written language* were severely disrupted in the lesion phase. Deficient scores

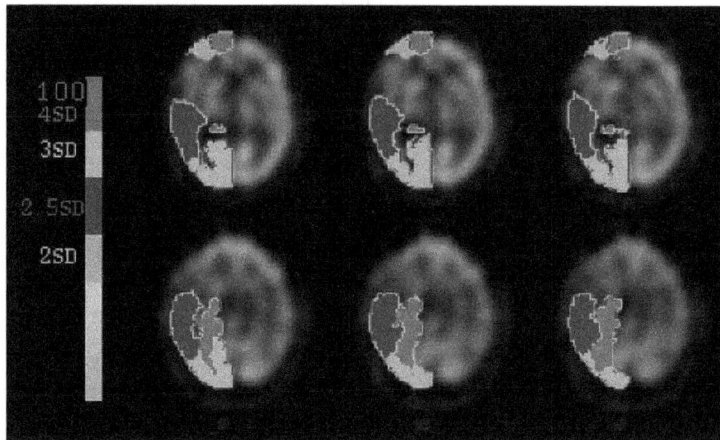

Fig. 2. Quantified Tc-99m-ethyl cysteinate dimmer SPECT performed 13 months post-onset revealing a relative cortical hypoperfusion in the fronto-temporo-parietal region associated with a marked aperfusion of the right thalamus.

were found for 'reading aloud' and 'composing on dictation'. Writing to dictation was characterized by neologistic jargonagraphia. During the late phase, writing had significantly improved: the patient obtained scores within the normal range for the AAT subtests 'composing' and 'writing to dictation'. Reading aloud remained impaired.

From the neurolinguistic assessment presented above, it can be concluded that the aphasia profile was consistent with a taxonomic diagnosis of transcortical sensory aphasia in the lesion phase of the stroke: speech was fluent with a high incidence of semantic and paragrammatic errors. In addition, language comprehension deficits, word-finding difficulties, lexical and graphical disturbances were found but repetition was intact. In the late phase, language comprehension, word-finding and reading had improved but remained defective. Only for writing, normal scores were obtained.

2.1.2. Neuropsychological investigations

As shown in Table 2 a severely deficient score of 18/30 was found on the MMSE [76]. The HDS revealed concentration deficits, a short-term memory disturbance, acalculia, left visual neglect, visuo-gnostic problems and ideomotor, ideational and constructional apraxia. The WMS-R revealed a pathological verbal memory index. Because of the left visuo-spatial neglect, assessment of visual memory functions was not carried out. The patient failed to copy the complex Figure of Rey. Severe left visuo-spatial neglect was also demonstrated on the BORB subtests 'length match task', 'size match task' and 'position of gap match task'.

Cognitive functions were formally re-investigated at 12 and 18 months post-onset. The MMSE score had improved but still remained defective. Verbal memory had normalized. The patient obtained percentile 40 on the CPM. The results on the HDS-subtests assessing 'concentration', 'registration', 'remote memory', 'arithmetics', 'gnosis' and 'ideational praxis' had also normalized. However ideomotor and constructional apraxia persisted. Copying the Rey-Osterrieth Figure was deficient. Re-evaluation of the visuo-spatial functions via the BORB, however, demonstrated remission of left visuo-spatial neglect.

The above-mentioned neurocognitive investigations initially revealed severe left visuo-spatial neglect in association with visuo-gnostic disturbances, constructional apraxia, ideomotor apraxia, ideational apraxia, acalculia, disturbance of concentration and verbal memory. With the exception of ideomotor and constructional apraxia, the cognitive deficits resolved after 12 months.

2.2. Discussion

Following a right thalamic ischemic infarction this patient presented in the lesion phase of the stroke a linguistic syndrome consistent with the diagnosis of crossed transcortical sensory aphasia with neologistic jargon agraphia and alexia. In association with these aphasic disturbances, severe left visuo-spatial neglect was found in conjunction with constructional, ideomotor and ideational apraxia. Although spontaneous speech had normalised at 18 months post-stroke, formal neuropsychological testing still revealed word-finding difficulties, alexia, ideomotor and constructional apraxia. With the exception of alexia, the neu-

Table 1
Neurolinguistic test results in the lesion and late phase of the stroke

Neurolinguistic tests	month 1	month 12	month 18	percentiles 1/12/18	max	mean	SD	ASD month 1	ASD month 12	ASD month 18
AKENSE APHASIA TEST										
Language comprehension total	41	67	–	4/24/-	120	108.5	10.24	−6.59	−4	–
auditory word comprehension	21	–	–	49/–/–	30	26.49	3.30	−1.66	–	–
auditory sentence comprehension	14	–	–	16/–/–	30	26.79	3.41	−3.75	–	–
total auditory comprehension	35	35	–	26/26/–	60	53.28	6.08	−3	−3	–
reading word comprehension	6	–	–	3/–/–	30	28.30	2.29	−9.74	–	–
reading sentence comprehension	0	–	–	1/–/–	30	26.91	3.39	−7.94	–	–
total reading comprehension	6	32	–	2/26/–	60	55.21	4.90	−10.04	−4.74	–
Token Test – number of errors	34	4	–	49/94/–	0					–
Spontaneous speech										
communicative behavior	–	5	–		5	4.63	0.54			–
articulation and prosody	–	5	–		5	4.63	0.67			–
automatisms	–	5	–		5	4.59	0.65			–
semantic structure	–	5	–		5	4.59	0.53			–
phonematic structure	–	5	–		5	4.54	0.56			–
syntactic structure	–	5	–		5	4.41	0.55			–
Imposed speech										
Repetition total	150	149	–	100/78/–	150	144.1	8.07	0.73	0.61	–
phonemes	30	30	–	88/88/–	30	28.91	2.09			–
one-syllable words	30	30	–	93/93/–	30	29.22	1.32			–
words of foreign origin	30	30	–	95/95/–	30	28.94	2.31			–
compound words	30	30	–	98/98/–	30	28.45	2.22			–
sentences	30	29	–	99/96/–	30	28.55	1.90			–
Naming total	62	110	–	38/96/–	120	109.3	8.42	−5.62	0.08	–
simple nouns	16	30	–	30/97/–	30	27.92	2.90	−4.11	0.72	–
colors	26	28	–	70/86/–	30	27.69	1.99	0.85	0.15	–
compound nouns	10	23	–	34/69/–	30	28.04	2.61	−6.91	−1.93	–
sentence construction	10	29	–	38/99/–	30	25.69	3.72	−4.21	0.89	–
Written language total	5	78	–	11/80/–	90	85.52	7.63	−10.55	0.98	–
reading aloud	4	24	–	15/56/–	30	28.95	1.93	−12.93	−2.56	–
composing on dictation	1	28	–	20/89/–	30	28.57	2.75	−10.03	0.21	–
writing on dictation	0	26	–	10/83/–	30	28	3.67		0.54	–
BOSTON NAMING TEST	–	25	34		60	51.60	5.87	–	−4.53	−2.99
VERBAL FLUENCY- semantic	–	21	29			43.40	11.76	–	−1.9	−1.20
animals		6	8							
vegetables		5	8							
clothing		3	6							
means of transport		7	7							

rolinguistic characteristics are semiologically compatible with the typical description of 'non-crossed thalamic aphasia' which is characterized by a fluent jargon aphasia in combination with hypophonia, normal repetition, normal lexical and graphical skills, auditory comprehension problems and word-finding difficulties (perseverations, neologisms, semantic and phonological paraphasias) [3,13,14,30,39,53,55,80,82]. Consequently, the anatomo-clinical configurations are compatible with 'mirror-image' CAD reflecting the expected lesion-behavior correlations [52,86].

The presence of ideomotor, ideational and constructional apraxia also corresponds with the neuropsychological expectations following a thalamic lesion of the dominant hemisphere [73]. Left visuo-spatial neglect in this patient corroborates the general assumption that extrapersonal and personal neglect follows from a non-dominant thalamic lesion. As a result it seems that the right thalamus in this patient subserves both typical dominant and non-dominant cognitive functions.

3. Further analysis of subcortical CAD

The structural lesion in our patient with CAD was located at the subcortical level in the right thalamus and was accompanied by a significantly decreased right hemisphere perfusion. Given the disruption of blood perfusion at the cortical level as evidenced by SPECT, the cognitive and linguistic dysfunctions cannot not easily be attributed exclusively to malfunctioning of subcortical structures. CAD was investigated in detail

Table 2
Neurocognitive test results in the lesion and late phase of the stroke

Neurocognitive tests	month 1	month 12	month 18	max	mean	SD	ASD month 1	ASD month 12	ASD month 18
Mini mental state examination	18	24	–	30	29	1.3	– 8.46	– 3.85	–
Hierarchic dementia scale (HDS)									
Total score	140	173	190	200					
item 1: orienting	10	10	10	10	10	0			
item 2: prefrontal	10	10	10	10	10	0			
item 3: ideomotor	8	8	8	10	9.89	0.31	– 6.10	– 6.10	– 6.10
item 4: looking	6	8	10	10	10	0	– 4	– 2	– 2
item 5: ideational	8	10	10	10	9.98	0.15	– 13.2	0.13	0.13
item 6: denomination	4	5	10	10	9.89	0.31	– 31.9	– 15.78	0.35
item 7: comprehension	5	9	9	10	9.93	0.25	– 19.72	– 3.72	– 3.72
item 8: registration	6	8	10	10	9.67	1.01	– 3.63	– 1.65	0.33
item 9: gnosis	7	8	9	10	9.80	0.40	– 7	– 4.5	– 2
item 10: reading	2	5	6	10	9.78	0.63	– 12.34	– 7.59	– 6
item 11: orientation	10	10	10	10	9.93	0.25			
item 12: construction	4	10	10	10	9.35	1.27	– 4.21	0.51	0.51
item 13: concentration	5	9	9	10	9.11	0.90	– 4.57	– 0.12	– 0.12
item 14: calculation	5	9	9	10	9.11	0.96	– 4.28	– 0.11	– 0.11
item 15: drawing	6	6	10	10	9.24	0.90	– 3.60	– 3.60	0.84
item 16: motor	10	10	10	10	9.61	1.34			
item 17: remote memory	10	10	10	10	9.91	0.59			
item 18: writing	6	10	10	10	9.72	0.58	– 6.41	0.48	0.48
item 19: similarities	8	10	10	10	9.26	1.22	– 1.03	0.61	0.61
item 20: recent memory	10	8	10	10	9.65	0.77			
Wechsler memory scale (WMS-R)									
Visual Memory Index		impossible				100	15		
Verbal Memory Index	68	84	–			100	15	– 2.13	– 1.01	–
Global Memory Index	–	–	–			100	15		
logical memory (A + B)	22	26	–		26				
verbal paired associates (I–III)	3	7	–						
Rey Osterrieth figure (Copy)	–	12	19		36	25	3		
BORB									
length match task – A	12	29	–	30	26.9	1.6	– 9.3	1.31	–
size match task – A	17	28	–	30	27.3	2.4	– 4.29	0.29	–
orientation match task – A	23	24	–	30	24.8	2.6	– 0.69	– 0.31	–
position of gap match task – A	22	36	–	40	35.1	4	– 3.28	0.22	–
minimal feature match	13	24	–	25	23.3	2	– 5.15	0.35	–
foreshortened match	–	24	–	25	21.6	2.6	–	0.92	–
object decision	–	26	–	32	27	2.2	–	– 0.45	–
Raven colored progressive matrices	–	–	19	36	pc 40				

in Mariën et al. [67], who systematically studied 152 CAD cases reported in the literature between 1975 and 2003. However, Mariën et al. [67] did not separately investigate the neurolinguistic and neuropsychological impact of subcortical lesions in CAD. In the remainder of this paper, the Mariën 2004-corpus is extended by all CAD cases reported between 2003 and 2007 (above-mentioned patient inclusive) and the neurolinguistic and nonverbal cognitive impairments associated with subcortical lesions will be reviewed.

3.1. Methods

Given the rarity of CAD, we are inclined to follow the plea of Coppens and Hungerford [61] to avoid un-

necessarily strict inclusion criteria. However, less stringent diagnostic criteria render several case-reports ambiguous and hence useless for drawing general conclusions, in spite of the often illuminating insights presented in the discussion of these cases. Therefore, it seems appropriate to adopt the more rigorous algorithm, defining the diagnostic criteria for CAD, as described by Mariën et al. [67] for the classification of 'vascular CAD' in adults. This algorithm is based on the following 5 criteria: 1) clear-cut evidence of aphasia, 2) evidence of natural (i.e. not shifted) right-handedness, documented by a formal test, 3) evidence of lesions strictly confined to the right hemisphere, leaving the left hemisphere structurally intact, 4) absence of familial left-handedness or ambidexterity, and 5) no his-

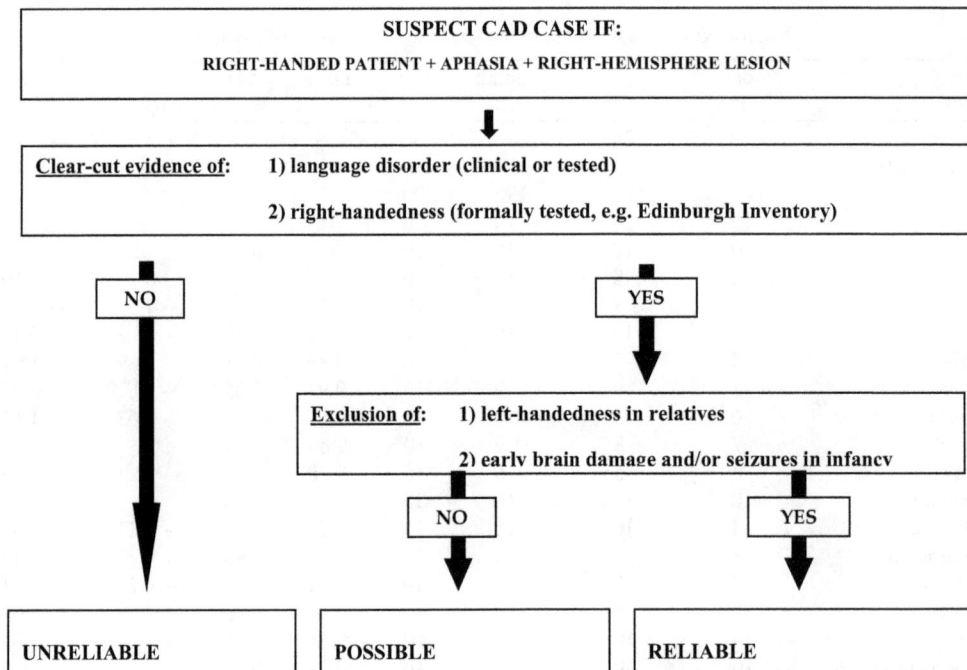

Fig. 3. Algorithm of diagnostic criteria for vascular CAD in adults [67].

tory of early brain damage and/or seizures in child-hood (Fig. 3). On the basis of this algorithm, Mariën et al. [67] classified 152 vascular CAD-cases for the period 1975–2003 into three categories: 1) unreliable CAD-cases ($n = 85$), 2) possible CAD-cases ($n = 18$) and 3) reliable CAD-cases ($n = 49$). For the present investigation, 23 vascular cases were added who were reported between 2003 and 2007 (this patient inclu-sive) and the same criteria were applied as in Mariën et al. [67] (cfr. Appendix 1: classification of adults CAD-cases with a vascular etiology 1975–2007).

From this corpus of 176 cases, only the CAD-cases with pure subcortical lesions were selected for fur-ther analysis. Subcortical lesion localisation was based on structural brain imaging data (CT/MRI). Unreliable subcortical CAD-cases were excluded from further in-vestigation because of: 1) absence of clear-cut evi-dence of right-handedness ($n = 15$) (case nrs. 1–3, 5–10, 12, 16–18, 20, 21) or 2) uncertainty about the structural integrity of the left hemisphere ($n = 1$) (case nr. 24) (see Appendix 2). A detailed analysis of neu-rolinguistic and nonverbal cognitive impairments was carried out in the group of 'possible' ($n = 2$) (case nrs. 11, 15) and 'reliable' ($n = 7$) (case nrs. 4, 13, 14, 19, 22, 23, 25) CAD with an isolated subcortical lesion (see Appendix 3, Appendix 4). Language was analyzed in terms of six linguistic parameters: 1) oral verbal fluency, 2) auditory-verbal comprehension, 3) repetition, 4) naming, 5) reading and 6) writing. The

degree of impairment was expressed on a four-point scale (severe $= +++$, moderate $= ++$, mild $= +$ and none $= 0$). The taxonomic diagnosis of the case-reports was also checked. Whenever the case-reports lacked a taxonomic label, it was attempted to classify the type of aphasia using the six linguistic parameters mentioned above. In the quantitative analysis of apha-sia, the following measures were considered: 1) total severity (range from zero to 18: 1 to 6 indicating mild aphasia, 7 to 12 moderate and 13 to 18 severe aphasia), 2) oral versus written language dissociation and 3) lan-guage recovery. Anatomo-clinical correlations were analysed in cases documented by linguistic data in the lesion phase. An attempt was made to divide the sub-cortical CAD-cases into 'mirror-image' and 'anoma-lous' cases [52,86]. Cases with a lesion-aphasia profile comparable to those following an analogous lesion in the left hemisphere were identified as 'mirror-image' cases. Cases with an unexpected lesion-aphasia corre-lation were considered as 'anomalous' cases. An anal-ysis of nonverbal disorders in a time frame model was not possible because the original case-reports did not systematically describe the deficits on a temporal basis. Consequently, analysis was restricted to a list marking the absence or presence of a deficit.

3.2. Results

On the basis of the paradigm developed in Mariën et al., 97 out of 176 cases ($= 55.1\%$) were identified as 'unreliable CAD', 22 (= 12.5%) were considered as 'possible CAD' and 57 (= 32.4%) emerged as 'reliable CAD' (Appendix 1). Out of the 176 cases, 151 cases (= 85.8%) (case nrs. 26–176) had cortico-subcortical lesions while 25 patients (= 14.2%) (case numbers 1–25) had isolated subcortical damage (Appendix 2). Focal thalamic damage was only found in four patients (= 2.3%) (case nrs. 6, 8, 21, 25). Sixteen pure subcortical CAD cases (= 64%) were classified as 'unreliable (case nrs. 1–3, 5–10, 12, 16–18, 20, 21, 24). Nine patients (= 36%) were identified as 'possible' ($n = 2$) (case nrs. 11, 15) or 'reliable' subcortical CAD-cases ($n = 7$) (case nrs. 4, 13, 14, 19, 22, 23, 25). The reliable subcortical CAD patients will be further analysed in terms of their demographic, neurolinguistic, and neuropsychologic characteristics.

3.2.1. Demographic characteristics

The nine reliable CAD cases with subcortical damage who were selected for further analysis (see Appendices 3 and 4) had a mean age of 65.5 years (range 38–79 years, SD = 12.06). Five out of 9 patients were men (= 55.5%) and four women (= 44.5%).

3.2.2. Neurolinguistic characteristics

Neurolinguistically, fluent aphasia ($n = 4$) (case nrs. 4, 14, 15, 25) was found almost as frequently as nonfluent aphasia ($n = 3$) (case nrs. 13, 19, 22). In two cases (case nrs. 11, 23), nonfluent aphasia was reported in the acute phase but no follow-up data were provided.

With respect to the clinical type of aphasia in the lesion phase, four patients (case nrs. 13, 19, 22, 25) presented with transcortical aphasia and one patient with Wernicke aphasia (case nr. 4). In two patients (case nrs. 14, 15) there was no indication of aphasia. The case of Deleval and Léonard (case nr. 11) presented with Broca-aphasia in the acute phase but no follow-up data were provided.

Quantitative analysis could be carried out for total severity of linguistic impairment and analysis of oral versus written language was possible in six cases (case nrs. 4, 14, 15, 19, 22 25). Out of six cases, three cases (case nrs. 11, 13, 23) were excluded because of the absence of lesion phase data.

Aphasia in the lesion phase was moderate in three cases (case nrs. 4, 22, 25) and severe in one case (case nr. 19). Two patients (case nrs. 14, 15) had no aphasia. In this small group of reliable subcortical CAD-cases, 3 patients (3/6) (case nrs. 19, 22, 25) were more severely impaired in written than oral language.

'Language recovery' could not be analysed because of the limited number of case-reports ($n = 4$) (case nrs. 4, 13, 22, 25) providing a complete description of the aphasia in the lesion and the late phase (Appendix 3).

As to the lesion site-aphasia correlation, four patients were excluded because of a lack of data (case nrs. 11, 23) and because of the absence of aphasia during the acute phase (case nrs. 14, 15). Out of the five remaining cases, four patients (case nrs. 13, 19, 22, 25) presented a 'mirror-image' type, consistent with the lesion-aphasia relationships in uncrossed aphasia. The case of Colombo et al. (case nr. 4) belongs to the 'anomalous' CAD group as it violates classical lesion-aphasia expectations.

3.2.3. Neuropsychological characteristics

As shown in Appendix 4, a variety of nonverbal disorders such as dysprosody, visual neglect, constructional, ideomotor, ideational and oral apraxia, acalculia as well as impairment of memory, orientation and nonverbal intelligence have been reported in the group of possible and reliable subcortical CAD-cases (case nrs. 4, 11, 13–15, 19, 22, 23, 25).

3.2.3.1. Prosody

In five (case nrs. 13, 14, 19, 22, 25) out of the nine subcortical CAD-cases, prosodic impairment was reported. Four cases (case nrs. 13, 14, 19, 22) presented dysprosodia.

3.2.3.2. Visuo-spatial neglect

Left-sided visuo-spatial neglect was investigated in eight patients (case nrs. 4, 11, 13-15, 19, 22, 25) of whom five (case nrs. 4, 13, 19, 22, 25) presented this disorder.

3.2.3.3. Constructional apraxia

Constructional apraxia was examined in six cases (case nrs. 4, 11, 15, 19, 22, 25) all of which presented this disorder with the exception of the case of Gomez-Tortosa et al. (case nr. 15).

3.2.3.4. Ideomotor, ideational and oral apraxia

Ideomotor praxis was assessed in eight subcortical CAD-cases (case nrs. 4, 11, 13, 14, 15, 19, 22, 25) of which three (case nrs. 4, 13, 25) demonstrated ideomotor apraxia. Ideational praxis was described in seven cases (case nrs. 4, 11, 13, 15, 19, 22, 25). In three (case nrs. 4, 19, 25) out of the seven cases, ideational apraxia was found. In seven (case nrs. 4, 13-15, 19, 22, 25) out of all subcortical CAD-cases, a specific statement was made about oral praxis. Two (case nrs. 4, 13) of them had oral apraxia.

3.2.3.5. Arithmetics

Arithmetics was only investigated in two patients (case nrs. 19, 25) of whom both presented acalculia.

3.2.3.6. Other cognitive domains

In five (case nrs. 4, 11, 13, 15, 25) out of the six cases (case nrs. 4,11, 13, 15, 22, 25) in which additional neuropsychological domains were investigated anosognosia, concentration and memory deficits were described.

3.3. Discussion

This review shows that subcortical vascular CAD ($n = 25$) occurs in 14.2% of the total corpus of vascular CAD cases ($n = 176$) published between 1975–2007. This finding strongly contradicts the hypothesis of Habib et al. [41] which postulates that pure subcortical lesions are overrepresented in the group of crossed aphasia patients. According to the paradigm of Mariën et al. [67], nine 'possible and reliable' subcortical CAD-cases were analyzed. The demographic data of this small group (mean age: 65.4; gender: 5 men, 4 women) are consistent with the general findings in the entire group of vascular CAD which show that CAD patients are not younger than non-crossed aphasics nor that CAD is more frequent in women than men [67]. In contrast with the most frequent aphasia type in the general CAD population, no Broca-like aphasia was found in subcortical CAD-cases. Transcortical aphasia was the most frequent type of aphasia in the subcortical CAD group ($n = 4/9$). This finding is consistent with the hypothesis suggesting similarity between subcortical and transcortical aphasia on the basis of the preservation of repetitive speech [2,14].

A quantitative analysis of the aphasia profiles in this study suggests some tentative conclusions. The fact that most subcortical CAD-patients (6/8, (case nrs. 4, 13, 19, 22, 25); one patient (case nr. 22) was excluded because of the lack of data in the lesion phase) were still aphasic in the lesion phase is in agreement with the findings in the general CAD-population which indicates that CAD is not a transient disorder. However, these findings contradict the general assumption that 'non-crossed subcortical aphasias' are characterised by a more rapid recovery than cortical aphasia [11,85,87] and have less severe impact on written language [45, 46]. In this review the oral versus written language dissociation was only examined in six cases (case nrs. 4, 14, 15, 19, 22, 25). In three (case nrs. 19, 22, 25) out of six cases, written language was more severely

impaired than oral language. Four cases (case nrs. 11, 13–15) had to be excluded from the lesion-behavior analysis because of the lack of data in the lesion phase and because of the normalisation of language during the acute phase.

As to the lesion-aphasia correlations, almost all subcortical CAD-cases (4/5) had a mirror-image profile (case nrs. 13, 19, 22, 25) which contrasts with the high incidence of 39.5% (15/38) of anomalous cases in the general vascular CAD-population [67]. This finding suggests a more consistent topographical organisation of neurolinguistic functions of the phylogenetically older subcortical structures. In-depth analysis of nonverbal disorders accompanying subcortical CAD was not possible since most cases were not systematically documented on a temporal basis. However, a variety of neuropsychological deficits such as dysprosody, visual neglect, constructional, ideomotor, ideational and oral apraxia, acalculia as well as impairment of memory, orientation and nonverbal intelligence have been reported in subcortical CAD-cases. Analogous to the patient reported in this paper, four of the eight subcortical CAD-cases presented the same association of crossed aphasia with left visuo-spatial neglect and apraxia (case nrs. 4, 13, 19, 22). With the exception of the first case-report of Cappa et al. [79], all cases (3/4) displayed left visuo-spatial neglect and constructional apraxia. Consequently, the combination of visuo-spatial neglect and constructional apraxia confirms the general assumption of both neglect and constructional apraxia as frequent nonverbal disorders in vascular subcortical CAD [27]. The subcortical lesion localisation of these four cases is quite different: Colombo et al. [1] recorded these symptoms after a lesion in the lentiform nucleus, while the patient of Cappa et al. [79] had a lesion in the lentiform nucleus in addition to lesions in the periventricular white matter. Mariën et al. [70] described a patient with a subcortical lesion involving the internal and external capsule, the pallidal globe, the putamen, the claustrum and the periventricular white matter. Laiacona et al. [43] reported a patient with a thalamic lesion and involvement of the internal capsule and putamen.

Among the explanations of the pathophysiological mechanism underlying reversed cerebral dominance for language in the CAD-population, Marie [64–66] and later Habib et al. [41] stated that language functions are not lateralized at the level of the subcortical structures. As a consequence of an absence of cerebral language dominance at the subcortical level, an overrepresentation of subcortical CAD was assumed [41].

In their review of subcortical CAD, Laiacona et al. [44] rejected this point of view because of the lack of confirmation of this hypothesis in population studies. As an alternative explanation, Laiacona et al. [44] proposed the view of 'crowding of functions' in the right hemisphere which implies that 'right deep structures are crucial for language and visual attention when the latter functions are both subserved by the right hemisphere'. This view was based on the fact that the incidence of crossed aphasia with unilateral neglect was higher in the subcortical than cortical CAD-group of Laiacona's study.

Our current observation in which a combination of dominant (aphasia, apraxia) and non-dominant hemisphere disorders (left visual neglect) is present, corroborates the view of ' a crowding of functions'. Moreover, stringent analysis of the reliable subcortical CAD-group resulted in almost two thirds ($5/8 = 62.5\%$) (case nrs. 4, 13, 19, 22, 25) of patients presenting with crossed aphasia in combination with visuo-spatial neglect. Analysis of anatomo-clinical configurations in these subcortical CAD-cases ($n = 5$) reveals that four out of five mirror-image cases displayed a combination of dominant and non-dominant hemisphere symptoms (case nrs. 13, 19, 22, 25).

4. General conclusion

The patient described in this paper incurred an ischemic lesion in the right thalamus. In the post-acute phase of the stroke, a unique combination of 'crossed thalamic aphasia' was found with left visuo-spatial neglect and constructional apraxia. As such, this patient represents the first reliable representative of CAD following an isolated lesion in the right thalamus. A further in-depth analysis of the linguistic and cognitive impairments of CAD-patients with a pure subcortical lesion reveals that the demographic data are consistent with the general findings of the entire group of vascular CAD cases. In addition, the neurolinguistic findings do not support the data in the general CAD-population with respect to the high prevalence of transcortical aphasia and the tendency towards a copresence of an oral versus written language dissociation and a 'mirror image' lesion-aphasia profile. Furthermore, subcortical CAD does not seem to be a transient phenomenon and the lesion-aphasia correlations are not congruent with the high incidence of anomalous cases in the general CAD population. Moreover, it was observed that subcortical CAD may be accompanied by neuropsychological impairments such as dysprosody, visual neglect, apraxia, acalculia and disturbance of orientation and memory. Finally, the frequent association of 'crossed subcortical aphasia' with left visual neglect, normally attributed to a lesion in the non-dominant hemisphere, corroborates the view of a crowding of functions. However, further investigation of subcortical CAD-cases is required to uncover the mechanism underlying the cerebral dominance of the diverse neuropsychological functions.

Appendix 1: Classification of adults CAD-cases with a vascular etiology 1975–2007 ($n = 176$)

unreliable CAD ($n = 97$)		possible CAD ($n = 22$)		reliable CAD ($n = 57$)	
absence clear-cut evidence of right handedness ($n = 83$)		presence of familial sinistrality ($n = 9$)			
1976	Kishida et al., case 3,	1976	Lozano and Clark	1977	April and Tse
	Kishida et al., case 4		Zangwill, case 2	1980	April and Han
	Wechsler	1981	Assal et al.	1981	Carr et al., case 2
1977	Sadavisam & Jaganathan	1983	Henderson, case 1		Carr et al., case 3
	Yamada et al.	1984	Demeurisse et al.		Denes and Caviezel
1978	Urbain et al.	1988	Kojima et al., case 2	1982	Assal
1979	Barroche et al.	1989	Alexander et al., case 1	1983	Habib et al.
	Goldstein et al., case 1	1992	Marshall and Halligan		Henderson, case 2
	Goldstein et al., case 2	1994	Gomez-Tortosa et al.		Henderson, case 3
	Hyodo et al.			1984	Colombo et al.
	Pillon et al., case 1	absence of information about familial sinistrality ($n = 6$)			Hindson et al.
	Pillon et al., case 2				Sartori et al.
	Tsuruoka et al., case 2			1985	Basso et al., case 1
	Tsuruoka et al., case 3	1987	Rapcsak et al. = Ochipa		Basso et al., case 2
	Zangwill, case 1		and Gonzalez Rothi (1989)		Basso et al., case 3
1980	Tanabe et al.	1991	Deleval and Léonard, case 3		Basso et al., case 4
	Donoso et al., case 2	1992	Coppens and Robey, case 1		Basso et al., case 5
1981	Yarnell, case 1		Coppens and Robey, case 2		Basso et al., case 6
	Yarnell, case 2	1994	Trojano et al.		Basso et al., case 7
	Yarnell, case 3	1996	Nédélec-Cicéri et al.		Sugimoto et al.
	Yokoyama et al., case 2			1987	Fournet et al.
1982	Brust et al.	absence of information of early brain damage and/or seizures in infancy ($n = 7$)			Perani et al., case 1
	Endo et al., case 1				Walker-Batson et al.
	Endo et al., case 2			1988	Kojima et al., case 1
	Endo et al., case 3			1989	Nagaraja et al.
	Endo et al., case 4	1982	Haaland and Miranda	1990	Faglia and Vignolo
	Endo et al., case 5	1986	*Youngjohn*	1991	Berndt et al.
	Endo et al., case 6	1994	Davous and Boller		Deleval and Léonard, case 1
	Endo et al., case 7	1999	Roebroek et al.		Deleval and Léonard, case 2
	Endo et al., case 8	2003	*Marangolo et al.*		Hadar et al.
	Endo et al., case 9		*Njemanze*	1992	Lanoë et al.
	Puel et al., case 1	2006	*Mansur et al.*		Sakurai et al.
	Wertz			1993	Cappa et al., case 1
1983	Donoso, case 2				Cappa et al., case 2
1984	Kapur & Dunkley				Cohen et al.
1985	Fromm et al., case 6			1994	Berthier and Starkstein
	Fromm et al., case 11				Ihori et al.
	Mendes and Benson, case 3				Rey et al.
1986	Gonzalo, Barrio et al.			1996	Laiacona et al.
	Sapir et al.			1997	Fujii et al.
1987	Berthier et al.			1998	Hashimoto et al.
	Castro-Caldas et al., case 1			1999	and 2001 Raymer et al.
	Castro-Caldas et al., case 2			2001	Mariën et al., case 1
	Castro-Caldas et al., case 3				Mariën et al., case 3
	Castro-Caldas et al., case 4				Mariën et al., case 4
	Gonzalez-Rothi et al				Mariën et al., case 5
	Hamasaki et al.				Mariën et al., case 6
	Klonoff et al.				Mariën et al., case 7
	Murdoch				Mariën et al., case 9
	Reinvang			2002	Paghera et al.
	Rétif et al., case 2			2003	*Diouf et al.*
	Schweiger et al.			2004	*Bartha et al., case 1*
1987	Washima et al.			2006	*Semenza et al., case 1*
1988	Perani et al., case 2				*Semenza et al., case 2*
1989	Delreux et al.				*Semenza et al., case 5*
	Tanridag and Ongel				*Semenza et al., case 6*

unreliable CAD ($n = 97$)		possible CAD ($n = 22$)	reliable CAD ($n = 57$)	
1991	Dobrzynska, case 1		2007	*current observation*
	Dobrzynska, case 2			
	Ferro et al.			
1992	Yamadori et al.			
1993	Shibati et al.			
1996	Alexander and Annett, case 4			
	Alexander and Annett, case 5			
	Alexander and Annett, case 6			
	Alexander and Annett, case 7			
	Alexander and Annett, case 8			
1996	Bakar et al., case 1			
	Bakar et al., case 2			
	Bakar et al., case 3			
	Melzi et al.			
1997	Stefanis et al.			
1998	Osmon et al.			
	Ozeren et al.			
1999	Nagaratnam et al.			
2000	*Gass et al.*			
2001	*Coppens and Hungerford, case 1*			
	Coppens and Hungerford, case 2			
	Maeshima et al.			
	Shintani et al.			
2004	*Seddoh et al.*			
	Sheehy & Haines			
2007	*Salis et al.*			
	Tabeling et al.			
presence of a left hemisphere lesion ($n = 9$)				
1980	Trojanowski et al.			
1981	Yokoyama et al., case 1			
1984	Sweet et al.			
1989	Alexander et al., case 2			
1990	Kitayama et al.			
1992	Le Gall et al.			
1994	Caramelli et al.			
1999	*Visch-Brink et al.*			
2001	Mariën et al., case 8			
left hemisphere integrity not ascertained ($n = 4$)				
1981	Carr et al., case 1			
	Carr et al., case 4			
2002	*Paparounas et al.*			
2006	*Bhatnagar et al.*			

Legend: References printed in cursive cases added till 2007.

Appendix 2: Classification of adult CAD-cases with pure subcortical and cortico-subcortical involvement (1975–2007) (n =176)

pure subcortical involvement (n = 25)			cortico-subcortical involvement (n = 151)					
[1]	1977	Sadavisam and Jaganatham	[26]	1976	Kishida et al., case 3	[89]	1986	Gonzalo, Barrio et al.
[2]	1979	Goldstein et al., case 1	[27]		Kishida et al., case 4	[90]		Sapir et al.
[3]		Pillon et al., case 1	[28]		Lozano and Clark	[91]		*Youngjohn*
[4]	1984	Colombo et al.	[29]		Wechsler	[92]	1987	Berthier et al.
[5]	1985	Fromm et al., case 6	[30]		Zangwill, case 2	[93]		Castro-Caldas et al., case 1
[6]		Fromm et al., case 11	[31]	1977	April and Tse	[94]		Castro-Caldas et al., case 2
[7]	1987	Hamasaki et al.	[32]		Yamada et al.	[95]		Castro-Caldas et al., case 3
[8]		Murdoch	[33]	1978	Urbain et al.	[96]		Castro-Caldas et al., case 4
[9]		Washimi et al.	[34]	1979	Barroche et al.	[97]		Fournet et al.
[10]	1988	Perani et al., case 2	[35]		Goldstein et al., case 2	[98]		Gonzalez-Rothi et al.
[11]	1991	Deleval and Léonard,case 3	[36]		Hyodo et al.	[99]		Klonoff et al.
[12]		Dobrzynska, case 2	[37]		Pillon et al., case 2	[100]		Rapcsak et al.=Ochipa et al.
[13]	1993	Cappa et al., case 1	[38]		Tsuruoka et al., case 2	[101]		Reinvang
[14]		Cappa et al., case 2	[39]		Tsuruoka et al., case 3	[102]		Rétif et al., case 2
[15]	1994	Gomez-Tortosa et al.	[40]		Zangwill, case 1	[103]		Schweiger et al.
[16]	1996	Alexander and Annett,case 6	[41]	1980	April and Han	[104]	1988	Kojima et al., case 1
[17]		Bakar et al., case 2	[42]		Tanabe et al. (japanese)	[105]		Kojima et al., case 2
[18]		Bakar et al., case 3	[43]		Trojanowski et al.	[106]		Perani et al., case 1
[19]		Laiacona et al.	[44]		Donoso et al., case 2	[107]		Walker-Batson, case 1
[20]	1998	Ozeren er al.	[45]	1981	Assal et al.	[108]		Alexander et al., case 1
[21]	2001	*Maeshima et al.*	[46]		Carr et al., case 1	[109]		Alexander et al., case 2
[22]		Mariën et al., case 3	[47]		Carr et al., case 2	[110]		Delreux et al.
[23]		Mariën et al., case 4	[48]		Carr et al., case 3	[111]		Nagaraja et al.
[24]	2006	Bhatnagar et al.	[49]		Carr et al., case 4	[112]		Tanridag and Ongel
[25]	2007	current observation	[50]		Denes and Caviezel	[113]	1990	Kitayama et al.
			[51]		Yarnell, case 1	[114]		Faglia and Vignolo
			[52]		Yarnell, case 2	[115]	1991	Berndt et al.
			[53]		Yarnell, case 3	[116]		Deleval and Léonard, case1
			[54]		Yokoyama et al., case 1	[117]		Deleval and Léonard, case 2
			[55]		Yokoyama et al., case 2	[118]		Dobrzynska, case 1
			[56]	1982	Assal	[119]		Ferro et al.
			[57]		Brust et al.	[120]		Hadar et al.
			[58]		Endo et al., case 1	[121]	1992	Coppens and Robbey,case 1
			[59]		Endo et al., case 2	[122]		Coppens and Robbey,case 2
			[60]		Endo et al., case 3	[123]		Lanoë et al.
			[61]		Endo et al., case 4	[124]		Le Gall et al.
			[62]		Endo et al., case 5	[125]		Marshall and Halligan
			[63]		Endo et al., case 6	[126]		Sakurai et al.
			[64]		Endo et al., case 7	[127]		Yamadori et al.
			[65]		Endo et al., case 8	[128]	1993	Cohen et al.
			[66]		Endo et al., case 9	[129]		Shibati et al.
			[67]		Haaland and Miranda	[130]	1994	Berthier and Starkstein
			[68]		Wertz	[131]		Caramelli et al.
			[69]	1983	Donoso, case 2	[132]		Davous and Boller
			[70]		Habib et al.	[133]		Ihori et al.
			[71]		Henderson, case 1	[134]		Rey et al.
			[72]		Henderson, case 2	[135]		Trojano et al.
			[71]		Henderson, case 3	[136]	1996	Alexander and Annett, case 4
			[74]	1984	Demeurisse et al.	[137]		Alexander and Annett, case 5
			[75]		Hindson et al.	[138]		Alexander and Annett, case 7
			[76]		Kapur and Dunkley	[139]		Alexander and Annett, case 8
			[77]		Puel et al., case 1	[140]		Bakar et al., case 1
			[78]		Sartori et al.	[141]		Melzi et al.
			[79]		Sweet et al.	[142]		Nédélec-Cicéri et al.
			[80]	1985	Basso et al., case 1	[143]	1997	Fujii et al.
			[81]		Basso et al., case 2	[144]		Stefanis et al.
			[82]		Basso et al., case 3	[145]	1998	Hashimoto et al.

pure subcortical involvement (n = 25)			cortico-subcortical involvement (n = 151)		
[83]		Basso et al., case 4	[146]		Osmon et al.
[84]		Basso et al., case 5	[147]		Nagaratnam et al.
[85]		Basso et al., case 6	[148]	1999	Raymer et al. (2001)
[86]		Basso et al., case 7	[149]		Roebroek et al.
[87]		Mendes and Benson, case 3	[150]		*Visch-Brink et al.*
[88]		Sugimoto et al.	[151]	2000	*Gass et al.*
[152]	2001	*Coppens and Hungerford, case 1*	[165]		*Marangola et al.*
[153]		*Coppens and Hungerford, case 2*	[166]	2003	*Njemanze et al.*
[154]		Mariën et al., case 1	[167]		*Semenza et al., case 1*
[155]		Mariën et al., case 2	[168]		*Semenza et al., case 2*
[156]		Mariën et al., case 5	[169]		*Semenza et al., case 5*
[157]		Mariën et al., case 6	[170]		*Semenza et al., case 6*
[158]		Mariën et al., case 7	[171]	2004	*Bartha et al.*
[159]		Mariën et al., case 8	[172]		*Seddoh et al.*
[160]		Mariën et al., case 9	[173]		*Sheehy and Haines*
[161]		*Shintani et al.*	[174]	2006	*Mansur et al.*
[162]	2002	Paghera et al.	[175]	2007	*Salis et al.*
[163]		*Paparounas et al.*	[176]		*Tabeling et al.*
[164]	2003	*Diouf et al.*			

Legend: References printed in cursive cases added till 2007.
References printed in bold reliable subcortical CAD-cases.

Appendix 3: Three epoch time-frame analysis of 9 possible/reliable subcortical CAD-cases with a vascular etiology

reference	age/gender	time post-onset	fluency	compreh	repetition	naming	reading	writing	severity score and aphasia type	lesion site
[4] Colombo et al., 1984	67/M	acute phase		+++	+++	+++	+++	+++	15 wernicke	basal ganglia
		lesion phase		++	+++	+++	++	+++	8 *wernicke*	
		late phase		+++	+++	+++	++	+++	8 *wernicke*	
[11] Deleval and Léonard, 1991, case 3	58/M	acute phase	+++	++	+++	+++	++	+	16 broca	anterior intern capsule, extern capsule and semi-oval centre
		lesion phase	?	?	+			+	?	
		late phase	?	?			?	?	?	
[13] Cappa et al., 1993, case 1	79/F	acute phase	+++	+++	+	+++	+++	+++	16 mixed transcortical	periventricular white matter and lenticular nucleus
		lesion phase	+++	+++	+	+++	++	?	12 mixed transcortical	
		late phase	++	+		++		+++	9 ?	
[14] Cappa et al., 1993, case 2	56/M	acute phase		+		++	+++	+++	4 *anomic*	periventricular region
		lesion phase							no aphasia	
		late phase							no aphasia	
[15] Gomez-Tortosa et al., 1994	38/F	acute phase							0 no aphasia	subcortical infarction involving lenticular branches of the middle cerebral artery
		lesion phase							0 no aphasia	
		late phase							0 no aphasia	
[19] Laiacona et al., 1996	68/M	acute phase	?	?	?	?	?	?	? global	genu and posterior limb of internal capsule, lateral and posterior parts of the thalamus and putamen
		lesion phase	+++	++	+	++	+++	+++	14 *transcortical motor*	
		late phase	?	?	?	?	?	?	?	
[22] Mariën et al., 2001, case 3	75/F	acute phase	++	+	+		+	++	7 transcortical motor	crus anterior of the internal capsule, globus pallidus, putamen, external capsule, claustrum and periventricular white matter
		lesion phase	+++	+	++		+++	+++	12 transcortical motor	
		late phase	+++	+	++			+	7 transcortical motor	
[23] Mariën et al., 2001, case 4	79/F	acute phase	+++	+++	+++	+++	+++	+++	18 global	parietal white matter and basal ganglia
	?	?	?	?	?	?	?	?	? ?	
		late phase	?	?	?	?	?	?	? ?	
[25] current observation, 2007	70/M	acute phase	?	++		+	+++	+++	10 transcortical sensory	thalamus
		lesion phase		++			++		5	
		late phase								

Legend: M male; F female; +++ severely disturbed; ++ moderately disturbed; + mildly disturbed; (blank) not disturbed; ? no information; severity scores (number of + signs) between 1 and 6 indicate mild aphasia, between 7 and 12 moderate aphasia, between 13 and 18 severe aphasia, zero score indicates absence of aphasia; aphasia type printed cursive: interpretation of the authors; reference printed bold and cursive: case added in 2007; compreh = comprehension.

Appendix 4: Neurocognitive symptoms of 9 possible/reliable subcortical CAD-cases with a vasuclar etiology

reference	age/ gender	dysprosodia	visual neglect	constructional apraxia	ideomotor apraxia	ideational apraxia	oral apraxia	acalculia	additional cognitive disturbances	lesion site
[4] Colombo et al., 1984	67/M	?	+	+	+	+	+	?	anosognosia	basal ganglia
[11] Deleval and Léonard,1991, case 3	58/M	?	-	+	-	-	?	?	Wechsler PIQ = 90	anterior intern capsule, extern capsule and semi-oval centre
[13] Cappa et al., 1993, case 1	79/F	+	+	?	+	-	+	?	anosognosia	periventricular white matter and lenticular nucleus
[14] Cappa et al., 1993, case 2	56/M	+	-	?	-	?	-	?	?	periventricular region
[15] Gomez-Tortosa et al., 1994	38/F	?	-	-	-	-	-	?	impaired immediate and delayed verbal and visual memory, decreased short term attention and concentration	subcortical infarction involving lenticular branches of the middle cerebral artery
[19] Laiacona et al., 1996	68/M	+	+	+	-	+	-	+	?	genu and posterior limb of internal capsule, lateral and posterior parts of the thalamus and putamen
[22] Mariën et al., 2001, case 3	75/F	+	+	+	-	-	-	?	none	crus anterior of the internal capsule, globus pallidus, putamen, external capsule, claustrum and periventricular white matter
[23] Mariën et al., 2001, case 4	79/F	?	?	?	?	?	?	?	?	parietal white matter and basal ganglia
[25] current observation, 2007	70/M	-	+	+	+	+	-	+	concentration and memory deficits	thalamus

Legend: M male; F female; '+ present'; - absent; ? no information; PIQ performal IQ; reference printed bold and cursive: case added in 2007.

References

[1]   A. Colombo, M.C. Guerzoni, G. Miscio and P. Panzetti, L'afasia crociata: considerazioni su un caso clinico, *Rivisto di Patologia Nervosa e Mentale* **105** (1984), 67–74.

[2]   A. Kreisler, O. Godefroy and C. Delmairg, The anatomy of aphasia revisited, *Neurology* **54** (2000), 1117–1123.

[3]   A.E. Hillis, P.B. Barker, R.J. Wityk, E.M. Aldrich, L. Restrepo, E.L. Breese and M. Work, Variability in subcortical aphasia is due to variable sites of cortical hypoperfusion, *Brain and Language* **89** (2004), 524–530.

[4]   A.M. Shintani, S. Maeshima and E. Nakai, Jargonagraphia with severe aphasia due to a right hemisphere lesion: case report, *Journal of Clinical Neuroscience* **8** (2001), 369–371.

[5]   B. Bramwell, On 'crossed' aphasia and the factors which go to determine whether 'leading' or 'drinving' speech-centres shall be located in the left or in the right hemisphere of the brain, with notes on a case of 'crossed' aphasia (aphasia with right-sided hemiplegia in a left-handed man), *The Lancet* **1** (1899), 1473–1479.

[6]   B. Clarke and O.L. Zangwill, A case of 'crossed aphasia' in a dextral, *Neuropsychologia* **3** (1965), 81–86.

[7]   B. Paghera, P. Marien and L.A. Vignolo, Crossed aphasia with left spatial neglect and visual imperception, *Neurological Sciences* **23** (2003), 317–322.

[8]   C. Gass, J. Whitney and A. Minagar, Crossed aphasia and cerebral localisation of a functional case study, *Archives of Clinical Neurpsychology* **15** (2000), 722.

[9]   C. Salis and S. Edwards, The manifestation of agrammatic comprehension in a case of crossed aphasia, *Brain and Language* **103**(1–2) (2005), 37–38.

[10] C. Semenza, M. Delazer, L. Bertella, A. Grana, I. Mori, F.M. Conti, R. Pignatti, L. Bartha, F. Domahs, T. Benke and A. Mauro, Is math lateralised on the same side as language? Right hemisphere aphasia and mathematical abilities, *Neuroscience Letters* **406** (2006), 285–288.

[11] C.W. Wallesch, H. Johanssen-Horbach, C. Bartels and M. Hermann, Mechanisms of and misconceptions about subcortical aphasia, *Brain and Language,* **58**(3) (1997), 403–409.

[12] D. Wechsler, *Manual for the Wechsler Memory Scale-Revised,* New York, The Psychological Corporation, 1987.

[13] D.C. Kuljic-Obradovic, Subcortical aphasia: three different language disorder syndromes? *European Journal of Neurology* **10** (2003), 445–448.

[14] D.F. Benson and A. Ardila, *Aphasia, a Clinical Perspective.* Oxford University Press, New York, 1996, 166–179.

[15] E. De Renzi and L.A. Vignolo, The Token Test: a sensitive test to detect receptive disturbances in aphasics, *Brain* **85** (1962), 665–678.

[16] E. Kaplan, H. Goodglass and S. Weintraub, *Boston Naming Test.* USA: Lea & Febiger, 1983.

[17] E. Visch-Brink, C. Niewold, T. Brouwer, R. Prins and F. Harskamp, Symptomatology of crossed aphasia after a second lesion in the left hemisphere, *Brain and Language* **69** (1999), 382–384.

[18] F. Mazzocchi and L.A. Vignolo, Localisation of lesions in aphasia: clinical CT-scan correlations in stroke patients, *Cortex* **15** (1979), 627–654.

[19] F. Moutier, *L'aphasie de Broca.* Paris: Steinheil, 1908.

[20] F.S. Diouf, J.P. Moly, M. De Seze, M. Barat and I.P. Ndiaye, Crossed aphasia with jargonagraphia in a right-handed patient, *Revue Neurologique* **159**(3) (2003), 316–318.

[21] G. Ettlinger, C.V. Jackson and O.L. Zangwill, Dysphasia following right temporal lobectomy in a right-handed man, *Journal of Neurology, Neurosurgery and Psychiatry* **18** (1955), 214–217.

[22] G. Marinesco, D. Grigoresco and S. Axente, Considérations sur l'aphasie croisée, *Encéphale* **33** (1938), 27–46.

[23] G. Milani, Le alterazioni del linguaggio nelle lesioni del cervello destro, *Il Policlinico, sez. Medica* **19** (1928), 321–333.

[24] G. Scollo, Sull'afasia motoria di Broca. A proposito di un interessante trauma del copo con complicazioni di ascesso cerebrale, *Il policlinico, sez. Pratica* **13** (1926), 437–441.

[25] H. Claude and H. Shaeffer, Un nouveau cas d'hémiplégie gauche avec aphasie chez un droitère, *Revue Neurologique* **37** (1921), 170–175.

[26] H. Goodglass and F. Quadfasel, Language laterality in left-handed aphasics, *Brain* **77** (1954), 521–548.

[27] J.C. Marshall and P.W. Halligan, Crossed aphasia in a dextral with minor hemisphere signs, *Behavioural Neurology* **5** (44) (1992), 247–250.

[28] J.C. Raven, J.H. Court and J. Raven, *Manual for Raven's progressive matrices and vocabulary scales.* Londen, 1983-1984.

[29] J.E. Holmes and R.L. Sadoff, Aphasia due to a right hemisphere tumor in a right-handed man, *Neurology* **16** (1996), 392–397.

[30] J.P. Neau and J. Bogousslavsky, The syndrome of posterior choroidal artery territory infarction, *Annals of Neurology* **39** (1996), 779–788.

[31] J.R. Youngjohn, Rapid recovery from crossed aphasia, *Archives of Clinical Neuropsychology* **1**(2) (1986), 165–174.

[32] J.W. Brown and H. Hecaen, Lateralisation and language representation: observation in aphasia in children, left-handers and 'anomalous' dextrals, *Neurology* **26** (1976), 183–189.

[33] Köster, 1900 (cited in Joffroy MA, 1903).

[34] K. Paparounas, D. Eftaxias and N. Akritidis, Dissociated crossed aphasia: a challenging language representation disorder, *Neurology* **59**(3) (2002), 441–442.

[35] K. Rotschild, The relation of Broca's center to lefthandedness, *American Journal of Medical Science* **182** (1931), 116–118.

[36] K. Willmes and K. Poeck, To what extent can aphasic syndromes be localized, *Brain* **116** (6), 1527–1540.

[37] L. Bartha, P. Marien, W. Poewe and T. Benke, Linguistic and neuro-psychological deficits in crossed conduction aphasia. Report of three cases, *Brain and Language* **88**(1) (2004), 83–95.

[38] L. De Lisi, Afasia crociate? *Riv Pat Nerv Ment* 1930, 4–31.

[39] L. De Witte and P. Marien, Subcorticale afasie: inzichten en casusbespreking, in: *Afasie (z)onder woorden,* E. Robert and P. Mariën, eds, Garant, Antwerpen-Apeldoorn, 2006, pp. 217–234.

[40] L.M. Sheehy and M.E. Haines, Crossed Wernicke's aphasia: a case report, *Brain and Language* **89**(1) (2004), 203–206.

[41] M. Habib, Y. Joanette, A. Ali-Cherif and M. Poncet, Crossed aphasia in dextrals: A case report with special reference to site of lesion, *Neuropsychologia* **21** (1983), 413–418.

[42] M. Humprhrey and O. Zangwill, Dysphasia in left-handed patients with unilateral brain lesions, *Journal of Neurology, Neurosurgery and Psychiatry* **115** (1952), 184–193.

[43] M. Laiacona, C. Stangalino and L. Lorenzi, Crossed aphasia. I: A case study with purely deep lesion, *Behavioural Neurology* **9** (1996), 155–162.

[44] M. Laiacona, E. Capitani, C. Stangalino and L. Lorenzi, Crossed aphasia. II: Why are deep lesions overrepresented with respect to standard aphasia? *Behavioural Neurology* **9** (1996), 163–170.

[45] M. Radanovic, L.L. Mansur, M.J. Azambuja, C.S. Porto and

M. Scaff, Contribution to the evaluation of language disturbances in subcortical lesions, *Arq Neuropsiquiatrica* **62** (2004), 51–57.

[46] M. Radanovic and M. Scaff, Speech and language disturbances due to subcortical lesions, *Brain and Language* **84** (2003), 337–352.

[47] M.A. Joffroy, Sur un cas d'aphasie sensorielle avec lésion temporo-pariétale droite, *Revue Neurologique* **16** (1903), 112–115.

[48] M.A. Souques, Aphasie avec hémiplégie gauche chez un droitier, *Revue Neurologique* **20** (1910), 547–549.

[49] M.G. Cole and D. Dastoor, A new hierarchic approach to the measurement of dementia, *Psychosomatics* **28** (1987), 298–305.

[50] M.I. Botez and N. Wertheim, Expressive aphasia and amusia following right frontal lesion in a right-handed man, *Brain* **82** (1959), 186–202.

[51] M.J. Riddioch and G.W. Humphreys, *BORB: Birmingham Object Recognition Battery.* Hove, UK: Erlbaum, 1993.

[52] M.P Alexander, Clinical-anatomical correlations of aphasia following predominant lesions, in: *Handbook of Neuropsychology*, F. Boller and J. Grafman, eds, Amsterdam: Elsevier Science Publishers, 1989.

[53] M.P. Alexander and D.F. Benson, The aphasia and related disturbances, in: *Clinical Neurology*, R.J. Joynt, ed., Philadelphia: Lippincott, 1991.

[54] M.P. Alexander and M. Annett, Crossed aphasia and related anomalies of cerebral organization: case reports and an genetic hypothesis, *Brain and Language* **112** (1996), 953–973.

[55] M.P. Alexander and S.R Lo Verme, Aphasia after left hemispheric intracerebral hemorrhage, *Neurology* **30** (1980), 1193–1202.

[56] M.S. Carr, T. Jacobson and F. Boller, Crossed aphasia: Analysis of four cases, *Brain and Language* **14** (1981), 190–202.

[57] M.S. Folstein, S.E. Folstein and P.R. Mc Hugh, Mini-Mental State: a practical method for grading the cognitive status of patients for the clinician, *Journal of Psychiatric Research* **12** (1975), 189–198.

[58] P. Ardin-Delteil, P. Levi-Valensi and M. Derrieu, Aphasie de Broca par lesion de l'hémisphère droit chez une droitière, *Revue Neurologique* **1** (1923), 14–21.

[59] P. Coppens and S. Hungerford, Crossed aphasia, in: *Aphasia in atypical populations,* P. Coppens, Y. Lebrun and A. Basso, eds, New Jersey: Lawrence Erlbaum Associates, 1998, pp. 203–260.

[60] P. Coppens and S. Hungerford, Crossed aphasia: two new cases, *Aphasiology* **15**(9) (2001), 827–854.

[61] P. Coppens, S. Hungerford, S. Yamaguchi and A. Yamadori, Crossed aphasia: An analysis of the symptoms, their frequency and a comparison with left-hemisphere aphasia symptomatology, *Brain and Language* **83** (2002), 425–463.

[62] P. Graetz, R. De Bleser and K. Willmes, *Akense Afasietest. Handleiding,* Lisse: Swets & Zetilinger, 1990.

[63] P. Marangolo, L. Picardi and M.C. Rinaldi, Dissociation between personal and extrapersonal neglect in a crossed aphasia study, *Neurocase* **9** (5) (2003), 414–420.

[64] P. Marie, Révision de la question de l'aphasie, *Semaine Médicale* **26** (1906), 241–246.

[65] P. Marie, Révision de la question de l'aphasie, *Semaine Médicale* **26** (1906), 493–500.

[66] P. Marie, Révision de la question de l'aphasie, *Semaine Médicale* **26** (1906), 565–571.

[67] P. Marien, B. Paghera, P.P. De Deyn and L.A. Vignolo, Adult crossed aphasia in dextrals revisited, *Cortex* **40** (2004), 41–74.

[68] P. Marien, E. Mampaey, A. Vervaet, J. Saerens and P.P. De Deyn, Normative data for the Boston naming test in native Dutch-speaking Belgian elderly, *Brain and Language* **65** (1998), 447–467.

[69] P. Marien, P. Paquier, S. Cassenaer and P.P. De Deyn, The history of crossed aphasia: early development of concepts and hypotheses, *Journal of Neurolinguistics* **15** (2002), 129–142.

[70] P. Marien, S. Engelborghs, L.A. Vignolo and P.P. De Deyn, The many faces of crossed aphasia in dextrals: Report of nine cases and review of the literature, *European Journal of Neurology* **8**(6) (2001c), 643–658.

[71] P.A. Osterrieth, Le test de copie d'une figure complexe: contribution à l'étude de l'aperception en de la mémoire, *Archives of Neurology* **30** (1944), 205–353.

[72] P.C. Njemanze, M. Hund-Georgiadis and D.Y. Von Cramon, Crossed aphasia in a dextral with right hemispheric lesion: a functional doppler study, *Stroke* **34** (2003), 213–214.

[73] P.P. Pramstaller and C.D. Marsden, The basal ganglia and apraxia., *Brain* **119** (1996), 319–340.

[74] R. Angelergues, H. Hecaen, R. Djindjian and N. Jarrie-Hazan, Un cas d'aphasie croisée, *Revue Neurologique* **107** (1962), 543–545.

[75] R.C. OLDFIELD, The assessment and analysis of handedness: the Edinburgh inventory, *Neuropsychologia* **9** (1971), 97–113.

[76] R.M. Crum, I.C. Anthony, S.S. Bassett and M.F. Folstein, Population-based norms for the min-mental state examination by age and educational level, *The Journal of the American Medical Association* **18** (1993), 2386–2391.

[77] S.A. Seddoh, Intonation perception in crossed aphasia, *Brain and Language* **91** (2004), 58–59.

[78] S.C. Bhatnagar, S. Imes, H.W. Buckingham and T. Puglishi-Creegan, Anomalous crossed aphasia in a patient with congenital lesion in the right hemisphere, *Brain and Language* **99**(1–2) (2006), 61–62.

[79] S.F. Cappa, D. Perani, S. Bressi, E. Paulesu, M. Francheschi and F. Fazio, Crossed aphasia: A PET follow-up study of two cases, *Journal of Neurology, Neurosurgery and Psychiatry* **56** (1993), 665–671.

[80] S.F. Cappa and L.A. Vignolo, Transcortical features of aphasia following left thalamic hemorrhage, *Cortex* **15** (1979), 121–130.

[81] S. Maeshima, F. Ozaki, R. Okita, H. Yamaga, H. Okada, K. Kakishita, H. Moriwaki and P. Roger, Transient crossed aphasia and persistent amnesia after right thalamic hemorrhage, *Brain Injury* **15**(10) (2001), 927–933.

[82] S. Nadeau and B. Crosson, Subcortical aphasia, *Brain and Language* **58** (1997), 355–402.

[83] S. Tabeling, B. Kopp, M. Braun, C. Moschner and K. Wessel, Crossed aphasia or Dysexecutive Syndrome? A Case Report, *Fortschritte der Neurologie und Psychiatrie* **75** (2007), 484–489.

[84] Touche 1899 (cited in Joffroy MA, 1903).

[85] T.S. Olsen, P. Bruhn and R.G. Oberg, Cortical hypoperfusion as a possible cause of subcortical aphasia, *Brain* **109** (1986), 393–410.

[86] V.W. Henderson, Speech fluency in crossed aphasia, *Brain* **106** (1983), 837–857.

[87] W.D. Heiss, J. Kessler and K. Herholz, Disturbance and recovery of language function: correlates in pet-activation-studies, *Neuroimage* **20** (2003), S42–S49.

[88] Y. Joanette, M. Puel, J.I. Nespoulos, A. Rascol and A. Roch Lecours, Aphasie croisée chez les droitiers. I Revue de la literature, *Revue Neurologique* **8–9** (1982), 575–586.

3

An overview on Primary Progressive Aphasia and its variants

Serena Amici[a,d,*], Maria Luisa Gorno-Tempini[a], Jennifer M. Ogar[a,b], Nina F. Dronkers[a,b,c] and Bruce L. Miller[a]

[a]*Memory and Aging Center, Department of Neurology, University of California, San Francisco, USA*
[b]*VA Northern California Health Care System, Martinez, CA, USA*
[c]*University of California, Davis, Davis, CA, USA*
[d]*Department of Neurosciences, University of Perugia, Perugia, Italy*

Abstract. We present a review of the literature on Primary Progressive Aphasia (PPA) together with the analysis of neuropschychological and neuroradiologic profiles of 42 PPA patients. Mesulam originally defined PPA as a progressive degenerative disorder characterized by isolated language impairment for at least two years. The most common variants of PPA are: 1) Progressive nonfluent aphasia (PNFA), 2) semantic dementia (SD), 3) logopenic progressive aphasia (LPA). PNFA is characterized by labored speech, agrammatism in production, and/or comprehension. In some cases the syndrome begins with isolated deficits in speech. SD patients typically present with loss of word and object meaning and surface dyslexia. LPA patients have word-finding difficulties, syntactically simple but accurate language output and impaired sentence comprehension. The neuropsychological data demonstrated that SD patients show the most characteristic pattern of impairment, while PNFA and LPA overlap within many cognitive domains. The neuroimaging analysis showed left perisylvian region involvement. A comprehensive cognitive, neuroimaging and pathological approach is necessary to identify the clinical and pathogenetic features of different PPA variants.

Keywords: Primary progressive aphasia, nonfluent progressive aphasia, semantic dementia, logopenic progressive aphasia, neuroimaging studies, language symptoms

1. Introduction

Neurodegenerative dementias represent an emergent worldwide problem, brought about in part by the aging of the population. The insidious onset and the heterogeneous clinical presentation represent a diagnostic dilemma for the clinician. Dementia is characterized by progressive cognitive deficits and/or behavioral changes that impair daily-life activity (DSM-IVR, 2003). Historically, memory deficits have been considered essential for the diagnosis of dementia. Nevertheless, many dementia patients experience memory deficits only in the later stage of the disease.

An example of a non-amnestic type of dementing condition is Primary Progressive Aphasia (PPA), a slowly progressive language impairment that remains isolated for at least two years [39]. Neuroimaging typically reveals greater atrophy and/or hypometabolism within the left hemisphere compared to the right. Imaging in PPA should be negative for focal lesions such as tumor, stroke or arterio-venous malformations. At pathology, the majority of clinically diagnosed PPA patients show non-Alzheimer's disease of three major subtypes. The majority of cases show tau or ubiquitin inclusions, although a minority have no inclusions (so-called dementia lacking distinctive histopathology) [60]. The three major tau aggregation disorders include Pick's disease (PiD) [29], progressive supranuclear palsy [10,24] or corticobasal degeneration (CBD) [16,41,45]. When ubiquitin-positive inclusions are present different authors have suggested

*Corresponding author: Serena Amici, 350 Parnassus Avenue, San Francisco, CA 94143-1207, USA.
E-mail: samici@memory.ucsf.edu.

different terminologies: frontotemporal dementia motor neuron disease (FTD-MND) if motor involvement is present; when motor involvement is not evident the various terms that have been used include frontotemporal lobar degeneration with ubiquitin-positive inclusions (FTLD-U) [48], frontotemporal lobar degeneration with inclusions that are tau and synclein-negative, ubiquitinated (FTLD with ITSNU) [30], and motor neuron disease inclusion dementia (MNDID) [23,57].

Non-FTLD pathologies have also been described in PPA patients such as Alzheimer's disease (AD) [12], Creutzfeldt-Jakob disease (CJD) and Lewy body disease (LBD) [5]. Similar to the imaging findings, left greater than right-sided pathological involvement is typical of PPA.

2. Symptomatology and diagnosis

2.1. Clinical presentation

According to current research criteria for PPA, symptoms such as apathy, disinhibition, forgetfulness, visuospatial symptoms, or sensori-motor dysfunction should not be prominent during the first two years of the illness [38]. Acalculia or ideomotor apraxia are the only disturbances that can be present along with the language deficits in the early stages of the disease. Remarkably, in one patient, isolated progressive language symptoms were reported for 14 years prior to the onset of other major cognitive deficits [53].

Neuropsychological testing in PPA patients can be particularly difficult to interpret for clinicians who are not experienced with this condition. It should be noted that language impairments may prevent reliable assessments of non-linguistic abilities, since nearly all neuropsychological tests require verbal instruction, verbal responses and covert verbal reasoning. Furthermore, often it is difficult to compare the variants described in the literature because different language tests have been used.

Word finding deficits are the most common initial symptom in PPA. They can be attributed to either semantic/lexical deficits or underlying speech output problems. In order to overcome these difficulties, the patient often uses different linguistic strategies such as *simplification* (the use of a generic and more common word instead of a more precise but less common one) *and circumlocutions* (talking around an idea when the exact word or set of words cannot be retrieved). Often, verbal comprehension is preserved in the initial stages

of PPA, but semantic memory deficits and difficulty comprehending specific types of sentences are apparent in different clinical variants when specific language tasks are performed.

Through the years, different terminology has been used to describe the heterogeneous clinical presentations of PPA and terms such as "nonfluent", "fluent", "PPA with agrammatism", "aphemic", "semantic dementia" (SD) and "logopenic aphasia" have been reported [40]. Based on current clinical criteria developed by Neary and colleagues, PNFA, (also referred to as "PPA with agrammatism") [40] is characterized by labored speech, agrammatism in production and/or comprehension, and, variable degrees of anomia, with relative sparing of single word comprehension. Sentence comprehension is impaired for the most difficult morphosyntactic constructions, such as negative passives and object negative clauses [21,44, 60,63]. Apraxia of speech (AOS), a motor speech disturbance characterized by impaired planning of the articulation of the words [64], is commonly found in this variant. Patients make inconsistent articulatory errors and prosody and fluency are typically disrupted [13]. In the early 1990s, an additional syndrome called progressive anarthria was described, in which patients presented primarily with articulatory errors, dysprosody and AOS [3]. Chapman and colleagues [6] have named a similar disorder "progressive isolated motor speech disorder", while Fukui and colleagues have called it "primary progressive apraxia" [11] and others "aphemic variant" [7,28]. Despite the variability of the nomenclature, all the authors emphasize AOS characteristics as a dominant symptom in these cases. Therefore, we have classified these patients as having classical PNFA [47]. Whether this presentation is a separate entity or one possible presentation of PNFA with mainly speech impairment is still a matter of debate.

In SD, also called "fluent" aphasia, spontaneous speech is fluent and grammatically correct, despite the loss of word and object meaning [22]. Semantic paraphasias (meaning the substitution of a more familiar exemplar within the same category: "dog" for "hyena") are common in this variant. In the initial stage, articulation, phonology, syntax and repetition remain intact [22,55]. As the disease progresses, language output can become "empty", poor in nouns, consisting primarily of vague fillers, such as "thing", and function words, such as "this" or "the". Spontaneous naming of objects is greatly impaired and performance does not usually improve when multiple choices are provided [13]. SD patients should show relative sparing of visual processing in the first two years from onset [40].

"Logopenic" language output, characterized by word-finding difficulties and decreased output with syntactically simple but correct output has also been described in PPA. Phonemic paraphasias (meaning sound substitutions within single words "tamp" instead of "lamp") are characteristic of this variant [28,63]. Recently, this clinical presentation has been suggested to be a distinct variant [13]. Sentence comprehension is severely impaired for all but the most simple morphosyntactic constructions and repetition is also below the normal limits. Naming is significantly impaired with spared recognition on multiple choices. Single-word comprehension and semantic memory are within normal limits. The core impairment in this variant is thought to be a short-term phonological memory deficit [13].

A consensus comprehensive classification of PPA has not yet been established. The use of different neuropsychological instruments and the fact that patients may present with different symptoms at different stages of the disease further complicates diagnosis. In Table 1, we summarize the clinical and language features of PPA variants described in the literature.

The heterogeneity of the clinical picture described in the literature is partially the result of the different assumptions and methodology applied to patient populations. Confounding factors include the variability in the use of specific language tests and the definition of fluency and agrammatism. In our view, the "pure progressive anarthria" should be considered together with PNFA, because often the two syndromes overlap and few cases remain purely anarthric with no evidence of language problems throughout the progression of the disease. The logopenic variant should include "PPA with conduction aphasia" [19]. Finally the "PPA with verbal comprehension deficits" should be considered as an early presentation of SD, when single word comprehension is significantly impaired. However, in the future, the heuristic value of these divisions will need to be determined validated with biological and neuropathological measures.

2.2. Associated symptoms

Behavioral problems are present to different degrees within the three variants. SD patients can show a wide variety of behavioral symptoms; the most frequent being depression, overeating or changes in food preferences, loss of insight, repetitive motor behaviors, al-

terations in social conduct and emotional blunting [52, 58]. PNFA patients are thought to develop behavioral symptoms similar to FTD later in the course of the disease, but usually remain polite and socially adept throughout the early stages of their illness. The logopenic variant has still not been neuropsychiatrically characterized, but these patients do not seem to show the severe behavioral disturbances that are common in the SD group.

On neurological examination, mild motor symptoms are common and usually localized in the right hand or the right side of the body, reflecting the focality of the left brain involvement [28,32]. PNFA cases showed more frequently diffuse motor slowing, reduced dexterity, and mild rigidity. Recently, a patient with PNFA who developed sudden-onset extrapyramidal symptoms with dystonia and alien hand has been described, providing further evidence that PNFA and cortico-basal syndrome can present in the same patient at different stages of the same disease [14]. In contrast, semantic dementia patients, apart for language impairment and agnosia, often have normal neurological examinations [13,37].

Limb apraxia is relatively common in PPA, being one of the two non-language symptoms that can be present early in the disease. In a small study, 14 patients had instrumental apraxia in imitation and/or with pantomiming [25]. This impaired gestural imitation is consistent with disruption of a left fronto-parietal network.

2.3. Pattern of language impairment and neuropathology

The pattern of language impairment does not easily allow the clinician to predict the etiology of underlying neuropathology. Indeed, many different neuropathology syndromes have been observed in PPA, including FTLD, CBD, PSP and AD. Clinical-pathological correlation is difficult in many cases because speech and language assessments were not sufficiently detailed to establish the presenting PPA variant [20,45]. Nonfluent aphasia (comprising isolated speech impairments) is often the first symptom of CBD, before the onset of extrapyramidal symptoms [15]. Dysarthria, buccofacial apraxia and AOS seem to be more common in cases of CBD [36,37,41,51], but other aphasia symptoms have also been reported. Attempts to link CBD pathology to a specific language pattern have, to date, been somewhat inconsistent. Nonfluent cases with AOS have also been associated with PSP pathology: tau inclusions were found in left fronto-temporal cortex (instead of

Table 1
Clinical and language characteristics of PPA variants

	Spontaneous Speech	Single Word Comprehension	Repetition	Naming	Sentence Comprehension	Reading	Associated Symptoms
Progressive Non-Fluent Aphasia (Hodges et al. 1996, Neary et al. 1998, Mesulam 2001, Grossman 2002, Gorno-Tempini 2004)	decreased fluency, articulatory errors and apraxia of speech ± agrammatism	spared	agrammatic errors	normal/variable anomia, greater for verbs	impaired only for complex sentences	impaired for both regular and irregular words	buccofacial and limb apraxia, mild controlateral motor symptoms
Semantic Dementia (Hodges et al. 1992, Snowden et al. 1992)	fluent and grammatically correct, semantic paraphasias	impaired	spared	impaired, greater for nouns	spared	impaired for irregular	multimodal semantic memory impairment (faces, objects, sounds); behavioural symptoms
Logopenic PPA (Gorno-Tempini et al. 2004)	word finding problem, phonemic paraphasia	spared	Impaired	impaired, but increased performance with recognition	impaired, also for the simple sentences	spared for single word	acalculia, apraxia
Progressive Anarhtria/Progressive Isolated Motor Speech Disorder (Broussulle et al. 1996, Fukui et al. 1996, Chapman et al.1997)	articulatory errors, stuttering, dysarthria, dysprosody	spared	Normal/decreased for articulatory errors	spared	mild impairment?	spared?	buccofacial apraxia
Progressive Aphasia with verbal comprehension deficits (Mesulam 2001)	fluent, with frequent word-finding pauses	Decreased	preserved/impaired	impaired (category-specificty e.g. animate vs inanimate)	NA	NA	NA

Table 2
Post-hoc analysis of neuropsychological test in the three variants

	SD N= 14 Mean (sd)	PNFA N= 17 Mean (sd)	LPA N= 11 Mean (sd)	NC N= 10 Mean (sd)
Demographic				
Age	63.8 (7.1)	67.3 (8.9)	68.0 (9.8)	66.4 (10.4)
Education	16.8 (2.4)	15.4 (2.3)	17.2 (3.3)	16.3 (2.7)
Gender (M/F)	9/5	5/12	7/4	4/8
Neuropsychological measures				
MMSE	23.8 (4.5)[a]	25.2 (4.9)	21.0 (6.0)[a]	29.7 (0.5)
Digit backward	4.5 (1.1)	2.9 (1.7)[a,d]	3.2 (1.2)[a]	5.0 (0.1)
Praxis	12.2 (1.8)[a]	11.5 (3.6)[a]	12.5 (1.8)	14 (0)
Calculation	4.4 (0.8)	4.4 (1.2)	2.5 (1.5)[a,b,c]	4.5 (0.5)
Speech and language production				
WAB speech fluency (10)	9.1 (0.7)[a]	6.1 (3.9)[a,d]	8.2 (1.5)[a]	10 (0)
Apraxia of speech rating (7 max deficit)	0 (0)	3.0 (2.3)	1.5 (1.7)	NA
Dysarthria rating (7 max deficit)	0 (0)	1.4 (2.0)	0 (0)	NA
WAB repetition (100)	91.5 (8.4)	79.2 (22.8)[a]	79.5 (20.7)[a]	99.5 (0.9)
Semantic fluency	4.57 (3.10)[a,b]	9.8 (4.9)[a]	7.4 (3.9)[a]	20.6 (4.5)
Phonetic fluency	6.35 (4.08)[a]	5.5 (4.7)[a]	7.9 (5.9)[a]	16.2 (5.1)
Lexical retrieval and word comprehension				
WAB word recognition total (60)	50.5 (9.9)[a,b,c]	59.6 (1.0)	58.5 (1.5)	60 (0)
Single categories (6)				
Real objects	4.7 (1.4)[a,b,c]	6 (0)	6 (0)	6 (0)
Drawn objects	5.3 (1.5)	5.9 (0.2)	6 (0)	6 (0)
Shapes	3.84 (1.99)[a,b,c]	5.88 (0.33)	5.9 (0.3)	6 (0)
Letters	6 (0)	5.4 (1.9)	6 (0)	6 (0)
Numbers	6 (0)	5.9 (0.2)	6 (0)	6 (0)
Colors	5.7 (0.6)	6 (0)	6 (0)	6 (0)
Furniture	5.5 (1.2)	6 (0)	6 (0)	6 (0)
Body parts	4.9 (1.2)[a,b,c]	6 (0)	6 (0)	6 (0)
Fingers	4.3 (1.7)[a,b]	5.8 (0.7)[a]	5.4 (0.7)	6 (0)
Left and right discrimination	4.1 (1.9)[a,b,c,]	5.82 (0.72)	5.20 (1.47)	6 (0)
BNT (15)	4.7 (3.7)[a,b,c]	12.5 (2.8)	9.18 (3.0)[a]	14.3 (1.2)
Sentence comprehension				
WAB sequential command (80)	74.5 (7.2)	71.9 (8.7)[a]	65.0 (18.9)[a]	80 (0)

[a] $p < 0.05$ vs Control.
[b] $p < 0.05$ vs NFPA.
[c] $p < 0.05$ vs LPA.
[d] $p < 0.05$ vs SD.

the "classical location" in precentral gyrus, subcortical areas and brainstem) [10,24]. The most common pathology in one study of 18 SD cases is MNDID (13 cases) [9], distantly followed by Pick's disease (3) and AD (2).

AD is probably the second most common neuropathology associated with PPA, and occurs with both fluent and nonfluent predominant clinical syndromes [33,49].

Recently two series of pathologically confirmed PPA cases have been described. One showed that "possible PPA" (because of early memory impairment) had AD pathology; while "probable PPA" cases were associated with FTLD pathology (MNDID, CBD and Pick's disease) [31]. The other [33] showed that nonfluent cases were more associated with tauopathies, while fluent cases showed predominantly MNDID; in both groups AD was the second most frequent diagnosis.

Future studies will need to include adequate samples to represent each PPA variant and a comprehensive language battery that can differentiate the variants during life. Finally, these batteries should be designed to detect patients with very mild impairments.

2.4. Neuroanatomy

Neuroimaging and neuropathology studies have shown left perisylvian involvement, affecting the language network, in most PPA patients [12,26,44]. SD patients, studied with Voxel Based Morphometry

(VBM), have significantly more atrophy in the medial and anterior temporal lobes than FTD [52] and AD [2]; these areas are involved in semantic memory. PET studies found left frontal hypometabolism in PNFA patients which might explain the agrammatism and AOS characteristics of these patients [17,46,61,62]. A recent study compared three PPA variants (PNFA, SD and LPA) in the same setting [13]. In addition to the areas previously reported, PNFA cases also showed atrophy in motor and premotor cortex. In our opinion, the involvement of motor cortex in PNFA provides further evidence that CBD could be the underlying pathology in some of these patients. Findings within the SD group showed atrophy in medial and lateral portions of the anterior temporal lobes bilaterally, confirming the results of previous studies. In the LPA group, atrophy was localized to the left inferior and medial parietal lobe, the posterior third of the middle temporal gyrus and the superior temporal sulcus and the left hippocampus. Atrophy in the LPA variant was more posterior than in the SD group, but the two variants overlapped in the middle and posterior thirds of the middle temporal gyrus. The temporo-parietal and hippocampal pattern of atrophy seen in LPA has previously been reported in AD patients [4,18], suggesting that AD pathology might be a common etiology in this variant.

Recent work compared a group of 11 PPA patients with 14 normal controls for studying the activation of the language network in this particular population (Sonty et al., 2003). They used phonological and semantic tasks with functional magnetic resonance imaging: PPA subjects showed overall increased activity in regions not typically activated by language tasks in normal subjects, such as left intraparietal sulcus, precentral gyrus and right fusiform gyrus. These results might be interpreted in two different ways: as compensatory neuronal strategies, with recruitment of areas outside the language network or defective inhibition, secondary to disintegration of specific neuronal pathways. In our view the first hypothesis is more plausible because subjects performed comparably to the controls, although with longer reaction times.

2.5. Hereditability

The hereditability of PPA is not well understood. Morris [42] described a family with four affected members with a clinical syndrome characterized by memory loss, language dysfunction, overeating and behavior and personality changes that he called Hereditary Dysphasic Disinhibition Dementia (HDDD1). Since

then, few families have been described with progressive aphasia as the dominant phenotype [1,34,35,43,45]. The families described by Basun, and coauthors [1] had autosomal dominant inheritance. Linkage to chromosome 17q21-22 in HDDD type 2 has been found [35], as well as to chromosome 17q21 [1], yet, the genetic mutation causing these aphasic syndromes still remains to be determined. The clinical phenotype of the family described by Lendon had onset with memory and language deficits such as decreased and hesitant output and dysnomia. Behavioral symptoms often occurred earlier, while parkinsonian symptoms started at different points during the disease.

In sporadic cases, the homozygosis for the allele H1 of the tau genotype confers a higher risk for PPA [56]. These cases might share the same genetic vulnerability of sporadic PSP and CBD where the association with the same allele is strong. Another possible explanation of these findings is that some of the cases will go on to show CBD pathology, especially those with PNFA or those PNFA patients who begin with pure progressive anarthria.

The frequency of the allele $\varepsilon 4$ of the genotype ApoE, a risk factor for AD, is higher in the logopenic, posterior predominant cases [13]. In that study, the frequency of ApoE $\varepsilon 4$ was 20 percent in PNFA, 0 percent in SD, and 67 percent in logopenic cases. This genetic finding strengthens the hypothesis that logopenic PPA could often be the clinical presentation of asymmetric, focal AD pathology. Unfortunately, these last two studies discussed cases not pathologically confirmed and it is difficult to draw definitive conclusions.

2.6. Treatment approaches

A specific treatment for this patient population has not yet been discovered. Cholinesterase inhibitors, the drugs used in Alzheimer's disease, seem to be ineffective and in some cases worsen the behavioral symptoms. Selective serotonin reuptake inhibitors (SSRIs) and atypical neuroleptics can be used to control behavioral and mood symptoms, but no study has directly addressed their efficacy for improving language symptoms in this group of patients. Recently, a small doubleblind, placebo-controlled cross over study, involving six PPA patients, tested bromocriptine for seven weeks: the dopamine agonist showed a mild slowing of language deterioration, but the benefits were limited [50].

3. Neuropsychological; language and neuroanatomical analysis of PPA

3.1. Cognitive results

We analyzed a sample of 42 consecutive PPA patients (17 PNFA, 14 SD and 11 LPA), (31 of them having already been described in a previous paper [13]) compared to 10 healthy elderly controls seen at the Memory and Aging Center at the University of California at San Francisco. All three PPA variants were determined based upon the criteria previously outlined. Our goal was to determine whether there were any distinguishing features related to demographic, neuropsychological or linguistic features of these three PPA subtypes.

Demographic variables were age, sex, education and disease duration. Neuropsychological variables were Mini Mental Status Examination (MMSE), digits backwards, phonemic and semantic fluency, praxis, calculation, 15 items from the Boston Naming Test, a spontaneous speech sample (fluency and information content), auditory word recognition, sequential commands and repetition subtests of the Western Aphasia Battery [27].

ANOVA or the Kruskal Wallis non-parametric test were used to determine overall group differences. Scheffe and Mann-Whithney tests were used to do post-hoc analysis on cognitive measures. These results are briefly described below.

Age, education and disease duration were not significantly different between patients and controls or within the three variants. As expected, results from neuropsychological testing showed significant differences when each PPA variant was compared to controls and to each other.

3.1.1. Progressive nonfluent aphasia

Patients with PNFA presented with halting, effortful spontaneous speech, AOS (14 out of 17) and/or dysarthria (6 out 17). (The most common dysarthria type was mixed (upper and lower motor neuron, 3 cases), while one case of each of the following types was also noted: lower motor neuron, upper motor neuron and hyperkinetic dysarthria. In some cases, AOS was so severe that a dysarthria classification could not be made. Information content was also significantly decreased, but this was clearly at least partially due to speech production impairments. Repetition subtest scores were significantly decreased. Semantic and phonemic fluency scores together with comprehension for complex commands were significantly lower than controls. Single word comprehension evaluated with

the WAB auditory word recognition was normal. Confrontation naming, often administered in the written rather than verbal modality, was relatively spared; additional improvement was noted when multiple choices were provided. MMSE scores were within normal limits. Performance on the digit backward task was significantly lower from the control and SD groups. On praxis, PNFA patients had the lowest scores, although not significantly different from the other two variants. Calculation was spared. Decreased fluency, speech impairment and working memory deficits were neuropsychological hallmarks of this group. These results suggest an involvement of left inferior frontal gyrus and anterior insula [13,46,60].

3.1.2. Semantic dementia

SD patients showed nearly normal fluency but decreased information content, because of poor naming of low frequency objects in the description of the picnic scene picture from the WAB. None of the SD patients had AOS and/or dysarthria; sentence comprehension was spared. Semantic fluency was significantly impaired compared to controls and PNFA; phonemic fluency was also significantly decreased. SD patients had significant difficulty with recognition of objects, body parts, fingers and shapes; and they were not able to discriminate the left and right side of the body. Repetition and sequential commands did not differ from controls. Confrontation naming scores were lowest in the SD group and significantly different than PNFA, LPA and controls; multiple choices did not improve their performance. MMSE scores were impaired, while scores on the digit backward task were within normal limits and significantly better than in the other two variants. Praxis was significantly impaired, perhaps due to difficulty with object recognition (e.g., hammer, saw), as previously mentioned. Calculation was normal. This neuropsychological profile reflects a loss of knowledge regarding objects, actions and words. These results suggest an involvement of anteroinferior-medial temporal gyrus, which has been verified with neuroimaging [8,13,59] and pathologic studies [9]. Knowledge of action might be more impaired when the disease progressed to the frontal lobe [54], although the atrophy is only mild in this area [9].

3.1.3. Logopenic progressive aphasia

LPA patients had spontaneous speech scores that fell between the other two variants. Speech output was slow and marked by word-finding difficulty. In some cases, phonemic paraphasias were difficult to differ-

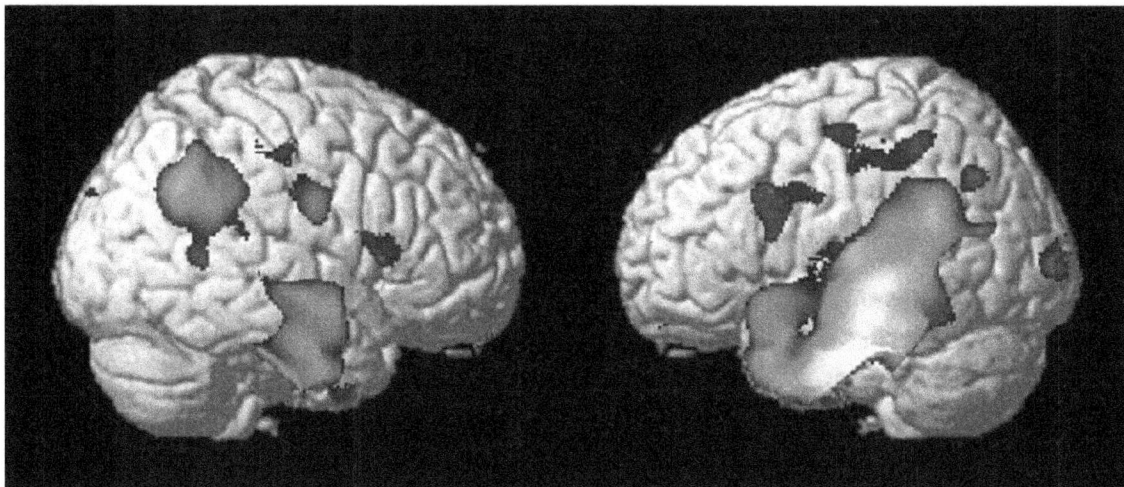

Fig. 1. Patients versus control. Involvement of a large network centered in the perysilvian region and left temporal lobe.

entiate from a "true" motor speech deficit, such as AOS. Phonemic and semantic fluency scores were significantly lower than controls, repetition scores were significantly decreased and the sequential commands subtest was more impaired than in the PNFA and SD groups. Single word comprehension was within normal limits. Confrontation naming test performance was impaired but, as opposed to SD, recognition on multiple choice partially improved the performance. Interestingly, this group was the only one in which calculation deficits were noted and MMSE scores were the lowest, although not significantly different than the other two variants. Scores on the digit backward task were also significantly impaired. Praxis scores were also significantly impaired. Overall, the LPA patients presented with prominent acalculia, and deficits in syntax comprehension and verbal rehearsal, suggesting left posterior temporal cortex and inferior parietal lobule atrophy [13].

In summary, SD patients showed the most consistent cognitive profile, easily distinguishable from the other two variants. PNFA and LPA performances overlapped in many cognitive tests. However, the mechanism behind the deficit was clearly different. For instance, while defective repetition was due to speech output difficulties and agrammatism in PNFA; phonological memory impairments probably accounted for poor repetition in LPA patients. Classic aphasia batteries such as the WAB, originally created for vascular aphasic patients, often fail to distinguish between variants of PPA.

3.2. Imaging results

We performed a structural MRI anatomical analysis of 51 MRI scans (39 images obtained from each patient described above and a group of 12 normal controls). Three patients were excluded from the analysis because they did not have an image acquired within six-months of the clinical and neuropsychological evaluation. MRI images were obtained on a 1.5T Magnetom VISION system (Siemens, Iselin, NJ). We analyzed the images with VBM, a technique for the detection of regional brain atrophy by voxel-wise comparison of gray matter volumes between groups of subjects. The technique includes an image preprocessing step (spatial normalization, segmentation, modulation, and smoothing) followed by statistical analysis. Grey matter volumes for each subject, age and gender were entered into the design matrix as nuisance variables. Regionally specific differences in gray matter volumes were assessed using the general linear model, and the significance of each effect was determined using the theory of Gaussian fields. Specific statistical analyses were performed to investigate the overall network of regions involved in PPA. We accepted a statistical threshold of $p < 0.05$ corrected for multiple comparisons for the whole brain, but we also report areas at $p < 0.001$ uncorrected if comprised in the left perysilvian language regions.

The results of the analysis (Fig. 1) showed that PPA diagnosis correlated with a large area in the left hemisphere that included inferior ($p < 0.05$, corrected), middle and superior temporal gyri ($p < 0.001$, uncorrected) together with left inferior frontal gyrus, ($p < 0.001$, uncorrected), insular ($p < 0.05$, corrected) and parietal inferior area ($p < 0.001$, uncorrected).

4. Conclusion

Isolated progressive speech and language difficulties are often the first symptom of left hemisphere focal forms of neurodegenerative diseases, particularly FTLD and CBD. AD patients also present with atypical focal cognitive manifestations, including fluent and nonfluent progressive aphasia. The variety of clinical presentations, anatomical areas involved and the multiple pathologies reflect the heterogeneity of the PPA population.

The clinical syndrome of PPA is associated with at least three distinct variants: PNFA, SD and LPA, but comprehensive language testing is often required to identify these anatomically, genetically and pathologically distinctive subtypes.

The heterogeneity of the clinical syndrome has relevance to neuropathology. We suspect that posterior variants of PPA will often show AD neuropathology, while frontally predominant cases will often show CBD at post-mortem. Language and neuroimaging testing help to separate these anatomical subgroups, although some patients will be difficult to classify into a single subtype.

Future studies should consider PPA variants as separate entities and use an integrated approach to collect longitudinal clinical, cognitive, and neuroimaging information as well as genetic and pathological data. Clinical, imaging and pathological information could then be correlated in order to better understand the pathogenesis and the specific etiology of the single variants. Since FTLD-like pathology might not be the underlying etiology in all variants, future studies investigating new treatments should also differentiate the three variants.

Acknowledgement

The authors are supported by the following grants: 1 P50 AG-03-006-01 NIH/NIA – Alzheimer's Disease Research Centers, Core A and Core B; 03-75271 DHS/ADP/ARCC – (Dr. Miller); 5 P01 AG019724-02 FTD PPG –, Core A and Project 4. Wessinger Foundation (Dr. Miller); NINDS 1R01AG22985 and 04-35516 DHS/ADP (Dr. Gorno-Tempini).

References

[1] H. Basun, O. Almkvist, K. Axelman, A. Brun, T.A. Campbell, J. Collinge, C. Forsell, S. Froelich, L.O. Wahlund, L. Wetterberg and L. Lannfelt, Clinical characteristics of a chromosome 17-linked rapidly progressive familial frontotemporal dementia, *Arch Neurol* **54**(5) (1997), 539–544.

[2] A.L. Boxer, K.P. Rankin, B.L. Miller, N. Schuff, M. Weiner, M.L. Gorno-Tempini and H.J. Rosen, Cinguloparietal atrophy distinguishes Alzheimer disease from semantic dementia, *Arch Neurol* **60**(7) (2003), 949–956.

[3] E. Broussolle, S. Bakchine, M. Tommasi, B. Laurent, B. Bazin, L. Cinotti, L. Cohen and G. Chazot, Slowly progressive anarthria with late anterior opercular syndrome: a variant form of frontal cortical atrophy syndromes, *J Neurol Sci* **144**(1–2) (1996), 44–58.

[4] A. Brun and E. Englund, Regional pattern of degeneration in Alzheimer's disease: neuronal loss and histopathological grading, *Histopathology* **5**(5) (1981), 549–564.

[5] R.J. Caselli, T.G. Beach, L.I. Sue, D.J. Connor and M.N. Sabbagh, Progressive aphasia with Lewy bodies, *Dement Geriatr Cogn Disord* **14**(2) (2002), 55–58.

[6] S.B. Chapman, R.N. Rosenberg, M.F. Weiner and A. Shobe, Autosomal dominant progressive syndrome of motor-speech loss without dementia, *Neurology* **49**(5) (1997), 1298–1306.

[7] L. Cohen, N. Benoit, P. Van Eeckhout, B. Ducarne and P. Brunet, Pure progressive aphemia, *J Neurol Neurosurg Psychiatry* **56**(8) (1993), 923–924.

[8] A. Damasio and D. Tranel, Nouns and Verbs are Retrieved with Differently Distributed Neural Systems *PNAS* **90**(11) (1993), 4957–4960.

[9] R.R. Davies, J.R. Hodges, J.J. Kril, K. Patterson, G.M. Halliday and J.H. Xuereb, The pathological basis of semantic dementia, *Brain* **128**(9) (2005), 1984–1995.

[10] T. Esmonde, E. Giles, J. Xuereb and J. Hodges, Progressive supranuclear palsy presenting with dynamic aphasia, *J Neurol Neurosurg Psychiatry* **60**(4) (1996), 403–410.

[11] T. Fukui, K. Sugita, M. Kawamura, J. Shiota and I. Nakano, Primary progressive apraxia in Pick's disease: a clinicopathologic study, *Neurology* **47**(2) (1996), 467–473.

[12] C.J. Galton, K. Patterson, J.H. Xuereb and J.R. Hodges, Atypical and typical presentations of Alzheimer's disease: a clinical, neuropsychological, neuroimaging and pathological study of 13 cases, *Brain* **123**(3) (2000), 484–498.

[13] M.L. Gorno-Tempini, N.F. Dronkers, K.P. Rankin, J.M. Ogar, L. Phengrasamy, H.J. Rosen, J.K. Johnson, M.W. Weiner and B.L. Miller, Cognition and anatomy in three variants of primary progressive aphasia, *Ann Neurol* **55**(3) (2004), 335–346.

[14] M.L. Gorno-Tempini, R.C. Murray, K.P. Rankin, M.W. Weiner and B.L. Miller, Clinical, cognitive and anatomical evolution from non-fluent progressive aphasia to corticobasal syndrome: a case report, *Neurocase* **10**(6) (2004), 426–436.

[15] N.L. Graham, T. Bak, K. Patterson and J.R. Hodges, Language function and dysfunction in corticobasal degeneration, *Neurology* **61**(4) (2003), 493–499.

[16] J.D. Greene, K. Patterson, J. Xuereb and J.R. Hodges, Alzheimer disease and nonfluent progressive aphasia, *Arch Neurol* **53**(10) (1996), 1072–1078.

[17] M. Grossman, F. Payer, K. Onishi, M. D'Esposito, D. Morrison, A. Sadek and A. Alavi, Language comprehension and regional cerebral defects in frontotemporal degeneration and Alzheimer's disease, *Neurology* **50**(1) (1998), 157–163.

[18] M. Grossman, F. Payer, K. Onishi, T. White-Devine, D. Morrison, M. D'Esposito, K. Robinson and A. Alavi, Constraints on the cerebral basis for semantic processing from neuroimaging studies of Alzheimer's disease, *J Neurol Neurosurg Psychiatry* **63**(2) (1997), 152–158.

[19] K. Hachisuka, M. Uchida, Y. Nozaki, S. Hashiguchi and M. Sasaki, Primary progressive aphasia presenting as conduction aphasia, *J Neurol Sci* **167**(2) (1999), 137–141.

[20] J.R. Hodges, R.R. Davies, J.H. Xuereb, B. Casey, M. Broe, T.H. Bak, J.J. Kril and G.M. Halliday, Clinicopathological correlates in frontotemporal dementia, *Ann Neurol* **56**(3) (2004), 399–406.

[21] J.R. Hodges and K. Patterson, Nonfluent progressive aphasia and semantic dementia: a comparative neuropsychological study, *J Int Neuropsychol Soc* **2**(6) (1996), 511–524.

[22] J.R. Hodges, K. Patterson, S. Oxbury and E. Funnell, Semantic dementia. Progressive fluent aphasia with temporal lobe atrophy, *Brain* **115**(6) (1992), 1783–1806.

[23] M. Jackson, G. Lennox and J. Lowe, Motor neurone disease-inclusion dementia, *Neurodegeneration* **5**(4) (1996), 339–350.

[24] K.A. Josephs, B.F. Boeve, J.R. Duffy, G.E. Smith, D.S. Knopman, J.E. Parisi, R.C. Petersen and D.W. Dickson, Atypical progressive supranuclear palsy underlying progressive apraxia of speech and nonfluent aphasia, *Neurocase* **11**(4) (2005), 283–296.

[25] A. Joshi, E.A. Roy, S.E. Black and K. Barbour, Patterns of limb apraxia in primary progressive aphasia, *Brain Cogn* **53**(2) (2003), 403–407.

[26] D. Kempler, E.J. Metter, W.H. Riege, C.A. Jackson, D.F. Benson and W.R. Hanson, Slowly progressive aphasia: three cases with language, memory, CT and PET data, *J Neurol Neurosurg Psychiatry* **53**(11) (1990), 987–993.

[27] A. Kertesz, *Western Aphasia Battery*, University of Western Ontario Press, London, Ontario, 1980.

[28] A. Kertesz, W. Davidson, P. McCabe, K. Takagi and D. Munoz, Primary progressive aphasia: diagnosis, varieties, evolution, *J Int Neuropsychol Soc* **9**(5) (2003), 710–719.

[29] A. Kertesz, L. Hudson, I.R. Mackenzie and D.G. Munoz, The pathology and nosology of primary progressive aphasia, *Neurology* **44**(11) (1994), 2065–2072.

[30] A. Kertesz, T. Kawarai, E. Rogaeva, P. St George-Hyslop, P. Poorkaj, T.D. Bird and D.G. Munoz, Familial frontotemporal dementia with ubiquitin-positive, tau-negative inclusions, *Neurology* **54**(4) (2000), 818–827.

[31] A. Kertesz, P. McMonagle, M. Blair, W. Davidson and D.G. Munoz, The evolution and pathology of frontotemporal dementia, *Brain* **128**(9) (2005), 1996–2005.

[32] A. Kertesz and D. Munoz, Relationship between frontotemporal dementia and corticobasal degeneration/progressive supranuclear palsy, *Dement Geriatr Cogn Disord* **17**(4) (2004), 282–286.

[33] J.A. Knibb, J.H. Xuereb, K. Patterson and J.R. Hodges, Clinical and pathological characterization of progressive aphasia, *Ann Neurol* **59**(1) (2006), 156–165.

[34] T.A. Krefft, N.R. Graff-Radford, D.W. Dickson, M. Baker and R.J. Castellani, Familial primary progressive aphasia, *Alzheimer Dis Assoc Disord* **17**(2) (2003), 106–112.

[35] C.L. Lendon, T. Lynch, J. Norton, D.W. McKeel, Jr., F. Busfield, N. Craddock, S. Chakraverty, G. Gopalakrishnan, S.D. Shears, W. Grimmett, K.C. Wilhelmsen, L. Hansen, J.C. Morris and A.M. Goate, Hereditary dysphasic disinhibition dementia: a frontotemporal dementia linked to 17q21-22, *Neurology* **50**(6) (1998), 1546–1555.

[36] P.J. Massman, K.T. Kreiter, J. Jankovic and R.S. Doody, Neuropsychological functioning in cortical-basal ganglionic degeneration: Differentiation from Alzheimer's disease, *Neurology* **46**(3) (1996), 720–726.

[37] P.S. Mathuranath, J.H. Xuereb, T. Bak and J.R. Hodges, Corticobasal ganglionic degeneration and/or frontotemporal dementia? A report of two overlap cases and review of literature, *J Neurol Neurosurg Psychiatry* **68**(3) (2000), 304–312.

[38] M.M. Mesulam, Slowly progressive aphasia without generalized dementia, *Ann Neurol* **11**(6) (1982), 592–598.

[39] M.M. Mesulam, Primary progressive aphasia – differentiation from Alzheimer's disease, *Ann Neurol* **22**(4) (1987), 533–534.

[40] M.M. Mesulam, Primary progressive aphasia, *Ann Neurol* **49**(4) (2001), 425–432.

[41] M. Mimura, T. Oda, K. Tsuchiya, M. Kato, K. Ikeda, K. Hori and H. Kashima, Corticobasal degeneration presenting with nonfluent primary progressive aphasia: a clinicopathological study, *J Neurol Sci* **183**(1) (2001), 19–26.

[42] J.C. Morris, M. Cole, B.Q. Banker and D. Wright, Hereditary dysphasic dementia and the Pick-Alzheimer spectrum, *Ann Neurol* **16**(4) (1984), 455–466.

[43] J.R. Murrell, M.G. Spillantini, P. Zolo, M. Guazzelli, M.J. Smith, M. Hasegawa, F. Redi, R.A. Crowther, P. Pietrini, B. Ghetti and M. Goedert, Tau gene mutation G389R causes a tauopathy with abundant pick body-like inclusions and axonal deposits, *J Neuropathol Exp Neurol* **58**(12) (1999), 1207–1226.

[44] D. Neary, J.S. Snowden, L. Gustafson, U. Passant, D. Stuss, S. Black, M. Freedman, A. Kertesz, P.H. Robert, M. Albert, K. Boone, B.L. Miller, J. Cummings and D.F. Benson, Frontotemporal lobar degeneration: a consensus on clinical diagnostic criteria, *Neurology* **51**(6) (1998), 1546–1554.

[45] D. Neary, J.S. Snowden and D.M. Mann, Familial progressive aphasia: its relationship to other forms of lobar atrophy, *J Neurol Neurosurg Psychiatry* **56**(10) (1993), 1122–1125.

[46] P.J. Nestor, N.L. Graham, T.D. Fryer, G.B. Williams, K. Patterson and J.R. Hodges, Progressive non-fluent aphasia is associated with hypometabolism centred on the left anterior insula, *Brain* **126**(11) (2003), 2406–2418.

[47] J. Ogar, H. Slama, N. Dronkers, S. Amici and M.L. Gorno-Tempini, Apraxia of speech: an overview, *Neurocase* **11**(6) (2005), 427–432.

[48] D.C. Paviour, A.J. Lees, K.A. Josephs, T. Ozawa, M. Ganguly, C. Strand, A. Godbolt, R.S. Howard, T. Revesz and J.L. Holton, Frontotemporal lobar degeneration with ubiquitin-only-immunoreactive neuronal changes: broadening the clinical picture to include progressive supranuclear palsy, *Brain* **127**(11) (2004), 2441–2451.

[49] S. Pogacar and R.S. Williams, Alzheimer's disease presenting as slowly progressive aphasia, *R I Med J* **67**(4) (1984), 181–185.

[50] D.A. Reed, N.A. Johnson, C. Thompson, S. Weintraub and M.M. Mesulam, A clinical trial of bromocriptine for treatment of primary progressive aphasia, *Ann Neurol* **56**(5) (2004), 750.

[51] J.O. Rinne, M.S. Lee, P.D. Thompson and C.D. Marsden, Corticobasal degeneration. A clinical study of 36 cases, *Brain* **117**(5) (1994), 1183–1196.

[52] H.J. Rosen, J.H. Kramer, M.L. Gorno-Tempini, N. Schuff, M. Weiner and B.L. Miller, Patterns of cerebral atrophy in primary progressive aphasia, *Am J Geriatr Psychiatry* **10**(1) (2002), 89–97.

[53] M. Schwarz, R. De Bleser, K. Poeck and J. Weis, A case of primary progressive aphasia. A 14-year follow-up study with neuropathological findings, *Brain* **121**(1) (1998), 115–126.

[54] W.W. Seeley, A.M. Bauer, B.L. Miller, M.L. Gorno-Tempini, J.H. Kramer, M. Weiner and H.J. Rosen, The natural history of temporal variant frontotemporal dementia, *Neurology* **64**(8) (2005), 1384–1390.

[55] J.S. Snowden, D. Neary, D.M. Mann, P.J. Goulding and H.J. Testa, Progressive language disorder due to lobar atrophy, *Ann Neurol* **31**(2) (1992), 174–183.

[56] M.J. Sobrido, A. Abu-Khalil, S. Weintraub, N. Johnson, B. Quinn, J.L. Cummings, M.M. Mesulam and D.H. Geschwind, Possible association of the tau H1/H1 genotype with primary progressive aphasia, *Neurology* **60**(5) (2003), 862–864.

[57] S. Taniguchi, A.M. McDonagh, S.M. Pickering-Brown, Y. Umeda, T. Iwatsubo, M. Hasegawa and D.M. Mann, The neuropathology of frontotemporal lobar degeneration with respect to the cytological and biochemical characteristics of tau protein, *Neuropathol Appl Neurobiol* **30**(1) (2004), 1–18.

[58] S.A. Thompson, K. Patterson and J.R. Hodges, Left/right asymmetry of atrophy in semantic dementia: behavioral-cognitive implications, *Neurology* **61**(9) (2003), 1196–1203.

[59] D. Tranel, C. Martin, H. Damasio, T.J. Grabowski and R. Hichwa, Effects of noun-verb homonymy on the neural correlates of naming concrete entities and actions, *Brain and Language* **92**(3) (2005), 288–299.

[60] R.S. Turner, L.C. Kenyon, J.Q. Trojanowski, N. Gonatas and M. Grossman, Clinical, neuroimaging, and pathologic features of progressive nonfluent aphasia, *Ann Neurol* **39**(2) (1996), 166–173.

[61] P.J. Tyrrell, L.D. Kartsounis, R.S. Frackowiak, L.J. Findley and M.N. Rossor, Progressive loss of speech output and orofacial dyspraxia associated with frontal lobe hypometabolism, *J Neurol Neurosurg Psychiatry* **54**(4) (1991), 351–357.

[62] P.J. Tyrrell, E.K. Warrington, R.S. Frackowiak and M.N. Rossor, Heterogeneity in progressive aphasia due to focal cortical atrophy. A clinical and PET study, *Brain* **113**(5) (1990), 1321–1336.

[63] S. Weintraub, N.P. Rubin and M.M. Mesulam, Primary progressive aphasia. Longitudinal course, neuropsychological profile, and language features, *Arch Neurol* **47**(12) (1990), 1329–1335.

[64] R. Wertz, L. LaPointe and J. Rosenbeck, *Apraxia of speech: The disorder and its management*, Grune and Stratton, New York, 1984.

4

Lexical-semantic variables affecting picture and word naming in Chinese: A mixed logit model study in aphasia

Davide Crepaldi[a,*], Wei-Chun Che[b], I.-Fan Su[c] and Claudio Luzzatti[a]

[a]*Department of Psychology, University of Milano-Bicocca, Milan, Italy*
[b]*Otorhinolaryngology Department, Taichung Veterans General Hospital, Taichung, Taiwan*
[c]*Division of Speech and Hearing Sciences, University of Hong-Kong, Hong-Kong, China*

Abstract. Lexical-semantic variables (such as word frequency, imageability and age of acquisition) have been studied extensively in neuropsychology to address the structure of the word production system. The evidence available on this issue is still rather controversial, mainly because of the very complex interrelations between lexical-semantic variables. Moreover, it is not clear whether the results obtained in Indo-European languages also hold in languages with a completely different structure and script, such as Chinese. The objective of the present study is to investigate this specific issue by studying the effect of word frequency, imageability, age of acquisition, visual complexity of the stimuli to be named, grammatical class and morphological structure in word and picture naming in Chinese. The effect of these variables on naming and reading accuracy of healthy and brain-damaged individuals is evaluated using mixed-effect models, a statistical technique that allows to model both fixed and random effects; this feature substantially enhances the statistical power of the technique, so that several variables – and their complex interrelations – can be handled effectively in a unique analysis. We found that grammatical class interacts consistently across tasks with morphological structure: all participants, both healthy and brain-damaged, found simple nouns significantly easier to read and name than complex nouns, whereas simple and complex verbs were of comparable difficulty. We also found that imageability was a strong predictor in picture naming, but not in word naming, whereas the contrary held true for age of acquisition. These results are taken to indicate the existence of a morphological level of processing in the Chinese word production system, and that reading aloud may occur along a non-semantic route (either lexical or sub-lexical) in this language.

Keywords: Chinese, aphasia, word naming, picture naming, imageability, age of acquisition, mixed-effects models, verbs, nouns

1. Introduction

The study of lexical-semantic variables such as word frequency, imageability, and age of acquisition (AoA) has a long history in neuropsychological and cognitive research as a tool to inform models of lexical processing [26]. For example, the discovery that word frequency affects the time necessary for identifying a word [29], reading it aloud [3], or retrieving a word name after the presentation of a picture [51] triggered a vivacious and still vigorous debate on models of lexical

selection [25,28,53,54]. Due to the strong intercorrelation of lexical-semantic variables [4,5], researchers have devoted substantial efforts in an attempt to disentangle the complex reciprocal relationships existing between word frequency, AoA, imageability, and morphological measures. For example, Lewis, Gerhand, and Ellis [41] provided evidence that both word frequency and AoA actually reflect a superordinate variable (cumulative frequency, i.e., the total number of times that a word has been encountered in life) and thus should not be considered as independent predictors of the behavior of brain-damaged and healthy individuals (see also [13]). The complex correlational structure of lexical-semantic variables has also been used to offer a direct cognitive interpretation of lexical effects: for example, based on the fact that frequency clustered

*Address for correspondence: Davide Crepaldi, MoMo Lab, Department of Psychology, University of Milano-Bicocca, piazza dell'Ateneo Nuovo 1, 20126 Milano, Italy.
E-mail: davide.crepaldi1@unimib.it.

with semantic measures in their lexical decision experiment, Baayen, Feldman, and Schreuder [2] suggested that word frequency effects arise primarily at the semantic level, rather than being exclusively related to the frequency with which specific word forms are seen or heard. Another reason that cognitive scientists made thorough investigation into the role of lexical-semantic variables is that some of these correlate with other linguistic factors, such as grammatical class. Indeed, great efforts have been made by cognitive neuropsychologists to understand whether imageability could explain the difference in the performance of aphasic patients in typical naming tasks of nouns (highly imageable) and verbs (relatively less imageable) [11,12, 23,57]. In this context, Luzzatti, Raggi, Zonca, Pistarini, Contardi, and Pinna [46] demonstrated that the performance of some – but not all – aphasic patients apparently showing noun-verb dissociation in picture naming could be explained in terms of word frequency or imageability; these authors went on to show that imageability was the most relevant predictor in verb-impaired patients, whereas in noun-impaired patients word frequency played this role.

This vast literature is still far from clearly determining the role of each lexical-semantic variable; however, it has provided substantial neuropsychological and psycholinguistic evidence showing that word frequency, imageability, and AoA play a crucial role in determining the performance of brain-damaged and healthy individuals in a variety of tasks, including lexical decision, reading aloud, and picture naming.

However, the literature currently available has one shortcoming; lexical-semantic variables have been studied predominantly in alphabetical languages, and it is far from clear whether these results can be straightforwardly generalized to languages with completely different structures, like Chinese. Indeed, there are many reasons why Chinese and a Western language such as English may differ substantially from a cognitive point of view, particularly as far as the processing needed to convert orthographic symbols into an ordered sequence of phonemes (as in reading) is concerned.

Chinese script is often characterized as morphosyllabic because most of its basic entities (the characters) are monosyllabic and represent morphemes [24]. The basic features of written Chinese are the strokes, which are typically arranged in a squared pattern to form a character. Characters may vary substantially in their visual complexity (the number of strokes they contain ranges from 1 to 36) [44] and are typically composite, i.e., are made up of a semantic radical and a phonetic

component. The semantic radical usually, but not always, provides an indication as to the semantic category of the character, whereas the phonetic component suggests its pronunciation; however, this is not always the case. Take for example the character 媽 (/ma1/- mother): it has the semantic radical 女 (/nu3/- woman) on the left and the phonetic component 馬 (/ma3/- horse) on the right; on the contrary, the character 猜 (/cai1/ – to guess) is made up of the semantic radical 犭 (/quan3/ – dog) – which is not related to the meaning of the whole character – and the phonetic component 青 (/qing1/ – young, green, or blue), which bears no relationship to the sound of the character. Xing [76] estimates that around 25% of Chinese composite characters are pronounced exactly as their phonetic component, indicating that the phonetic component is not an effective cue to guess the pronunciation of the composite character. In Chinese, reliable print-to-sound correspondences cannot be established at the sub-component level either, as single strokes do not correspond to any phonemic unit. In addition, the tone of a character is not orthographically marked [38], thus highlighting again that proficient reading in Chinese must be heavily based on a lexical route.

In addition to its script, Chinese has other distinguishing features that are more general and thus likely to impact not only on orthographic identification and reading aloud, but also on other cognitive tasks such as lexical retrieval and naming. For example, unlike English and other Western languages, Chinese has very few inflectional and derivational morphemes and the morphological system is almost exclusively based on compounding, being the vast majority of the words morphologically complex; therefore the linguistic system of native speakers of Chinese might be closely bound to morphological analysis, which is not necessary in English or Dutch for example.

Despite these differences between Chinese and Western languages, the results that emerge from Chinese studies on lexical-semantic variables do not seem to differ substantially from those reported in studies on Indo-European languages. Bates et al. [8] and Zhang and Yang [73] found that word frequency is a predictor for the picture naming latency in healthy Chinese speakers (see also [44]). Weekes and colleagues [68], however, did not find significant impact of word frequency on picture naming latency, which is not uncommon in studies when other factors, such as AoA, are controlled [34,38]. When taking into consideration reading aloud, results are more clear-cut; as in other languages, characters with higher frequency are named more quickly and more accurately [33].

Several studies on Chinese, as those conducted in Western languages, have shown that words typically learned at a younger age are processed faster than words acquired later in life in a number of different tasks, including lexical decision on written words [15,16,64, 67], reading aloud [16,18,69], and semantic categorization [17,18,69]. It has also been suggested that AoA plays a role independently of word frequency both in lexical decision [64,67] and in reading aloud [34,38]. The effect of AoA has also been reported to influence aphasic patients' performance in reading aloud and picture naming [34,36,38]. In these studies, a patient (FWL) who suffered from severe semantic deficits was described; her condition was so severe that her word reading only relied on a non-semantic pathway. The authors also described a second patient (TWT) whose reading was clearly mediated by the semantic route as he made several semantic errors. They used a logistic regression analysis to investigate the ability of these two patients to read 260 characters aloud, and found that AoA was a significant predictor of the reading accuracy of both, indicating that AoA affects both the semantic and the non-semantic reading route. All the other variables that were considered in this study (e.g., character frequency, imageability, number of strokes, and semantic radical consistency) were not significant predictors. Although this study was seminal in considering several variables at the same time, it only focused on two brain-damaged individuals and did not consider healthy speakers, which hinders the generality of its results. Law et al. [36] investigated the picture naming performance of five anomic aphasic patients in a study where also object familiarity, naming agreement, visual complexity, and word length were considered; AoA turned out to be the strongest predictor.

Results of studies focusing on familiarity were much less clear-cut. Whereas some studies on Cantonese aphasic speakers report that familiarity does not play a role in picture naming accuracy [36], Weekes and colleagues [68] found that familiarity predicts picture naming reaction times in healthy speakers of Cantonese even after AoA is partialled out (see also [73]).

Studies exploring the number of strokes in a character as an indicator of visual complexity have also produced mixed results. Liu et al. [43] found that characters with fewer strokes were named faster, thus suggesting that the number of strokes in a character contributes significantly to naming speed in healthy speakers, but Law et al. [34,36] did not find a number of strokes effect in a word naming task performed by dyslexic readers.

Several studies have highlighted the importance of imageability in written lexical processing of Chinese and Kanji characters in Japanese. These studies focused on tasks as diverse as silent reading [32], recall of words [52], reading aloud [10], lexical decision [72], and semantic judgment on written words [61]. Some of these studies employed neurophysiological methodologies and showed imageability effects both in behavioral responses and in brain activity patterns. Notably, imageability correlates strongly with grammatical class, as nouns tend to be much more imageable than verbs, at least in picture naming; it is in fact no easy matter to disentangle these two effects. Zhang et al. [72] and Tsai et al. [61] provided solid evidence that imageability effects hold independently of grammatical class. In Zhang et al.'s study, for example, the imageability effect at the N400 was broader for nouns than for verbs as evidenced by the ERP topography. Tsai and colleagues [61] went on to show that concrete nouns and verbs elicit a greater N400 than abstract nouns and verbs in both lexical decision and semantic judgment tasks. Data are much less clear with regards to the impact of imageability on aphasic patients' behavior. For example, Bi et al. [10] reported an imageability effect in the reading performance of WJX, a patient who suffered from dementia. However, Law et al. [34] showed that, once other variables had been taken into consideration (e.g., AoA, character frequency, number of strokes), imageability was irrelevant for the reading performance of their two dyslexic patients (FWL and TWT).

To sum up, most of the lexical and lexical-semantic variables that have been shown to affect the performance of healthy and brain-damaged speakers in Western languages are also relevant in Chinese. Data are generally clearer on unimpaired individuals than on aphasic/dyslexic patients, most likely because the variables that best predict the performance of language impaired individuals may differ substantially depending on the specific cognitive impairment. What seems to be lacking is a study that takes this issue into consideration and thus focuses on a large group of brain-damaged individuals suffering from different types of aphasia, and differing widely on other dimensions, like lesion localization, deficit severity, age and education. In addition, most recent studies [2] have highlighted that the strong collinearity between lexical and lexical-semantic predictors makes it very difficult – perhaps impossible – to test a few of them without considering the others in the same design, which is another limitation of the studies conducted so far on Chinese; most of them, in fact, have focused on a small number of predictors (but see [34]). Finally, some variability has emerged in the various tasks that have been used in the literature, possibly reflecting the different cognitive levels they tap on. The core aim of the present study is therefore to address these problems:

(i) Addressing the role of several lexical-semantic variables simultaneously;

(ii) In two different tasks (picture and word naming) that require different cognitive processes;

(iii) In a large sample of healthy and aphasic speakers of different types.

As in the literature regarding Western languages, picture naming tasks were used to identify noun-verb dissociation in Chinese aphasic speakers [7,19]. Bates et al. [7] tested the noun-verb dissociation in Broca's and Wernicke's aphasic speakers of Chinese and reported that the former group performs better on object naming than action naming, whereas the contrary holds for the latter group. On the basis of these results, the authors suggested that nouns and verbs are represented differently at the lexical level in Chinese. Although lexical-semantic variables were not taken into consideration in the analyses of the data in this study, Chen and Bates [19] did provide additional evidence that grammatical class is likely to be an organizing principle of the lexical production system in Chinese. For this reason – and also to provide a further assessment of whether grammatical class explains speakers' performance over and above other lexical-semantic variables – the set of items for the present study will include both nouns and verbs and the data will be analysed also on the basis of grammatical class.

Although shown to be a strong determinant of behavior both in aphasic patients [8] and in healthy speakers [60], morphological structure has been somewhat neglected in the literature on Chinese. Interestingly, several psycholinguistic studies have been carried out in Chinese on written compound recognition [61,74,75], but much less attention has been paid to lexical production (see [50]). Chen and Chen [20] carried out implicit priming experiments where participants learned arbitrary associations between pairs of compound words, and were subsequently asked to produce one item of the pair after being cued with the other one. Response times were shown to be equivalent on pairs where compound words shared a morpheme in the initial position (e.g., 家事, jia1-shi4, household, and 家電, jia1-dia4, household appliances) and on pairs where compound words shared only a homophonic, non-homographic syllable in the same position (e.g., 家事, jia1-shi4, household, and 佳餚, jia1-yao2, delicacy). As morphological

priming was equivalent to phonological priming in this experiment, the authors suggested that morphology is not an organizing principle of the word production system over and above phonology. This conclusion received further support from other experiments [20,31], showing that in a number of tasks (including picture naming) the frequency of the individual constituents does not influence the time necessary for producing a compound. This body of evidence is very intriguing because it seems to deny a level of morphological processing in a language where over 70% of words are compounds [75].

The role of morphology in Chinese is also debated in the literature on language and literacy acquisition. For example, McBride and colleagues [47,48] have shown that morphological awareness is associated with vocabulary knowledge in Chinese-speaking second graders, and also correlates with character recognition in preschoolers and second graders after controlling for age, phonological awareness, speed of processing, and vocabulary size. These results suggest that morphology contributes to language acquisition and the development of literacy skills over and above phonology. Sensitivity to the morphological structure of Chinese words was also found later in development among fourth-graders by Liu and colleagues [42]. However, Chung and Hu [21] have shown that morphological awareness is not associated to the ability to read Chinese characters once vocabulary knowledge had been partialled out; the authors concluded from these data that morphological knowledge in reading does not facilitate performance in the very initial stages of reading acquisition.

As we have illustrated, there seems to be substantial disagreement as to the role of morphology in the Chinese word identification and word production system. For this reason, we included both simple (i.e., monosyllabic, monomorphemic and one-character) and complex (bisyllabic, bimorphemic and two-character) words in our set of stimuli, and considered morphological structure as a further potential predictor of speakers' performance in our analyses.

2. Materials and methods

2.1. Participants

Twenty Taiwanese speakers suffering from aphasia after a vascular left-hemisphere brain damage (12 suffering from Broca's aphasia, 2 from Wernicke's

Table 1
Examples of the types of items used in this paper

Categories	Constituents	Example	Transcription and English translation
Simple noun		箭	*jian4*, arrow
Simple verb		哭	*ku1*, to cry
Nominal compound			
[NN]$_N$	N+N	奶瓶	*nai3-ping2*, "milk + bottle", feeding-bottle
[NV]$_N$	N+V	沙漏	*sa1-lou4*, "stand + to leak" hourglass
[VN]$_N$	V+N	剪刀	*jian3-dao1*, "to cut + knife", scissors
[VV]$_N$	V+V	裁判	*cai2-pan4*, "to judge + to decide" (the) referee
Verbal compound			
[NV]$_V$	N+V	肩負	*jian1-fu4*, "shoulder + to carry something on the back", to bear
[VN]$_V$	V+N	拔河	*ba2-he2*, "to pull out + river", to do a tug of war
[VV]$_V$	V+V	賽跑	*sai4-pao3*, "to compete + to run", to race

Notes. N, noun; V, verb.

aphasia, 3 from anomic aphasia, and 3 from a non-classifiable form of aphasia) were recruited for the study. Prior to brain damage they were proficient in Mandarin Chinese, which they used for everyday communication.[1] None suffered from severe dysarthria, severe apraxia of speech, auditory problems, visual problems, or more general cognitive impairments. All aphasic patients were at least six months post-onset. They participated in both a picture naming and a reading task, with the exception of participant A13, who could not complete the reading task. Twenty neurologically healthy individuals also participated in this study; they were matched in gender, age, and education level with the aphasic patients and were all proficient in Mandarin Chinese.

2.2. Materials

Two tasks – a picture naming and a reading task – were specifically designed to test the participants' ability to retrieve morphologically simple and complex nouns and verbs. Both tasks contained simple nouns, simple verbs, verbal compounds and nominal compounds. The items for nominal and verbal compounds were further divided into groups according to the grammatical category of their constituents. Nominal compounds were composed of a noun plus a noun ([NN]N), or a noun plus a verb ([NV]N), or a verb plus a noun ([VN]N), or a verb plus a verb ([VV]N). Verbal compounds were composed of a verb plus a verb ([VV]V), or a verb plus a noun ([VN]V), or a noun plus a verb ([NV]V). There were six categories and 95 items in total for the picture naming task: 20 simple nouns, 20

[NN]N, 20 [VN]N, 10 simple verbs, 15 [VN]V, and 10 [VV]V. Three categories, [NV]N, [VV]N, and [NV]V, were not included in the picture naming task because too few depictable testing items could be found. There were nine categories of stimuli in the reading task: simple nouns, [NN]N, [NV]N, [VN]N, [VV]N, simple verbs, [NV]V, [VN]V, and [VV]V) (see Table 1 for examples). Each category contained 20 items, for a total of 180 items for the whole task. [VN]V compounds are notoriously difficult to distinguish from verbal phrases. The criteria described by Packard [55] were adopted to define this type of verbal compounds in the present study. Verb+object elements (V-O) were thus considered as verbal compounds when:

(i) One of the constituents was a bound morpheme;
(ii) The V-O could be followed by an object;
(iii) The meaning of the V-O compound could not be inferred from the meaning of its constituents.

For the picture naming task, naming agreement was estimated for each item on the basis of the naming performance of 30 healthy participants, aged from 21 to 33. Only pictures whose naming agreement was above 70% were retained for the final version of the test: alternative answers that were given by at least 10% of the healthy participants were considered to be correct if produced by the aphasic patients. In order to avoid unnecessary collinearity among predictors, the word frequency, familiarity, imageability, and AoA of the items used in the picture naming and the reading aloud task were matched as closely as possible (see Table 2). Because no data are available on oral word frequency in Chinese, written frequency was considered in both the picture and the word naming task; this does not limit the generality of our findings because written and oral word frequency have been shown to correlate strictly [2]. Frequency values were obtained by con-

---

[1]Taiwanese is still very diffused in Taiwan, particularly among older people; therefore, some of the participants in this study also used Taiwanese extensively for everyday communication.

Table 2

Word frequency (*WF*), familiarity (*Fam*), imageability (*Img*), and age of acquisition (*AoA*) values for the different types of stimuli used in the present study (mean ± standard deviation)

		N	WF	Fam	Img	AoA
(a) Picture naming						
Nouns						
	Simple	20	5.40 ± 0.93	5.37 ± 1.23	6.62 ± 0.32	2.32 ± 0.62
	NN	20	3.45 ± 0.94	5.10 ± 1.03	6.69 ± 0.17	3.02 ± 0.77
	VN	20	2.91 ± 1.50	4.92 ± 1.25	6.57 ± 0.30	3.23 ± 0.79
Verbs						
	Simple	10	5.12 ± 1.45	5.63 ± 0.66	5.58 ± 0.56	2.38 ± 0.52
	VN	15	1.14 ± 1.14	4.92 ± 1.31	5.78 ± 0.49	3.40 ± 1.06
	VV	10	3.53 ± 0.69	4.73 ± 1.01	5.51 ± 0.60	3.96 ± 0.87
(b) Reading aloud						
Nouns						
	Simple	20	4.93 ± 0.69	5.03 ± 1.17	6.44 ± 0.63	2.56 ± 0.58
	NN	20	4.72 ± 1.07	4.63 ± 0.76	4.13 ± 2.06	4.51 ± 1.11
	NV	20	3.23 ± 1.61	4.42 ± 0.71	4.26 ± 1.88	5.15 ± 0.97
	VN	20	3.91 ± 1.69	4.92 ± 1.06	4.19 ± 1.96	4.43 ± 1.16
	VV	20	4.35 ± 1.45	4.69 ± 0.79	3.04 ± 1.40	5.15 ± 0.84
Verbs						
	Simple	20	4.86 ± 1.08	5.36 ± 0.70	5.41 ± 0.88	2.41 ± 0.57
	NV	20	2.76 ± 0.93	3.64 ± 0.56	2.40 ± 1.03	5.85 ± 0.39
	VN	20	3.74 ± 1.58	4.74 ± 0.83	2.97 ± 0.90	4.99 ± 0.86
	VV	20	4.27 ± 1.36	4.58 ± 0.76	3.10 ± 1.08	4.86 ± 0.69

sulting the Academia Sinica Balanced Corpus of Modern Chinese (*http://www.sinica.edu.tw/SinicaCorpus*). The corpus is based on about 5 millions written words taken from various sources, such as newspapers, play scripts, and essays. Ratings of word familiarity and imageability were obtained by using a 7-point scale ranging from 1 (not familiar/imageable) to 7 (very familiar/imageable); for the imageability ratings, participants were asked to score each word according to the ease with which it evoked a mental image. The ratings of AoA were estimated on a 9-point scale: 1 corresponded to acquisition within the second year of life, 2 within the third year of life and so on until 9 (13 years of age or later). The ratings for each variable were made by at least 23 volunteer participants (age ranged from 19 to 33), none of which had participated in the naming agreement study. The number of strokes making up each character was also computed at this stage; this variable ranged from 4 to 20 in simple words (average = 11.95), and from 2 to 25 (for each character) in complex words (average = 10.62).

Certain words or characters occurred twice across the tests: in the picture naming task, one character was repeated twice among nouns, one was repeated twice among verbs, and 1 character was repeated twice across nouns and verbs. In the reading aloud task, 29 characters appeared twice. Overall, 18 characters were repeated across tasks, all among simple nouns and verbs. Specific care was thus taken to arrange

the stimuli in separate sessions, so that none of the participants saw the same character twice in the same session (see below).

2.3. General procedures

Pictures and written words were shown one by one to the participants on a 15 × 20 cm paper sheet. Objects and actions were presented in two separate blocks in a semi-randomized order; the items with repeated characters were kept apart as much as possible. In the reading aloud task, nouns and verbs were instead tested together and were semi-randomized into two blocks, so that no repeated characters occurred in the same block. Participants were presented with a first block of the reading aloud task, then with the two blocks of picture naming task, and finally with a second block of the reading aloud task. The presentation order of the noun and verb blocks in the picture naming task was counterbalanced across subjects. The four testing sessions were carried out on different days for most patients. Healthy control speakers were tested following exactly the same procedure used with the aphasic patients, except that they were tested first on the picture naming blocks, and then on the word naming blocks. This was done in order to avoid repetition effects in the picture naming task on those items that were also included in the reading task; these effects were thought to have no impact on the reading task, as healthy speakers were expected to perform at ceiling in reading aloud, while the same assumption was not justified *a priori* for the picture naming task (as demonstrated by the imperfect naming agreement on several drawings).

In both tasks participants were given standard instructions ("please name the following pictures" or "please, read aloud the following words") followed by practice trials on words/pictures that were not included in the experimental sets. The tasks were administered in a quiet room by a speech and language pathologist (W-CC). Each session lasted about 45 minutes; participants could ask for a break at any time of the session. All the answers were recorded, transcribed, and scored after testing.

Responses were counted as correct only when participants responded appropriately and promptly, i.e., less than 3 seconds after the stimulus presentation. Taiwanese and Hakka dialects are still very common in Taiwan together with Mandarin Chinese, so target words named in either dialect were counted as correct.

2.4. Data analysis

Data were analyzed using Mixed Logit Models (MLM) [30]. MLM are similar to Logistic Regression Analysis (LRA) [49] because they study the relationship between several continuous or non-continuous independent predictors and one dichotomous dependent variable. However, MLM distinguish between *fixed effects*, i.e., effects that hold across the whole sample of patients, and *random effects*, i.e., patient-specific effects that are added to the fixed effects to provide a better account of the overall variability of the data. On the strength of this differentiation, MLM can address the question of whether any specific predictor has an impact on the performance of the whole sample of patients, as well as the question of whether patients differ in their sensitivity to this predictor.

MLM were fitted and analysed using the free statistical software R (version 2.10.1; *http://www.r-project. org/*), and in particular using the *lmer* function from the *lme4* package (*http://cran.r-project.org/web/packages /lme4/index.html*). The R code is available from the authors on request. Before fitting the models we analysed the correlational structure of the predictors and took the steps necessary to reduce collinearity (see below). An initial model was built up that included all main effects and second-level interactions as fixed effects; higher-level interactions were not considered because they seriously affect the sensitivity of the analyses of main effects and second-level interactions. This model

also had a random intercept for subjects and for items; these effects are not related to any specific predictor, but account for the general variability related to the random selection of subjects (e.g., some people are generally more accurate than others) and items (e.g., some items are intrinsically more difficult than others). The initial model was then progressively simplified by removing stepwise non-significant fixed effects until the deletion of any additional effect caused a significant loss of fit to the model (as tested by a Chi-square test). Then the structure of the random effects specifically related to each predictor (*random slopes*) was examined, i.e., the parameters that indicate whether the effect of each specific predictor varies substantially across patients. The same stepwise procedure was applied here: each individual random effect was added to the model and its impact on the goodness of fit was tested. When the fit improved significantly, the specific random slope was retained in the model, otherwise it was removed. The analysis of the random slopes is also very useful because it captures variability that would be considered as error variance in standard regression or in ANOVA, thus limiting the sensitivity of the statistical test on fixed effects.

Grammatical class (nouns vs. verbs; *GC*), morphological structure (simple vs. complex; *Morph*), familiarity (*Fam*), age of acquisition (*AoA*), imageability (*Img*), and log-transformed word frequency (*WF*) were considered as possible predictors in the analysis of the healthy speakers' performance. Aphasia type (fluent vs. non-fluent vs. non-classified; *AT*) was added to the set of predictors for the analysis of the performance of the brain-damaged participants.

3. Results

3.1. Picture naming

3.1.1. Correlation between predictors

The correlation matrix between the predictors in the picture naming task is shown in Table 3. A useful index to investigate the degree of collinearity among predictors is the condition number k [9]. This index equals 16.46 in the matrix, thus indicating medium collinearity [1]. This can be attributed to the correlation between:

(i) *Img* and *GC* (nouns are more imageable than verbs);
(ii) *Morph* and *AoA* (simple words are judged to be learned earlier in life than complex words);

(iii) *Morph* and *WF* (simple words are more frequent than complex words);

(iv) *WF* and *AoA* (frequent words are judged to be learned earlier in life);

(v) *AoA* and *Fam* (words that are judged to be learned earlier in life are also judged as more familiar).

We tried to reduce collinearity by using factorial analysis, but no factorial solution was satisfying, i.e., factors were neither clearly interpretable theoretically nor allowed a consistent reduction of collinearity. We then tried to exclude the factors that were involved in the strongest correlations. The highest correlation index in the matrix is between *GC* and *Img*; however, we could not drop either of these variables because they clearly map onto separate theoretical concepts, both of which were of interest to us. We then turned our attention to the second strongest correlation in the matrix, which is between *AoA* and *Fam*. The theoretical constructs underlying these variables are not clearly distinguishable; no one can really remember as an adult when s/he has learned a specific word, and thus the subjective AoA ratings might reflect some sort of "introspective feeling of strength" about the representation of any given word, which might really be what Fam ratings are also based on. If this is the case, *Fam* and *AoA* are two different measures of the same construct: we thus felt that we could drop either of these variables without a significant loss of theoretical strength for our study. Fam was excluded rather than AoA because this latter variable has received substantial attention in the relevant literature and was thus more important to allow a meaningful comparison between our results and those obtained in past studies. The removal of *Fam* was sufficient for k to drop to 6.62, indicating that the following analyses could be carried out safely [1].

3.1.2. Healthy participants

The overall average accuracy of the healthy participants is reported in Table 4 (upper part). Not all the participants performed at ceiling, particularly on verbs. The sub-optimal performance of the healthy speakers provided the opportunity of conducting a statistical analysis of the impact of the predictors on response accuracy. MLM analyses indicated that the speakers' performance was influenced by *GC*, *Morph*, *Img*, and by the joint effects of *GC* and *Morph* (see Table 5). In MLM, the *Beta* parameters indicate either a correlation between the predictor and the probability of success (if the predictor is continuous), or a change in probabil-

Table 3

Correlation matrix between the predictors in the picture naming task. Spearman's r – rather than Pearson's r – was used because morphological structure and grammatical class are dichotomous variables

	GC	Morph	Fam	Img	AoA	WF
GC	1					
Morph	−0.05	1				
Fam	−0.04	0.20	1			
Img	−0.78	0.03	0.31	1		
AoA	0.20	−0.49	−0.73	−0.41	1	
WF	0.02	0.64	0.45	0.00	−0.53	1

Notes. *GC*, grammatical class; *Morph*, morphological structure; *Fam*, familiarity; *Img*, imageability; *AoA*, age of acquisition; *WF*, word frequency.

ity of success with respect to a reference level (if the predictor is dichotomous). So, for example, the reference level for *GC* is noun; thus, the positive *Beta* for *GC* indicates that the probability of success is higher in verbs as compared to nouns.[2] Because the reference level for *Morph* is complex words, the positive *Beta* for this factor indicates that simple words are easier to name than complex words. The positive *Beta* for *Img* shows that high-imageability words are easier to name than low-imageability words. Since the reference levels for *GC* and *Morph* are nouns and complex words respectively, the interaction between these variables indicates a drop in probability of success (*Beta* is negative) when the word to be named is a verb and is morphologically simple; this suggests that the general advantage for simple over complex words revealed by the *Morph* main effect is less for verbs as compared to nouns (see Fig. 1 for a complete illustration of the *GC* × *Morph* interaction). Because no random slope determined a significant increase in the model goodness of fit, the fixed effects described above can be taken to be constant across subjects. The overall goodness of fit of the model, measured by the Somers' *Dxy*, is very satisfactory: this index quantifies the correlation between predicted and observed accuracy and equals 0.80 in the final model [1].

3.1.3. Brain-damaged patients

The overall average accuracy achieved by the brain-damaged participants in the picture naming task is reported in Table 4 (lower part) and shows that patients vary greatly in their pattern of performance. In certain patients (e.g., A01, A13), the picture naming ability is dramatically impaired, whereas others (e.g., A15, A18)

---

[2]This main effect of grammatical class is better qualified by the GC × Morph interaction that emerges in these analyses and in the subsequent MLMs.

Table 4
Mean accuracy (proportion of correct responses) shown by healthy speakers and brain-damaged patients in the picture naming task

Sbj ID	Age	Ed	Group	Nouns			Verbs			Grand Tot
				S	C	Tot	S	C	Tot	
C01	21	14	Healthy	1	0.95	0.97	1	1	1	0.98
C02	36	12	Healthy	1	0.93	0.95	1	0.92	0.94	0.95
C03	21	14	Healthy	0.95	0.95	0.95	0.90	0.96	0.94	0.95
C04	30	16	Healthy	0.95	1	0.98	1	0.68	0.77	0.91
C05	39	14	Healthy	1	0.98	0.98	1	0.84	0.89	0.95
C06	42	14	Healthy	0.95	0.85	0.88	0.90	0.88	0.89	0.88
C07	43	14	Healthy	1	0.88	0.92	0.80	1	0.94	0.93
C08	42	16	Healthy	0.95	0.93	0.93	0.90	0.96	0.94	0.94
C09	44	16	Healthy	1	0.95	0.97	1	0.96	0.97	0.97
C10	51	16	Healthy	0.95	0.83	0.87	1	0.80	0.86	0.86
C11	57	6	Healthy	1	0.70	0.80	0.80	0.60	0.66	0.75
C12	57	16	Healthy	1	0.85	0.90	1	0.92	0.94	0.92
C13	35	14	Healthy	1	0.95	0.97	1	0.84	0.89	0.94
C14	84	12	Healthy	1	0.70	0.80	0.50	0.80	0.71	0.77
C15	52	18	Healthy	0.95	0.80	0.85	0.80	0.68	0.71	0.80
C16	59	8	Healthy	0.85	0.55	0.65	0.30	0.40	0.37	0.55
C17	67	12	Healthy	0.90	0.73	0.78	0.80	0.80	0.80	0.79
C18	36	16	Healthy	0.95	0.98	0.97	1	0.92	0.94	0.96
C19	45	16	Healthy	1	0.80	0.87	1	0.76	0.83	0.85
C20	42	14	Healthy	1	0.98	0.98	0.60	0.84	0.77	0.91
A01	22	13	AnF	0.30	0.15	0.20	0.10	0.28	0.23	0.21
A02	38	12	AnF	0.80	0.68	0.72	0.50	0.60	0.57	0.66
A03	20	13	AnF	0.45	0.25	0.32	0.10	0.20	0.17	0.26
A04	33	16	AnF	0.60	0.38	0.45	0.20	0.32	0.29	0.39
A05	40	14	AnF	0.95	0.33	0.53	0.90	0.44	0.57	0.55
A06	41	12	AnF	0.70	0.35	0.47	0.20	0.44	0.37	0.43
A07	42	14	AnF	0.95	0.55	0.68	0.60	0.36	0.43	0.59
A08	42	14	AnF	0.60	0.15	0.30	0.10	0.16	0.14	0.24
A09	45	16	AnF	0.55	0.48	0.50	0.20	0.28	0.26	0.41
A10	55	16	AnF	0.90	0.53	0.65	0.50	0.40	0.43	0.57
A11	55	6	AnF	0.80	0.25	0.43	0.50	0.24	0.31	0.39
A12	60	18	AnF	0.95	0.40	0.58	0.70	0.52	0.57	0.58
A13	35	12	AF	0.40	0.15	0.23	0.10	0.08	0.09	0.18
A14	79	16	AF	0.70	0.23	0.38	0.50	0.40	0.43	0.40
A15	48	18	AF	0.95	0.75	0.82	0.50	0.76	0.69	0.77
A16	65	6	AF	0.60	0.40	0.47	0.10	0.16	0.14	0.35
A17	66	12	AF	0.85	0.33	0.50	0.60	0.44	0.49	0.49
A18	40	16	AnC	0.90	0.83	0.85	0.70	0.88	0.83	0.84
A19	42	16	AnC	0.95	0.70	0.78	0.70	0.64	0.66	0.74
A20	45	14	AnC	0.85	0.28	0.47	0.70	0.32	0.43	0.45

Notes. Ed, education; *Healthy*, healthy speakers; *AF*, aphasic patient suffering from fluent aphasia; *AnF*, aphasic patient suffering from non-fluent aphasia; *AnC*, aphasic patient suffering from a form of aphasia that could not be classified; *C*, simple words; *C*, complex words.

show only mild impairment; some (e.g., A09, A16) perform very different on nouns and verbs, whereas others (e.g., A01, A12) behave similarly on the two word classes; some (e.g., A20) are very sensitive to the morphological structure of the target words, whereas others (e.g., A09) are not. However, as this paper focuses specifically on the role of lexical-semantic variables, our attention was concentrated on the MLM analyses.

The final model described in Table 6 shows that the patients' performance mainly depends on grammatical class, morphological structure, imageability, spo-

ken word frequency, aphasia type, and on the joint effect of grammatical class and morphological structure. Regarding main effects, it was seen that:

(i) Verbs have a higher probability of being retrieved correctly than nouns;
(ii) Simple words have a higher probability of success than complex words;
(iii) High-imageability words are easier than low-imageability words;
(iv) *WF* correlates positively with probability of success;

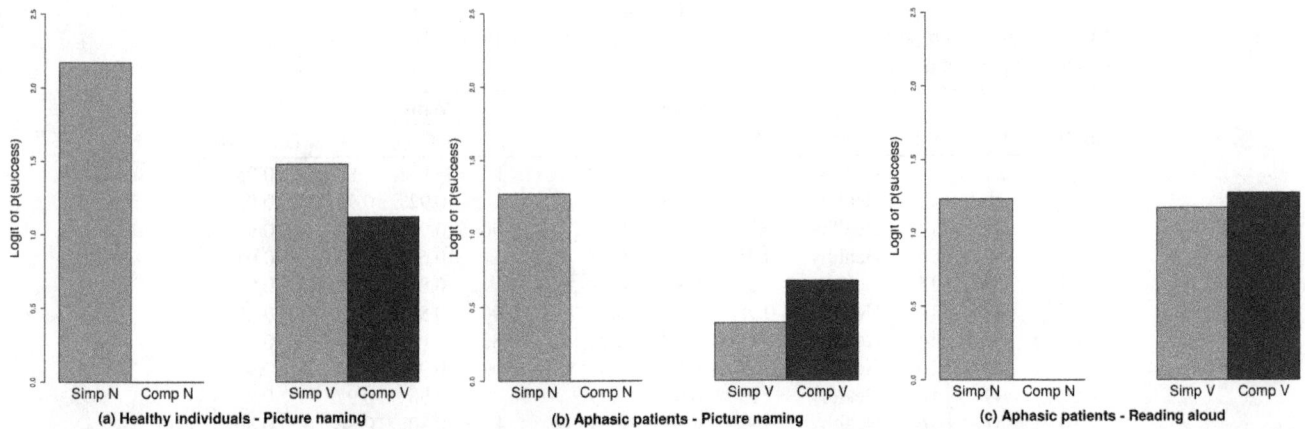

Fig. 1. Schematic representation of the $GC \times Morph$ interaction that emerged in the analysis of the performance of (a) healthy speakers in picture naming, (b) aphasic patients in picture naming, (c) aphasic patients in reading aloud. The performance of normal speakers in the reading task is not included in the figure because it was virtually at ceiling. Change in probability of success as measured against a reference level – i.e., complex nouns – is represented on the Y axis. This variable is calculated on the basis of the *Beta* parameters estimated by the MLM; this ensures that figures refer to the genuine effects of *GC* and *Morph*, i.e., once the contribution of all other predictors has been taken out. Because *Beta* parameters are additive, figures for each class are calculated by simply adding the relevant Betas; for example, the value for simple nouns is obtained by adding the parameter for simple words ($Beta(Morph) = 2.17$) to the parameter for nouns (0, because nouns are the reference level for the variable *GC*); similarly, the value for complex verbs is calculated by adding the parameter for complex words (0, because complex words are the reference level for the variable *Morph*) and the parameter for verbs ($Beta(GC) = 1.12$). Probability of success is expressed in the logit space; higher values mean higher probability of success.

Table 5

MLM offering the best fit to the observed performance of healthy speakers in the picture naming task

Fixed effects	Beta	Std. error	z value	p
Intercept	−8.06	2.61	−3.08	0.002
GC	1.12	0.54	2.07	0.04
Morph	2.17	0.55	3.95	< 0.001
Img	1.62	0.39	4.14	< 0.001
$GC \times Morph$	−1.81	0.78	−2.33	0.02
Random effects	Variance			
Sbj (intercept)	1.04			
Item (intercept)	1.52			
Log Likelihood = −563.4			*Dxy = 0.80*	

Notes. *GC*, grammatical class; *Morph*, morphological structure; *Img*, imageability. Reference levels are nouns for *GC* and complex words for *Morph*. *Dxy* refers to Somer's rank correlation between predicted probabilities and observed responses; this index varies from 0 (the model has no predictive value) to 1 (the model predicts the data perfectly).

(v) Non-fluent patients were as compromised as fluent patients (*Beta* for *AT* (*non-fluent*) is non-significant), whereas non-classified patients had a better overall performance than fluent patients (*Beta* for *AT* (*non-classified*) is significant and positive).

In the brain-damaged participants, the interaction between *GC* and *Morph* indicates that the probability of success decreases for simple verbs (*Beta* is negative and the reference levels are nouns and complex words as above); this shows that the difference between simple verbs and complex verbs is less than the difference

Table 6

MLM offering the best fit to the observed performance of brain-damaged speakers in the picture naming task

Fixed effects	Beta	Std. error	z value	p
Intercept	−7.58	1.71	−4.47	< 0.001
GC	0.68	0.33	2.04	0.04
Morph	1.27	0.37	3.45	< 0.001
Img	0.90	0.25	3.66	< 0.001
WF	0.29	0.08	3.57	< 0.001
AT (non-fluent)	0.04	0.49	0.08	0.94
AT (non-classified)	1.37	0.69	2.06	0.04
$GC \times Morph$	−1.56	0.44	−3.56	< 0.001
Random effects	Variance	Correlation		
Item (intercept)	0.57			
Sbj (intercept)	0.81			
Sbj (Morph slope)	0.71	−0.20		
Log Likelihood = −1050			*Dxy = 0.70*	

Notes. *GC*, grammatical class; *Morph*, morphological structure; *Img*, imageability; *WF*, log-transformed word frequency. Reference levels are nouns for *GC*, complex words for *Morph*, and fluent aphasic patients for *AT*. *Dxy* refers to Somer's rank correlation between predicted probabilities and observed responses; this index varies from 0 (the model has no predictive value) to 1 (the model predicts the data perfectly).

between simple nouns and complex nouns. It is interesting to note that the last two fixed effects removed from the model were $AT \times GC$ and $AT \times Img$. Although they do not contribute significantly to the model fit, these effects were close to significance before being removed ($Beta = −0.63$; $z = −1.48$; $p = 0.14$ for $AT \times GC$; $Beta = −0.66$; $z = −1.84$; $p = 0.06$ for $AT \times Img$), indicating that non-fluent patients were less suc-

Table 7
Correlation matrix between the predictors in the reading task. Spearman's r – rather than Pearson's r – was used because morphological structure and grammatical class are dichotomous variables

	GC	Morph	Fam	Img	AoA	WF
GC	1					
Morph	0.06	1				
Fam	−0.06	0.30	1			
Img	−0.24	0.54	0.28	1		
AoA	0.06	−0.69	−0.55	−0.76	1	
WF	−0.12	0.30	0.46	−0.02	−0.30	1

Notes. *GC*, grammatical class; *Morph*, morphological structure; *Fam*, familiarity; *Img*, imageability; *AoA*, age of acquisition; *WF*, word frequency.

cessful in naming verbs than nouns (*Beta* was negative on $AT \times GC$) as well as in naming high-imageability words than low-imageability words (*Beta* was negative on $AT \times Img$). Quite surprisingly, no random slope was necessary for *GC* (Chi^2 between the model including this effect and the model without this effect is 0.89 on 2 degrees of freedom; $p = 0.64$), *Img* ($Chi^2 = 0.69$; $df = 3$; $p = 0.88$), and *WF* ($Chi^2 = 0.52$; $df = 3$; $p = 0.92$). The sensitivity shown to these factors by individual patients did not vary substantially within the participant sample. On the contrary, the introduction of a random slope for *Morph* in the model determined an increase in the model goodness of fit ($Chi^2 = 19.95$; $df = 2$; $p < 0.001$), showing that some patients – but not all – were sensitive to the morphological structure of words (some patients were better at naming simple words than complex words; e.g., A05, A12, and A20).

The overall goodness of fit of the model was quite good for the brain-damaged speakers too, as indicated by the fact that predicted and observed values correlate 0.70 (see the *Dxy* index in Table 4).

3.2. Reading aloud

3.2.1. Correlation between predictors

The correlation matrix between the predictors in the reading task in shown in Table 7 and is quite similar to that observed in the picture naming task. The most relevant differences are that *GC* and *Img* entertained a much weaker correlation (as stimuli did not need to be depicted, and so low-imageability nouns could be introduced into the battery), whereas *AoA* and *Img* are more strongly correlated (most imageable words are acquired earlier) in the reading task than in the picture naming task. As the theoretical constructs underlying *AoA* and *Img* are quite different, and both variables have been reported as important predictors in reading performance [2,41], neither were excluded from the

subsequent analyses. *Fam* was excluded, as it was for the picture naming task, because it correlates strongly with both *AoA* and *WF*. The condition number k [9] was 25.24 in the final set of predictors, thus indicating the existence of some collinearity, which, however, is not high enough to hinder the reliability of the MLM [1].

3.2.2. Healthy participants

The performance of the healthy participants in the reading task is described in Table 8 (upper part). Unlike the picture naming task, nearly all healthy participants performed at ceiling level in the reading aloud task. It is important to note that this was not due to a sampling bias; target words had comparable lexical-semantic characteristics in the two tasks (see above) given all other constraints (e.g., naming agreement). This asymmetry is most likely due to a particular feature of Chinese, in that pictures may be generally named through more alternative lexical labels [8] than in Western languages, and are thus more likely to elicit non-standard responses, particularly from the elderly and/or less educated. Critically, the fact that the performance of the healthy speakers was at ceiling in reading, but not in picture naming, does not affect the reliability and generality of our findings; subject-specific variability is absorbed by random effects in MLM, and thus the evaluation of the more general fixed effects is not compromised by this additional variance. One unfortunate aspect of the healthy speakers being at ceiling was that it was not possible to run MLM on their performance and so it was impossible to compare the impact of lexical-semantic variables on reading in healthy vs. brain-damaged participants.

3.2.3. Brain-damaged patients

The overall average accuracy of the brain-damaged participants in the reading task is reported in Table 8 (lower part). The final model is described in Table 9, and shows that:

(i) Verbs were marginally easier than nouns (*Beta* is positive, but just outside the significance threshold);

(ii) Simple words were read better than complex words;

(iii) *AoA* correlated positively with probability of success, but the effect is only marginally significant;

(iv) High-frequency words were more likely to be read correctly than low-frequency words;

(v) AT had no role in the prediction of accuracy;

Table 8
Mean accuracy shown by healthy speakers and brain-damaged patients in the reading aloud task

Sbj ID	Age	Ed	Group	Nouns			Verbs			Gran Tot
				S	C	Tot	S	C	Tot	
C01	21	14	Healthy	1	0.99	0.99	1	1	1	0.99
C02	36	12	Healthy	1	0.99	0.99	1	1	1	0.99
C03	21	14	Healthy	1	1	1	1	0.97	0.98	0.99
C04	30	16	Healthy	1	1	1	1	1	1	1
C05	39	14	Healthy	1	1	1	1	1	1	1
C06	42	14	Healthy	1	1	1	1	1	1	1
C07	43	14	Healthy	1	0.99	0.99	1	0.97	0.98	0.98
C08	42	16	Healthy	1	1	1	1	1	1	1
C09	44	16	Healthy	1	1	1	1	1	1	1
C10	51	16	Healthy	1	1	1	1	0.98	0.99	0.99
C11	57	6	Healthy	1	0.97	0.97	1	0.98	0.99	0.98
C12	57	16	Healthy	1	0.99	0.99	1	1	1	0.99
C13	35	14	Healthy	1	1	1	1	1	1	1
C14	84	12	Healthy	1	0.99	0.99	1	0.98	0.99	0.99
C15	52	18	Healthy	1	1	1	1	1	1	1
C16	59	8	Healthy	1	0.98	0.98	1	0.97	0.98	0.98
C17	67	12	Healthy	0.95	0.97	0.96	1	0.93	0.95	0.96
C18	36	16	Healthy	1	0.98	0.98	1	0.98	0.99	0.98
C19	45	16	Healthy	1	0.98	0.98	1	0.95	0.96	0.97
C20	42	14	Healthy	1	1	1	1	0.95	0.96	0.98
A01	22	13	AnF	0.95	0.54	0.62	0.95	0.53	0.63	0.63
A02	38	12	AnF	0.90	0.69	0.73	0.85	0.65	0.70	0.72
A03	20	13	AnF	0.85	0.31	0.42	0.80	0.27	0.40	0.41
A04	33	16	AnF	1	0.78	0.82	1	0.82	0.86	0.84
A05	40	14	AnF	0.95	0.88	0.89	0.90	0.87	0.88	0.88
A06	41	12	AnF	0.90	0.87	0.87	0.90	0.83	0.85	0.86
A07	42	14	AnF	1	0.73	0.78	0.95	0.67	0.74	0.76
A08	42	14	AnF	0.80	0.12	0.25	0.55	0.12	0.23	0.24
A09	45	16	AnF	0.75	0.65	0.67	0.60	0.77	0.73	0.69
A10	55	16	AnF	0.95	0.95	0.95	1	0.95	0.97	0.96
A11	55	6	AnF	0.95	0.81	0.84	0.95	0.82	0.85	0.84
A12	60	18	AnF	0.95	0.66	0.72	0.90	0.53	0.63	0.68
A13	35	12	AF	NA	NA	NA	NA	NA	NA	NA
A14	79	16	AF	1	0.81	0.85	0.95	0.80	0.84	0.85
A15	48	18	AF	1	1	1	1	0.97	0.98	0.99
A16	65	6	AF	1	0.86	0.89	0.95	0.85	0.88	0.88
A17	66	12	AF	1	0.86	0.89	0.85	0.87	0.86	0.88
A18	40	16	AnC	0.95	0.98	0.97	1	1	1	0.98
A19	42	16	AnC	0.95	0.91	0.92	0.90	0.92	0.91	0.92
A20	45	14	AnC	0.90	0.44	0.53	0.80	0.38	0.49	0.51

Notes. *Ed*, education; *Healthy*, healthy speakers; *AF*, aphasic patient suffering from fluent aphasia; *AnF*, aphasic patient suffering from non-fluent aphasia; *AnC*, aphasic patient suffering from a form of aphasia that could not be classified; *S*, simple words; *C*, complex words; NA, not available.

(vi) The advantage of simple over complex words was higher in nouns than in verbs (as in the picture naming task, *Beta* for *GC* × *Morph* is positive and once again the reference levels are nouns and complex words);

(vii) The effect of AoA is weaker in verbs than in nouns (*Beta* for *GC* × *AoA* is negative), although this effect is only marginally significant;

(viii) *AoA* interacts with *WF*, indicating that words with high *AoA* and *WF* have lower probability of success;

(ix) *WF* has reduced impact on the performance of non-fluent and non-classified patients compared to fluent patients.

The goodness of fit of the model benefits from the addition of a random slope for *Morph* ($Chi^2 = 25.34$, $df = 2$, $p < 0.001$), thus indicating that patients differ in their sensitivity to morphological structure. Also, the random slopes for *AoA* and *WF* improve the model fit, but not significantly so (*AoA*: $Chi^2 = 4.70$, $df = 3$, $p = 0.20$; *WF*: $Chi^2 = 3.87$, $df = 3$, $p = 0.28$). On the contrary, there is no evidence at all for the insertion of random slopes for either *GC* or *GC* × *Morph*; patients

Table 9
MLM offering the best fit to the observed performance of brain-damaged speakers in the reading task

Fixed effects	Beta	Std. error	z value	p
Intercept	0.03	0.99	0.03	0.97
GC	1.27	0.76	1.68	0.09
Morph	1.23	0.39	3.12	0.001
AoA	0.28	0.15	1.81	0.07
WF	0.76	0.19	4.09	< 0.001
AT (non-fluent)	-0.39	0.76	-0.51	0.61
AT (non-classified)	0.12	1.00	0.12	0.90
GC × Morph	-1.33	0.51	-2.63	0.008
GC × AoA	-0.26	0.15	-1.77	0.07
AoA × WF	-0.10	0.04	-2.92	0.003
WF × AT (non-fluent)	-0.25	0.09	-2.79	0.005
WF × AT (non-classified)	-0.23	0.12	-1.96	0.04
Random effects	Variance			
Item (intercept)	0.18			
Sbj (intercept)	1.87			
Sbj (Morph slope)	0.79			
Log Likelihood $= -1418$		$Dxy = 0.70$		

Notes. *GC*, grammatical class; *Morph*, morphological structure; *AoA*, age of acquisition; *WF*, word frequency. Reference levels are nouns for *GC*, complex words for *Morph*, and fluent patients for *AT*. *Dxy* refers to Somer's rank correlation between predicted probabilities and observed responses; this index varies from 0 (the model has no predictive value) to 1 (the model predicts the data perfectly).

are thus quite homogeneous regarding these factors. The final model has a satisfactory predictive power as shown by the fact that Somer's $Dxy = 0.70$.

3.3. Separate analyses on simple and complex nouns and verbs

The MLM analyses described above show consistent effects of grammatical class, morphological structure, and an interaction between these variables. In order to investigate this interaction more in depth, separate MLM analyses were carried out on (a) simple nouns, (b) complex nouns, (c) simple verbs, and (d) complex verbs, in both picture naming and reading. Because the effects of *GC*, *Morph*, and *GC × Morph* were found in the healthy participants as well as in brain-damaged patients in the previous analyses on picture naming, data from these two populations were analyzed jointly.

In the subsequent analyses on the picture naming task, the starting model included *Group* (brain-damaged individuals – which is the reference level – vs. healthy speakers), *AoA*, *Img*, *WF*, and the interaction between *Group* and these three latter variables as fixed effects. The grammatical class of the constituents (*ConstGC*; noun-noun vs. noun-verb vs. verb-noun vs. verb-verb) was also included in the analyses of the performance on compound words. Random intercepts for items and subjects were included in the initial model.

The starting model was identical with that used for the reading aloud data, except that the analyses were carried out on the aphasic speakers only, and thus *Group* was not among the predictors. Moreover, an index of the visual complexity of the characters to be read (i.e., the number of strokes they are composed of) was also included in the reading aloud analyses.

3.3.1. Picture naming
Simple nouns
The final MLM included *AoA* (*Beta* $= -0.91$; $z = -2.37$; $p = 0.02$), *WF* (*Beta* $= 0.30$; $z = 1.52$; $p = 0.13$), *Group* (*Beta* $= 7.73$; $z = 3.20$; $p = 0.001$), and the interaction between this latter factor and *AoA* (*Beta* $= -1.70$; $z = -2.33$; $p = 0.02$) as fixed effects; moreover, the model included a random slope for *AoA*, showing that participants differ in their sensitivity to this factor. This model indicates that the probability of success for simple nouns:

(i) Increases as *AoA* decreases, even if this effect is less evident in neurologically intact speakers;
(ii) Is only marginally higher for high-frequency compared to for low-frequency words;
(iii) Is higher in healthy individuals than in brain-damaged participants.

Simple verbs

The final MLM for simple verbs in picture naming included only two fixed effects: *Group* (brain-damaged individuals vs. healthy participants; *Beta* = 3.13; z = 5.740; $p < 0.001$) and *AoA* (*Beta* = -1.27; $z = -3.23$; $p = 0.001$). Not surprisingly, this indicates that healthy participants performed better than brain-damaged individuals, and that words learnt early in life were the easiest to retrieve overall. No random slope determined a significant increase in the goodness of fit of the model.

Complex nouns

Due to the constraints posed on the item selection, complex nouns only included noun-noun and verb-noun compounds; the variable *ConstGC* thus included these two levels only (with noun-noun compounds taken as the reference level). The final model included *Group* (*Beta* = -5.84; $z = -1.52$; $p = 0.12$), *Img* (*Beta* = 1.76; $z = -3.23$; $p = 0.001$), *WF* (*Beta* = 0.28; $z = 1.99$; $p = 0.04$), and *Group* × *Img* (*Beta* = 1.37; $z = 2.36$; $p = 0.02$) as fixed effects, and no additional random slopes. Interestingly, the grammatical class of the constituents did not play any role in complex noun retrieval.

Complex verbs

Items in this category included verb-noun and verb-verb compounds; the former group constituted the reference level for the variable *ConstGC*. The final model included Group (*Beta* = 2.67; $z = 8.12$; $p < 0.001$), *ConstGC* (*Beta* = -0.42; $z = -1.43$; $p = 0.15$), *Img* (*Beta* = 0.51; $z = 1.53$; $p = 0.12$), and *AoA* (*Beta* = -0.36; $z = -2.19$; $p = 0.03$) as fixed effects, and a random slope for *Img*. This model shows that healthy participants performed better than brain-damaged individuals. It also indicates that performance was slightly better on verb-noun compounds as opposed to on verb-verb compounds, and confirms the effect of imageability observed on complex nouns, even if this effect did not interact with participant group in this analysis.

3.3.2. Reading aloud

Only data regarding the reading aloud performance of the brain-damaged participants were analysed as all healthy participants performed at ceiling.

Simple nouns

The final MLM included only the intercept as a fixed effect; there was no statistic justification for introduc-

ing any of the predictors into the model as none determined a significant improvement of the goodness of fit. The final model did not include any random slope. This produced a rather unusual MLM, which might be partially attributed to the fact that the brain-damaged patients too performed close to ceiling on simple nouns (the proportion of correct responses varied from 0.75 to 1; median = 0.95; see Table 6).

Simple verbs

The final MLM included *Img* (*Beta* = -0.59; $z = -2.06$; $p = 0.04$) and *AoA* (*Beta* = -1.11; $z = -3.06$; $p = 0.002$) as fixed effects; the absence of a random slope produced a significant increase in the model goodness of fit. Interestingly, the negative *Beta* for this *Img* indicates that the performance of brain-damaged individuals on simple verbs increases as imageability decreases (reverse imageability effect). However, caution must be used when interpreting the results of this MLM analysis because the reading performance was nearly at ceiling on simple verbs (range of proportion correct = 0.55–1; median = 0.925; see Table 6).

Complex nouns

The final MLM only included the fixed-effect of the number of strokes of the first constituent (*Beta* = -0.04; $z = -2.03$; $p = 0.04$) and the random intercepts for items and subjects; no lexical-semantic predictor determined a significant increase in the goodness of fit of the model. Thus, the performance of the brain-damaged participants on complex noun reading was unaffected by the grammatical class of the constituents, imageability, AoA, and frequency. The overall goodness of fit of the model improved when a random slope for *Img* was included into the model, thus showing cross-subject variability for sensitivity to this factor.

Complex verbs

The final MLM fit to these data included *AoA* as a fixed effect (*Beta* = -0.37; $z = -2.81$; $p = 0.004$), but no random slopes. It is worth noting that written frequency was close to being significant (*Beta* = 0.10; $z = 1.56$; $p = 0.12$) before being excluded from the model; moreover, its contribution to the model goodness of fit was not entirely negligible – although non-significant (*Chi*^{2} between the model including this effect and the model without this effect is 2.34 on 1 degree of freedom; $p = 0.13$). As for the simple words – and contrary to the nominal compounds –, the number of strokes making up the characters does not seem to influence the patients' performance in word naming.

4. Discussion

The objective of the present study is to investigate the impact of lexical-semantic variables on picture and word naming in healthy and aphasic Chinese speakers, with a particular focus on the role of written word frequency, familiarity, age of acquisition (AoA), imageability, morphological structure, and grammatical class. Five main findings emerged:

(i) An interaction exists between grammatical class and morphological structure in both tasks and in both groups of participants, indicating that complex nouns were far more difficult to retrieve than simple nouns, but the effect of complexity was greatly reduced (or absent) in verbs;

(ii) The effect of morphological complexity varied substantially across the sample of patients in both tasks, as indicated by the by-subject random slope for morphological structure in the relevant Mixed Logit Models (*MLM*);

(iii) Imageability was a significant predictor of picture naming accuracy in both healthy and aphasic speakers, whereas it did not predict either the patients' or the healthy participants' performance in word naming;

(iv) Word frequency was a significant predictor in both picture and word naming, but only for the aphasic participants;

(v) Finally, AoA contributes to the explanation of the patients' performance in the word naming task, but not in the picture naming task.

4.1. Morphology and grammatical class

As illustrated in the Introduction, some results suggest minimal involvement of morphological encoding in the lexical production of Chinese [20,31], which is very interesting considering the extreme productivity of compounding in this language. The results obtained in the present study are clearly in conflict with Chen et al.'s [20] and Janssen et al.'s [31] results. Retrieval of simple words, at least for nouns, was consistently better than that of complex words. This might be attributed to an effect of difficulty, but certain considerations suggest otherwise:

(i) In the present study, the effect of morphological structure emerged independently of word frequency, imageability, AoA, and other lexical-semantic variables (which were taken into account independently in the MLM);

(ii) The interaction between morphology and grammatical class was very consistent (i.e., in both tasks and in both healthy and brain-damaged participants); this is difficult to explain if one considers morphological effects just as due to difficulty.

Intriguingly, evidence for morphological decomposition is available in the literature on Chinese word recognition. However, the morphological effects described in this paper cannot be interpreted as being due to the word recognition system because they also emerge in picture naming, in which no written word identification process is involved. Therefore, data seem to point to a morphological level of representation in the Chinese word production system, in analogy to what has been suggested for Indo-European languages [39, 45].

How can the present data be reconciled with the lack of morphological effects in Chen and Chen's [20] and Janssen et al.'s [31] studies? One possibility is that these experiments may have failed to detect morphological effects in spite of the existence of a morphological level of representation in the Chinese word production system. In Chen and Chen's [20] experiment, for example, participants were trained to associate cue and target words that were semantically related in the vast majority of cases; the morphological effect was thus likely to add on a baseline semantic effect, which may have made morphological priming more difficult to detect. In line with this hypothesis, the morphological facilitation highlighted by Chen and Chen [20] was indeed greater than the phonological facilitation, but this difference fell short of reaching significance (Experiment 3: $p = 0.16$ in the by-subject analysis). As far as the lack of morpheme frequency effects in picture naming [31] and in Chen and Chen's [20] task is concerned, results indicate the absence of a morphological level of representation *only if* the morpheme frequency effect and the whole-word frequency effect are assumed to be *additive*. In an interactive system where a morphological level of representation exists, but morpheme and whole-word selection overlap in time and influence each other, it might well be the case that word frequency effects hide morpheme frequency effects, or vice versa. Taft [59] demonstrated this point elegantly in a lexical decision experiment. Using the same experimental items, he showed both equivalent and completely opposite effects of morpheme and whole-word frequency by manipulating the filler trials; these results cast serious doubts on the assumption that morpheme and whole-word frequency effects are necessarily additive, and were in fact interpreted as evidence for two interactive systems, one involved in morpheme processing and the other involved in whole-word processing. This proposal might also be applicable to the word production system in Chinese, which would in fact nicely reconcile our results with those found by Chen and Chen [20] and by Janssen et al. [31].

Our results also demonstrate that morphology interacts with grammatical class: the difference between simple and complex words is in fact much more pronounced among nouns than among verbs. Therefore, it appears that nouns and verbs have different morphological representations and/or undergo different types of morphological processing. This result – and its theoretical interpretation – is in line with evidence obtained from studies on aphasic speakers of Indo-European languages. Shapiro, Shelton, and Caramazza [58], for example, described the case of a fluent aphasic patient who was better at producing the third-person singular form of verbs (or of nonwords inflected as verbs) than at producing the plural form of nouns (or of nonwords inflected as nouns; see also [62]). The difference in morphological processing between nouns and verbs in Chinese might be related to the specific distributional properties of Chinese compounds. In fact, the constituents that appear more frequently in nominal compounds tend to be rather high in frequency also as free-standing words; this might encourage segmentation, which would explain why compound nouns are more difficult to process than monomorphemic nouns. On the contrary, the constituents that appear more frequently in compound verbs tend to be used predominantly as bound morphemes; it is often the case, then, that the frequency of a verb compound is higher than the frequency of its constituents, which should make segmentation less likely, thus reducing the gap in difficulty between compound and simple verbs.

4.2. The number of strokes

The number of strokes composing the characters to be read is not a predictor of the performance of Chinese dyslexic readers. This variable was far from being significant in all analyses of simple words and compound verbs; it only turned out to be significant for the first constituent in nominal compounds, but this evidence palls given the null results on simple words and compound verbs. Our data thus confirm those reported by Law et al. [34] and are in contrast to the findings of Liu et al. [43]. The present results seem to imply

that the visual complexity of the characters to be read does not impact substantially on reading accuracy; this might indicate that character recognition in Chinese is a holistic procedure based on the overall visual pattern of the whole character, rather than an analytic process that requires a detailed analysis of each stroke.

4.3. Lexical-semantic variables

It is not surprising that imageability influences the speakers' performance in picture naming, as this task clearly requires semantic processing of the depicted stimuli [10]. Moreover, imageability effects have been found in a number of picture naming experiments, particularly when they investigated the performance of brain-damaged individuals [12,46]. Similar results have also been obtained in studies on Chinese, both in healthy [43] and aphasic speakers [38]; this shows once again that in Chinese the semantic system is involved in picture naming. On the contrary, imageability is *not* a relevant predictor in word naming. This result is in strong contrast with the hypothesis that picture and word naming engage the same lexical-semantic pathway in Chinese because of its logographic writing system; since Chinese characters are not made up of phonologically interpretable subunits, one might in fact argue that just like people access the semantic (and phonological) representation of an object when they see its pictorial representation, similarly they might access the meaning and the phonological counterpart of a Chinese character. However, this hypothesis would also predict imageability effects in word naming, which was not found in the present study.

The inconsistent effect of imageability might be accounted for by assuming that different types of conceptual knowledge are activated when looking at a picture and looking at a character. A drawing usually activates visual semantic knowledge, whereas a character may activate lexical, functional and abstract semantic knowledge from the earliest processing phase; this would predict imageability effects predominantly in the former case, as observed in the present study. Alternatively, it could be suggested that our Chinese aphasic patients were reading along a non-semantic route. This would be in agreement with the results reported by Bi et al. [10], who described a patient with severe lexical-semantic impairment (as shown by his several semantic errors in word-to-picture matching), but spared word naming (where no semantic errors were observed). Quite intriguingly, this patient could easily read aloud words that he could not match to the corresponding pictures. These results – and those reported in the present study – suggest that reading in Chinese is also based on a dual-route system, where characters are read both by accessing their meaning (i.e., involving the conceptual system) and through a conceptually-blind procedure that bypasses the lexical-semantic store (see also [35,66]). Our data do not address the question of whether non-semantic reading takes the form of a direct association between written and spoken words (similar to the direct route of reading described in alphabetic languages), or rather of a sub-lexical routine whereby words are read on the basis of their phonetic component [10].

The proposal that reading aloud in Chinese is not necessarily mediated by the semantic system is also supported by psycholinguistic data. In a recent study, Verdonschot, Heij, and Schiller [63] carried out a picture-word interference task where healthy Chinese readers were equally fast in reading aloud words when these were superimposed on semantically related vs. unrelated pictures. It is difficult to explain these results without hypothesizing that the participants were reading aloud words non-semantically. Interestingly, when the same subjects were asked to name the pictures – rather than the written words – the typical picture-word interference effect emerged, thus indicating that the lack of semantic effect in the reading task was not due to some particular aspect of the items/subjects studied in this experiment, but was indeed due to the fact that participants were reading via a non-semantic route.

Age of acquisition seems to play the same role in reading as played by Imageability in picture naming; this result is consistent with findings recorded in the previous literature in English and in Chinese [27,38]. The nature of the AoA effect has been debated for years. Lewis [40], for example, suggested that both frequency and AoA effects depend on the total number of times that a word has been encountered in life; words acquired in the early childhood are likely to be processed (heard, read, written, or articulated) more often in someone's life than words acquired later, and thus their processing becomes faster and more accurate. Perhaps more relevantly for the present work, Barry and Gerhand [6] suggested that AoA effects arise when retrieving lexical phonology, because words acquired early in life have "more complete" explicit representations in the phonological output lexicon than words acquired later [14]. Our data are problematic for this interpretation of AoA effects, because the phonological lexicon is addressed in both picture and word naming, but in our study the AoA effect is only observed in this

latter task. In fact, other studies have found AoA effects in picture naming [68], even if with a different dependent variable (response time rather than accuracy) and a different type of analysis (linear regression rather than mixed-effects models); this indicates that indeed AoA effects may arise at the level of lexical phonology. However, our data also suggest that this might not be the whole story and AoA effects might also emerge at some processing level involved in word naming, but not in picture naming. There are two available candidates:

(i)   The direct route that connects the orthographic input lexicon to the phonological output lexicon by-passing the semantic system;
(ii) A sub-lexical routine whereby characters are converted into syllables on the basis of associations between phonetic components and their dominant pronunciation.

The first option appears to be more straightforward. There is no doubt about the existence of a lexical, non-semantic route for reading in Chinese [66]; moreover, Liu et al. [43] suggest that AoA reflects the mapping between orthography and phonology along this route, which of course supports oral reading only. Also considering the frequency-based interpretation of AoA described above (but see [64] for evidence against this account of AoA), it seems plausible to suggest that associations between orthographic and phonological lexical representations are stronger when words were acquired earlier in life. This proposal would also be compatible with some data obtained in English; Zevin and Seidenberg [70,71] reported that the AoA effect in reading aloud is larger for irregular words, which lead them to suggest that this effect emerges as a consequence of arbitrary mapping between orthography and phonology in the lexical network (the Arbitrary Mapping Hypothesis).

However, the second alternative cannot be discarded. Although the existence of a sub-lexical routine in Chinese has been questioned [22] on the basis of the fact that only 25% of the Chinese written words can be read correctly on the basis of their phonetic component, there is evidence that something similar to the GPC route in alphabetic languages may emerge occasionally in Chinese dyslexic patients [10]. Weekes and Chen [65], for example, have described patients with surface dyslexia who read aloud regular words better than irregular words and, perhaps more surprisingly, made errors on irregular words by producing the syllable corresponding to the dominant pronunciation of their phonetic component (LARC errors) [56]. These results could be explained in terms of a lexical (non-semantic) route for the phonetic components that are free-standing words in themselves. In this case, the phonetic component might activate its corresponding entry in the orthographic input lexicon and, subsequently, in the phonological output lexicon [74]; when the contribution of the semantic reading route is severely reduced and/or the frequency of the target is quite low, the pronunciation of the phonetic component might predominate over the correct pronunciation of the whole character, thus giving rise to a LARC error. This account, however, is clearly not applicable for the phonetic components that are not free-standing words [36, 37]; in these cases, there is no entry for the phonetic component in the orthographic lexicon and, thus, the syllable corresponding to the dominant reading of the phonetic component can only be activated from a sub-lexical reading route.

5. Conclusions

The results of the present study suggest the existence of a morphological level of representation in the Chinese word production system. Although our data do not support strong conjectures on where this level of representation should be placed (e.g., within the lexicon vs. post-lexically), they suggest that the process of morpheme selection and the process of word selection overlap in time and influence each other, explaining why previous studies failed to report morphological effects in word production experiments. Grammatical class is also shown to be a relevant factor in morphological processing, so that this latter may impinge differently on nouns and verbs. Finally, it has been shown that imageability does not influence the performance of brain-damaged individuals in word naming, thus suggesting that reading in Chinese aphasic patients may also occur via a non-semantic route; however, our data do not provide direct evidence as to whether this non-semantic route is lexical (i.e., comparable to the direct route of reading in Indo-European languages) or non-lexical (i.e., based on associations between non-freestanding phonetic components/characters and syllables).

Acknowledgments

We thank Brendan Weekes, Na'ama Friedmann and an anonymous reviewer for their helpful suggestions on a previous draft of this manuscript. This work has been conducted by the second author in partial fulfillment of the requirements for the European Master in Clinical Linguistics (EMCL), an EU-supported Erasmus Mundus Excellence Program. This work has also benefited from a grant (PRIN 20074EKLSX_002) awarded to Claudio Luzzatti by the Italian Ministry of Education, University and Research (MIUR).

References

[1] R.H. Baayen, *Analyzing linguistic data. A practical introduction to statistics using R*, Cambridge University Press, Cambridge, UK, 2008.

[2] R.H. Baayen, L.B. Feldman and R. Schreuder, Morphological influences on the recognition of monosyllabic monomorphemic words, *Journal of Memory and Language* **55** (2006), 290–313.

[3] D.A. Balota and J.I. Chumbley, The locus of word-frequency effects in the pronunciation task: Lexical access and/or production?, *Journal of Memory and Language* **24** (1985), 89–106.

[4] D.A. Balota, M.J. Cortese, S.D. Sergent-Marshall, D.H. Spieler and M.J. Yap, Visual Word Recognition of Single-Syllable Words, *Journal of Experimental Psychology: General* **133** (2004), 283–316.

[5] L. Barca, C. Burani and L.S. Arduino, Word naming times and psycholinguistic norms for Italian nouns, *Behavior Research Methods, Instruments and Computers* **34** (2002), 424–434.

[6] C. Barry and S. Gerhand, Both concreteness and age-of-acquisition affect reading accuracy but only concreteness affects comprehension in a deep dyslexic patient, *Brain and Language* **84** (2003), 84–104.

[7] E. Bates, S. Chen, O.J. Tzeng and P. Li, The noun-verb problem in Chinese aphasia, *Brain and Language* **41** (1991), 203–233.

[8] E. Bates, S. D'Amico, T. Jacobsen et al., Timed picture naming in seven languages, *Psychonomic Bulletin and Review* **10** (2003), 344–380.

[9] D. Belsley, E. Kuth and R. Welsch, *Regression Diagnostics. Indentifying Influential Data and Sources of Collinearity*, Wiley, New York, 1980.

[10] Y. Bi, Z. Han, B. Weekes and H. Shu, The interaction between semantic and the nonsemantic systems in reading: Evidence from Chinese, *Neuropsychologia* **45** (2007), 2660–2673.

[11] H. Bird, D. Howard and S. Franklin, Why is a verb like an inanimate object? Grammatical category and semantic category deficits, *Brain and Language* **72** (2000), 246–309.

[12] H. Bird, D. Howard and S. Franklin, Noun-verb differences? A question of semantics: A response to Shapiro and Caramazza, *Brain and Language* **76** (2001), 213–222.

[13] P. Bonin, C. Barry, A. Meot and M. Chalard, The influence of age of acquisition in word reading and other tasks: A never ending story? *Journal of Memory and Language* **50** (2004), 456–476.

[14] G.D. Brown and F.L. Watson, First in, first out: Word learning age and spoken word frequency as predictors of word familiarity and word naming latency, *Memory and Cognition* **15** (1987), 208–216.

[15] B. Chen, K. Dent, W. You and G. Wu, Age of acquisition affects early orthographic processing during Chinese character recognition, *Acta Psychologica* **130** (2009), 196–203.

[16] B. Chen, L. Wang, L. Wang and D. Peng, The influence of age of acquisition and word frequency on word recognition, *Psychological Science* **27** (2004), 1060–1064.

[17] B. Chen, W. You and H. Zhou, Age of acquisition effects in reading Chinese: Evidence in favor of the semantic hypothesis, *Acta Psychologica Sinica* **39** (2007), 9–17.

[18] B.G. Chen, H.X. Zhou, S. Dunlap and C.A. Perfetti, Age of acquisition effects in reading Chinese: Evidence in favour of the arbitrary mapping hypothesis, *British Journal of Psychology* **98** (2007), 499–516.

[19] S. Chen and E. Bates, The dissociation between nouns and verbs in Broca's and Wernicke's aphasia: Findings from Chinese, *Aphasiology* **12** (1998), 5–36.

[20] T.-M. Chen and J.-Y. Chen, Morphological encoding in the production of compound words in Mandarin Chinese, *Journal of Memory and Language* **54** (2006), 491–514.

[21] W.-L. Chung and C.-F. Hu, Morphological awareness and learning to read Chinese, *Reading and Writing* **20** (2007), 441–461.

[22] M. Coltheart, K. Rastle, C. Perry, R. Langdon and J. Ziegler, DRC: A dual route cascaded model of visual word recognition and reading aloud, *Psychological Review* **108** (2001), 204–256.

[23] D. Crepaldi, S. Aggujaro, L.S. Arduino et al., Noun-verb dissociation in aphasia: The role of imageability and functional locus of the lesion, *Neuropsychologia* **44** (2006), 73–89.

[24] J. DeFrancis, *Visible speech: the diverse oneness of writing systems*, University of Hawaii Press, Honolulu, HI, 1989.

[25] K. I. Forster, Accessing the mental lexicon, in: *New Approaches to Language Mechanisms*, R.J. Wales and C.T. Walker, eds, North Holland, Amsterdam, 1976.

[26] H. Gardner, The naming of objects and symbols by children and aphasic patients, *Journal of Psycholinguistic Research* **3** (1974), 133–149.

[27] S. Gerhand and C. Barry, When does a deep dyslexic make a semantic error? The roles of age-of-acquisition, concreteness, and frequency, *Brain and Language* **74** (2000), 26–47.

[28] J. Grainger and A.M. Jacobs, Orthographic processing in visual word recognition: A multiple read-out model, *Psychological Review* **103** (1996), 518–565.

[29] D.H. Howes and R.L. Solomon, Visual duration threshold as a function of word-probability, *Journal of Experimental Psychology* **41** (1951), 401–410.

[30] T.F. Jaeger, Categorical data analysis: Away from ANOVAs (transformation or not) and towards logit mixed models, *Journal of Memory and Language* **59** (2008), 434–446.

[31] N. Janssen, Y. Bi and A. Caramazza, A tale of two frequencies: Determining the speed of lexical access for Mandarin Chinese and English compounds, *Language and Cognitive Processes* **23** (2008), 1191–1223.

[32] K. Kansaku, I. Shimoyama, Y. Nakajima et al., Functional magnetic resonance imaging during recognition of written words: Chinese characters for concrete objects versus abstract concepts, *Neuroscience Research* **30** (1998), 83–86.

[33] W. Kuo, Frequency effects of Chinese character processing in the brain: an event-related fMRI study, *Neuroimage* **18** (2003), 720–730.

[34] S.-P. Law, Age-of-acquisition effects on reading aloud in two Chinese dyslexic individuals, *Brain and Language* **103** (2007), 107–108.

[35] S.-P. Law and B. Or, A case study of acquired dyslexia and dysgraphia in Cantonese: Evidence for nonsemantic pathways for reading and writing Chinese, *Cognitive Neuropsychology* **18** (2001), 729–748.

[36] S.-P. Law, B.S Weekes, O. Yeung and K. Chiu, Age of acquisition effects on picture naming in Chinese anomia, in: *Language Disorders in Speakers of Chinese*, B.S. Weekes and W. Wong, eds, Multilingual Matters, Clevedon, UK, 2009, pp. 222–239.

[37] S.-P. Law, B.S. Weekes and W. Wong, Naming of real and pseudo-characters with free-standing and non-free-standing phonetic radicals, *Brain and Language* **99** (2006), 29–30.

[38] S.-P. Law, W. Wong, O. Leung and B. Weekes, The effect of age-of-acquisition on reading aloud in Chinese dyslexia, *Neurocase* **14** (2008), 276–289.

[39] W.J.M. Levelt, A. Roelofs and A.S. Meyer, A theory of lexical access in speech production, *Behavioral and Brain Sciences* **22** (1999), 1–75.

[40] M.B. Lewis, Age of acquisition in face categorisation: Is there an instance-based account? *Cognition* **71** (1999), 23–39.

[41] M.B. Lewis, S. Gerhand and H.D. Ellis, Re-evaluating age-of-acquisition effects: Are they simply cumulative-frequency effects? *Cognition* **78** (2001), 189–205.

[42] P.D. Liu, K.K. Chung, C. McBride-Chang and X. Tong, Holistic versus analytic processing: Evidence for a different approach to processing of Chinese at the word and character levels in Chinese children, *Journal of Experimental Child Psychology* **107** (2010), 466–478.

[43] Y. Liu, M. Hao, H. Shu, L.H. Tan and B.S. Weekes, Age-of-acquisition effects on oral reading in Chinese, *Psychonomic Bulletin and Review* **15** (2008), 344–350.

[44] Y. Liu, H. Shu and P. Li, Word naming and psycholinguistic norms: Chinese, *Behavior Research Methods* **39** (2007), 192–198.

[45] C. Luzzatti, S. Mondini and C. Semenza, Lexical representation and processing of morphologically complex words: Evidence from the reading performance of an Italian agrammatic patient, *Brain and Language* **79** (2001), 345–359.

[46] C. Luzzatti, R. Raggi, G. Zonca et al., Verb-noun dissociation in aphasic lexical impairments: the role of word frequency and imageability, *Brain and Language* **81** (2002), 432–444.

[47] C. McBride-Chang, J.-R. Cho, H. Liu et al., Changing models across cultures: Associations of phonological awareness and morphological structure awareness with vocabulary and word recognition in second graders from Beijing, Hong Kong, Korea, and the United States, *Journal of Experimental Child Psychology* **92** (2005), 140–160.

[48] C. McBride-Chang, H. Shu, A. Zhou, C.P. Wat and R.K. Wagner, Morphological Awareness Uniquely Predicts Young Children's Chinese Character Recognition, *Journal of Educational Psychology* **95** (2003), 743–751.

[49] P. McCullagh and J. Nelder, *Generalised linear models*, Chapman and Halls, London, 1983.

[50] J. Myers, Processing Chinese compounds: A survey in the literature, in: *The Representation and Processing of Compound Words*, G Libben and G Jarema, eds, Oxford University Press, Oxford, UK, 2006, pp. 169–196.

[51] F.B. Newcombe, Object-naming by dysphasic patients, *Nature* **207** (1965), 1217.

[52] H. Nittono, M. Suehiro and T. Hori, Word imageability and N400 in an incidental memory paradigm, *International Journal of Psychophysiology* **44** (2002), 219–229.

[53] D. Norris, The Bayesian reader: Explaining word recognition as an optimal Bayesian decision process, *Psychological Review* **113** (2006), 327–357.

[54] D. Norris, Putting it all together: A unified account of word recognition and reaction-time distributions, *Psychological Review* **116** (2009), 207–219.

[55] J. Packard, *The morphology of Chinese: A linguistic and cognitive approach*, Cambridge University Press, New York, 2000.

[56] K. Patterson, Progressive aphasia and surface alexia in Japanese, *Neurocase* **1** (1995), 155–165.

[57] K. Shapiro and A. Caramazza, Language is more than its parts: A reply to Bird, Howard, and Franklin, *Brain and Language* **78** (2001), 397–401.

[58] K. Shapiro, J. Shelton and A. Caramazza, Grammatical class in lexical production and morphological processing: Evidence from a case of fluent aphasia, *Cognitive Neuropsychology* **17** (2000), 665–682.

[59] M. Taft, Morphological decomposition and the reverse base frequency effect, *The Quarterly Journal of Experimental Psychology A: Human Experimental Psychology* **57A** (2004), 745–765.

[60] M. Taft and K.I. Forster, Lexical storage and retrieval of polymorphemic and polysyllabic words, *Journal of Verbal Learning and Verbal Behavior* **15** (1976), 607–620.

[61] P.-S. Tsai, B. H.-Y. Yu, C.-Y. Lee et al., An event-related potential study of the concreteness effect between Chinese nouns and verbs, *Brain Research* (2009), 149–160.

[62] K. Tsapkini, G. Jarema and E. Kehayia, A morphological processing deficit in verbs but not in nouns: A case study in a highly inflected language, *Journal of Neurolinguistics* **15** (2002), 265–288.

[63] R.G. Verdonschot, U. La Hei and N.O. Schiller, Semantic context effects when naming Japanese kanji, but not Chinese hanzi, *Cognition* **115** (2010), 512–518.

[64] B.S. Weekes, AoA effects on Chinese language processing: An fMRI study, *Brain and Language* **91** (2004), 33–34.

[65] B. Weekes, Surface dyslexia in Chinese, *Neurocase* **5** (1999), 161–172.

[66] B. Weekes, Anomia without surface dyslexia in Chinese speakers, *Brain and Language* **60** (1997), 140–143.

[67] B.S. Weekes, A. Chan and L.-H. Tan, Effects of age of acquisition and word frequency on brain activation during Chinese character recognition, *Neuropsychologia* **46** (2008), 2086–2090.

[68] B.S. Weekes, H. Shu, M. Hao, Y. Liu and L.H. Tan, Predictors of timed pictured naming in Chinese, *Behavior Research Methods* **39** (2007), 335–342.

[69] W. You, B. Chen and S. Dunlap, Frequency trajectory effects in Chinese character recognition: Evidence for the arbitrary mapping hypothesis, *Cognition* **110** (2009), 39–50.

[70] J.D. Zevin and M.S. Seidenberg, Age of acquisition effects in word reading and other tasks, *Journal of Memory and Language* **47** (2002), 1–29.

[71] J.D. Zevin and M.S. Seidenberg, Age-of-acquisition effects in reading aloud: Tests of cumulative frequency and frequency trajectory, *Memory and Cognition* **32** (2004), 31–38.

[72] Q. Zhang, C.-Y. Guo, J.-H. Ding and Z.-Y. Wang, Concreteness effects in the processing of Chinese words, *Brain and Language* **96** (2006), 59–68.

[73] Q. Zhang and Y. Yang, The Determiners of Picture-Naming Latency, *Acta Psychologica Sinica* **35** (2003), 447–454.

[74] X. Zhou and W. Marslen-Wilson, The nature of sublexical processing in reading Chinese characters, *Journal of Experimental Psychology: Learning, Memory, and Cognition* **25** (1999), 819–837.

[75] X. Zhou, W. Marslen-Wilson, M. Taft and H. Shu, Morphology, orthography, and phonology in reading Chinese compound words, *Language and Cognitive Processes* **14** (1999), 525–565.

[76] H. Xing, Analysis of phonetics of semantic-phonetic compound characters in elementary school textbooks and a self-organizing connectionist model of character acquisition in Chinese, 2002. Unpublished Ph.D. tesis.

5

Adaptation and validation of standardized aphasia tests in different languages: Lessons from the Boston Diagnostic Aphasia Examination – Short Form in Greek

Kyrana Tsapkini[a,b,*], Christina Helen Vlahou[b] and Costantin Potagas[c]

[a]*Department of Neurology, Johns Hopkins Medical Institutions, Baltimore, MD, USA*
[b]*Department of Psychology, Aristotle University of Thessaloniki, Thessaloniki, Greece*
[c]*Department of Neurology, University of Athens, Eginition Hospital, Athens, Greece*

Abstract. The aim of the current study was to adapt the Boston Diagnostic Aphasia Examination – Short Form (BDAE-SF) [1] to the Greek language and culture, determine the influence of demographic variables on performance and in particular the effects of age and education, develop normative data, and examine the discriminative validity of the test for acute stroke patients. A sample of 129 community healthy adults participated in the study (66 women), covering a broad range of ages and education levels so as to maximize representation of the Greek population and be able to examine the effects of age and education in language performance. Regression models showed that, overall, younger and more educated individuals presented higher performance on several subtests. Normative data for the Greek population are presented in percentile tables. Neurological patients' performance was compared to that of the neurologically intact population using Wilcoxon's rank sum test and for the most part was found to be significantly inferior, indicating good discriminant validity of the test. Qualitative errors of patients diagnosed with aphasia on the test are presented, and limitations and generalizable strengths of this adaptation are discussed.

Keywords: Aphasia testing, BDAE, Greek, normative data, educational effects, cross-cultural neuropsychology

1. Introduction

The Boston Diagnostic Aphasia Examination (BDAE -3 [1,2]) is extensively used in clinical evaluations for the measurement of aphasic patients' performance in all aspects of language functions, identifying the specific language deficits and the exact profile of differential aphasic syndromes. Further, this test is widely used in research protocols. Initially developed in English, efforts have also been made to adapt this test and create norms for non-English populations [3–6]. A previous study has also presented normative data on the Boston Naming Test, which, in its extended form, comprises a subtest of the BDAE [7]. There has also been a preliminary attempt to provide some normative data of the previous full version of BDAE-2 [8] without, however, providing any data from aphasic patients' performance that would assess the discriminant validity of the full-test adaptation.

A short form of its third edition (BDAE-SF) was designed as a brief assessment tool for several language aspects in the 3rd version of the BDAE [1,2]. Given the need for screening tools that could be administered under the time limits frequently imposed in medical settings and determine the need for further referral to a

*Corresponding author: Kyrana Tsapkini, Ph.D., Department of Neurology, Johns Hopkins University School of Medicine, 600 North Wolfe Street, Meyer 6-113, Baltimore, MD 21287, USA. E-mail: tsapkini@jhmi.edu.

neurolinguist, speech pathologist, neurologist, or other health clinicians, we decided to adapt the *short form* of the original test to the Greek language and culture, mainly for the use of clinicians.

The importance of avoiding direct translation of items, but rather modifying existing tests so that they are culturally relevant and appropriate to use in each different cultural context has been repeatedly stressed [9], and progressively more and more efforts in Greece focus on this endeavor [10]. In language tests, the issue of cultural adaptation is critical, as the cognitive ability of language is impacted by the particular characteristics and linguistic properties of the individual's native tongue as has been particularly shown to be the case in Greek aphasia [11–13]. It is thus important to avoid pitfalls such as concepts being misinterpreted in the process, or use of test items that are not culturally pertinent for language assessment.

The BDAE-SF includes five functional subsections: (1) conversational and expository speech such as simple social responses, free conversation, and picture description; (2) auditory comprehension including word comprehension, commands, and complex ideational material; (3) oral expression, such as automatized sequences, single word repetitions, repetitions of sentences, responsive naming, the Boston Naming Test – Short Form (BNT-SF), screening of special categories; (4) reading, including letter and number recognition, picture-word matching, basic oral word reading, oral reading of sentences with comprehension, reading comprehension of sentences and paragraphs; and (5) writing, including mechanics, dictation writing of primer words, regular phonics and common irregular forms, written naming, narrative writing – mechanics, written vocabulary access, syntax, and adequacy of content.

The aims of the current study were to administer each subtest of the Greek version of the BDAE-SF to a Greek sample in order to: (1) determine the influence of demographic characteristics on performance, as scores on language tasks are clearly related to age and education [1]; (2) create a normative database and use minimum normal controls' scores as indicators of the differentiating cutoff between aphasics with mild deficits and normal controls; (3) compare the performance of normal controls to neurological patients in order to determine that test's ability to discriminate between normal functioning and aphasia. We also aimed to discuss the qualitative errors presented by aphasics in the first section of the test assessing conversational and expository speech.

2. Method

2.1. Participants

Our sample consisted of 129 community healthy adults (66 women) including a broad range of age and education level. Age and education categories were chosen in accord with the existing literature. In particular, we followed the categories in previous adaptations of the BDAE in other languages such as Spanish [4] as well as in previous normative studies of neuropsychological tests in Greek (see [10], for the adaptation of verbal fluency test into Greek). Specifically, our normal sample was divided into three different age groups (younger adults: 18–39 years old ($N = 37$, or 28.7%); middle-aged adults, 40–59 years old ($N = 43$, or 33.3%); older adults, 60–81 years old ($N = 49$, or 38%); $M = 51.4$, $SD = 16.6$) and three different education groups according to the Greek school system (low education group: 1–9 education years, i.e. mandatory schooling ($N = 25$, or 19/4%); middle education group, i.e. Lyceum: 10–12 education years ($N = 53$, or 40.3%); high education group, i.e. college and postgraduate studies: 13–21 education years ($N = 52$, or 40.3%). We conducted a brief screening interview in order to exclude individuals with a history of a neurological or psychiatric diagnosis, closed head injury, or any condition that might indicate cognitive impairment. Genders did not differ significantly in age or education level achieved. All participants reported that Greek was their first and dominant language and the majority reported that right hand was their dominant hand preference.

Participants in the normative sample were recruited from a large metropolitan area in Northern Greece. The criterion for participant selection was the recruitment of a stratified sample representing a range of age and education levels. Participants were approached in the community (sample of convenience) by trained psychology undergraduates and graduate students and offered their participation voluntarily. Students were trained and supervised during the data collection process by the first author (K.T.). The test was administered individually, in a quiet, private setting in the community. Administration instructions and procedures followed closely those of the English version of the test. Neurological patients who were hospitalized and treated for a left hemisphere CVA and clinically diagnosed with aphasia subsequent to the stroke were offered participation in a medical setting and tested at bedside by a trained psychology graduate student supervised by the last author (C.P.). Written consent was obtained from all control participants and oral consent from all patients. All data were collected in compliance with the Helsinki declaration.

In addition to the normative sample, a sample of 16 neurological patients who had been previously diagnosed with aphasia secondary to a stroke was recruited for comparison in performance scores. The patients' age ranged from 47 to 87 years old ($M = 65.8$, $SD = 12.5$), and their education level from 4 to 20 years of education.

2.2. Procedure

Given the specific characteristics of the Greek language, we adapted the BDAE-SF (3rd Ed.) to the need of an appropriate test for the assessment of aphasic disorders in Greek, and developed a version of the BDAE-SF for the Greek population. Examples of the adjustments made include replacing names of US cities (e.g., New York) with Greek cities of similar proportion (i.e., Athens), or providing as multiple choice options Greek words that follow the rationale of the word selection in the original test (e.g., selection of options for the target word included a word that rhymes, a semantically-related word, and a phonologically related word, all in the Greek language, following the example of the English version of the test). The Greek version of the BDAE-SF includes the same five language functional subsections and subtests as the English one.

3. Results

3.1. Contribution of age, education and sex in the variation of subtests

We examined the contribution of age, education, and sex in explaining the variation of each language subtest. All results were analyzed using the free statistical software 'R' (http://cran.cnr.berkeley.edu/). Understanding the contribution of each factor is easier if the factors do not interact with each other. For this reason, for each language subset, first we assessed the fit of a linear regression model that included all three factors (age, education, and sex) additively with no interaction, compared to the saturated model with all interactions (3 levels for age $\times$ 3 levels for education $\times$ 2 levels for sex).

For the reading subtest, the additive model for the three explanatory factors was found to be very good

(the additional R^2 of the saturated model was 0.0%, $F(10, 123) = 0.985$, $p = 0.460$)). The results of the additive model, given in Table 1, show that education explains close to 17% ($p < 0.001$) of the variation in the subtest, and this is due to the people with 1–9 yrs of education scoring lower on average than the others. The other factors were not numerically or statistically significant.

For the auditory comprehension subtest, the additive model for the three explanatory factors had a relatively good fit compared to the saturated model (the additional R^2 of the saturated model was 5.0%, $F(10, 123) = 1.763$, $p = 0.075$)). The results of the additive model, given in Table 2, show that education explains 8.3% ($p < 0.001$) of the variation in the subtest, and, as with reading, this is due to the people with 1–9 yrs of education scoring lower on average than the others. The other factors did not explain any variation in the subtest.

For the oral expression subtest, the difference in fit between the additive model and the saturated model was statistically significant but again relatively small (the additional R^2 of the saturated model was 5.2%, $F(10, 123) = 1.939$, $p = 0.047$)). For this reason, the results of the additive model (given in Table 3) are still useful, and show that age and education together explain 36.4% of the variation. Specifically, in this additive model: (i) people with only 9 yrs of education perform lower than those with 12 yrs of education, and the latter perform lower than those with higher education (contrasts significant at 0.05); and (ii) people older than 40 yrs performed lower than the others. Figure 1 depicts the sources of these differences in the saturated (full interaction) model. As it is shown, older people with low education performed significantly worse than their age group peers with mid- and high education. Furthermore, education did not differentiate the performance in the middle age group but it did in the younger group, i.e. young people with high education performed significantly better than their peers with mid education and better than any other age and education group.

For the writing subtest, as with oral comprehension, the difference in fit between the additive model and the saturated model was statistically significant but relatively small (the additional R^2 of the saturated model was 5.3%, $F(10, 123) = 2.90$, $p = 0.003$)). The results of the additive model (given in Table 4) show that age and education together explain 60.3% of the variation. In the additive model: (i) people with low education perform worse than the others; and (ii) older women

Table 1
Predictors of the reading subtest

	Overall results			Contribution of each factor		
	R^2(1)	F	p	Coef (2)	t(df)	p
all factors	19.6%	7,23 (5, 123)	< 0.0001			
age	0.0%	0.74 (2, 125)	0.48			
18–39 (ref)				–	–	–
40–60				−0.14	−1.13 (123)	0.261
60+				−0.004	−0.29 (123)	0.771
education	17.1%	14.3 (2,125)	< 0.0001			
> 12 (ref)				–	–	–
10–12				0.05	0.45 (123)	0.654
1–9				−0.65	−4.71 (123)	< 0.0001
gender	0.0%	1.68(1,124)	0.197			
male (ref)				–	–	–
female				−0.12	−1.30(123)	0.197

(1) R-squares are relative to not having that factor when the others are present; these R-squares do not add up to the total.
(2) Residual standard deviation: 0.53.

Table 2
Predictors of the auditory comprehension subtest

	Overall results			Contribution of each factor		
	R^2(1)	F	p	Coef(2)	t(df)	p
all factors	8.3%	3.32 (5, 123)	0.01			
age	0.0%	0.93 (2, 125)	0.40			
18–39 (ref)				–	–	–
40–60				0.15	0.63 (123)	0.53
60+				0.32	1.35 (123)	0.18
education	8.3%	8.27 (2, 125)	< 0.001			
> 12 (ref)				–	–	–
10–12				−0.18	−0.90 (123)	0.37
1–9				−1.05	−4.00 (123)	0.001
gender	0.0%	0.04 (1, 124)	0.85			
male (ref)				–	–	–
female				0.03	0.19	0.085

(1) R-squares are relative to not having that factor when the others are present; these R-squares do not add up to the total.
(2) Residual standard deviation: 1.01.

Table 3
Predictors of the oral expression subtest

	Overall results				Contribution of each factor		
	R^2(1)	F	p		Coef (2)	t(df)	p
all factors	36.4%	15.62 (5, 123)	< 0.0001				
age	4.6%	5.49 (2, 125)	0.005				
18–39 (ref)					–	–	–
40–60					−0.56	−2.06 (123)	0.04
60+					−0.92	−3.31 (123)	0.001
				contrast	0.36	1.69 (123)	0.094
education	19.8%	20.48 (2,125)	< 0.0001				
> 12 (ref)					–	–	–
10–12					−1.97	−6.40 (123)	< 0.0001
1–9					−0.60	−2.56 (123)	0.012
				contrast	−1.37	−5.37 (123)	< 0.0001
gender	0.0%	1.14(1, 124)	0.289				
male (ref)					–	–	–
female					0.22	1.07(123)	0.289

(1) R-squares are relative to not having that factor when the others are present; these R-squares do not add up to the total.
(2) Residual standard deviation: 1.19.

Table 4
Predictors of the writing subtest

	Overall results			Contribution of each factor		
	R^2 (1)	F	p	Coef (2)	t(df)	p
all factors	60.3%	39.9 (5, 123)	< 0.0001			
age	0.0%	0.54 (2, 125)	0.585			
18–39 (ref)				–	–	–
40–60				0.21	0.45 (123)	0.653
60+				−0.24	−0.50 (123)	0.617
education	50.3%	80.17 (2, 125)	< 0.0001			
> 12 (ref)				–	–	–
10–12				−0.24	−0.60 (123)	0.548
0–9				−6.3	−11.8 (123)	< 0.0001
gender	1.9%	6.88 (1, 124)	0.009			
male (ref)				–	–	–
female				0.95	2.62 (123)	0.010

(1) R-squares are relative to not having that factor when the others are present; these R-squares do not add up to the total.
(2) Residual standard deviation: 2.05.

Age	Edcation	men	women
60+	1-9yrs	44	44
	10-12	46	46
	>12	46	47
40-59	1-9yrs	45	46
	10-12	46	47
	>12	46	46
18-39	1-9yrs		
	10-12	46	47
	>12	48	47

Fig. 1. Interaction between age and education in the oral expression subtest. Numbers in cells are average scores. Cells of common shade have average scores that are not statistically significantly different from each other. The averages (standard errors) for different shades are: 47.5 (0.3) for clear shade; 46.1 (0.1) for light grey; 43.9 (0.3) for dark grey; and black cells are empty.

performed better than older men. Figure 2 depicts the sources of these differences in the saturated (full inter-action) model. As it is shown, not only people with lower education performed differently from those with mid- and high-education in all age groups, but men with lower education performed worse than women from their education group as well.

3.2. Normative data and discriminant validity

Percentiles were calculated after compiling data into four major categories, i.e. auditory comprehension, oral expression, reading and writing, each of which resulted from the summation of subcategory scores. Percentiles and descriptive statistics of normals' performance are

presented in Table 5 (for auditory comprehension and oral expression) and Table 6 (for reading and writing).

To test discriminant validity of this test, we compared the performance of normals to that of stroke patients with the same education, age and sex group. Because within these groups, the scores of the subtests were not normally distributed, we used Wilcoxon's rank sum test with a two-sided type I error of 5%. The maximal number of normals within each group was 10, so a minimum of 2 patients is required to have non-zero power with this test. Below, we present the Wilcoxon test results (W, p-value) for the comparisons that had at least 2 patients.

a) Old (60+), low-education (1–9 years), men (n{aphasics} = 7; n{normals} = 9): Audito-ry comprehension: $W = 56.5$, $p = 0.009$; oral

Table 5
Normative data for auditory comprehension (AC) and oral expression (OE) stratified by age and education

	Age 18–39 years Education (years)						Age 40–59 years Education (years)						Age 60–81 years Education (years)					
	1–9 (n = 0)		10–12 (n = 17)		13–21 (n = 20)		1–9 (n = 8)		10–12 (n = 18)		13–21 (n = 17)		1–9 (n = 17)		10–12 (n = 17)		13–21 (n = 15)	
%ile	AC	OE	AC	OE	AC	OE	AC	OE	AC	OE	AC	OE	AC	OE	AC	OE	AC	OE
100			32.0	48.0	32.0	48.0	32.0	48.0	32.0	48.0	32.0	48.0	32.0	46.0	32.0	47.0	32.0	48.0
90	—	—	32.0	48.0	32.0	48.0	32.0	48.0	32.0	48.0	32.0	48.0	32.0	45.0	32.0	47.0	32.0	48.0
80	—	—	32.0	48.0	32.0	48.0	32.0	46.4	32.0	47.2	32.0	47.4	32.0	45.0	32.0	46.4	32.0	47.0
70	—	—	32.0	47.0	32.0	48.0	32.0	46.0	32.0	47.0	32.0	47.0	32.0	44.0	32.0	46.0	32.0	47.0
60	—	—	32.0	47.0	32.0	48.0	32.0	45.4	32.0	46.4	32.0	47.0	31.4	44.0	32.0	46.0	32.0	47.0
50	—	—	32.0	47.0	32.0	48.0	31.8	45.0	32.0	46.0	32.0	46.0	31.0	44.0	32.0	46.0	32.0	47.0
40	—	—	32.0	46.0	32.0	47.0	31.1	45.0	32.0	46.0	32.0	46.0	30.6	44.0	32.0	45.3	32.0	46.0
30	—	—	32.0	46.0	32.0	47.0	30.4	44.7	32.0	46.0	31.5	46.0	30.2	43.0	32.0	45.0	32.0	46.0
20	—	—	30.5	44.6	32.0	47.0	29.8	44.0	31.4	45.0	30.6	44.6	29.0	43.0	32.0	45.0	32.0	46.0
10	—	—	28.4	45.6	31.0	47.0	29.0	44.0	30.5	44.0	29.9	42.8	28.5	42.0	31.5	45.0	32.0	45.0
M	—	—	31.2	46.3	31.9	47.5	31.1	45.4	31.7	46.2	31.5	46.1	30.1	43.9	31.1	45.8	32.0	46.5
SD	—	—	2.0	1.2	0.3	0.76	1.6	1.3	0.6	1.2	0.85	1.7	1.3	1.1	0.2	0.75	0.0	0.9

Table 6
Normative data for reading (R) and writing (WR) stratified by age and education

	Age 18–39 years Education (years)						Age 40–59 years Education (years)						Age 60–81 years Education (years)					
	1–9 (n = 0)		10–12 (n = 17)		13–21 (n = 20)		1–9 (n = 8)		10–12 (n = 18)		13–21 (n = 17)		1–9 (n = 17)		10–12 (n = 17)		13–21 (n = 15)	
%ile	R	WR	R	WR	R	WR	R	WR	R	WR	R	WR	R	WR	R	WR	R	WR
100	—	—	39.0	84.0	39.0	84.0	39.0	84.0	39.0	84.0	39.0	84.0	39.0	83.0	39.0	84.0	39.0	84.0
90	—	—	39.0	84.0	39.0	84.0	39.0	84.0	39.0	84.0	39.0	84.0	39.0	81.4	39.0	84.0	39.0	84.0
80	—	—	39.0	84.0	39.0	84.0	39.0	83.2	39.0	84.0	39.0	84.0	39.0	80.4	39.0	84.0	39.0	84.0
70	—	—	39.0	84.0	39.0	84.0	39.0	82.3	39.0	84.0	39.0	84.0	39.0	79.6	39.0	84.0	39.0	84.0
60	—	—	39.0	84.0	39.0	84.0	38.4	80.2	39.0	84.0	39.0	84.0	39.0	79.0	39.0	84.0	39.0	84.0
50	—	—	39.0	84.0	39.0	84.0	38.0	78.5	39.0	84.0	39.0	84.0	39.0	78.0	39.0	84.0	39.0	84.0
40	—	—	39.0	84.0	39.0	84.0	38.0	77.6	39.0	84.0	39.0	83.2	38.2	75.4	39.0	84.0	39.0	84.0
30	—	—	39.0	83.4	39.0	84.0	37.7	76.7	39.0	84.0	39.0	83.0	38.0	74.4	39.0	83.4	39.0	84.0
20	—	—	39.0	83.0	39.0	84.0	36.8	75.8	39.0	83.0	38.0	83.0	38.0	71.4	39.0	83.0	39.0	84.0
10	—	—	39.0	82.2	39.0	84.0	36.0	75.0	39.0	81.8	38.0	81.0	36.6	68.6	37.8	82.0	39.0	84.0
M	—	—	39.0	83.5	39.0	83.9	38.0	79.3	39.0	83.5	38.8	83.4	38.4	76.4	38.8	83.6	39.0	84.0
SD	—	—	0.0	1.2	0.2	0.5	1.1	3.4	0.0	1.0	0.44	1.0	1.1	4.7	0.5	0.7	0.0	0.0

Age	Education	men	women
60+	1-9yrs	74	79
	10-12	83	84
	>12	84	84
40-59	1-9yrs	79	80
	10-12	83	84
	>12	83	84
18-39	1-9yrs		
	10-12	83	84
	>12	84	84

Fig. 2. Interaction between age and education and sex and education in the writing subtest. Cells of common shade have average scores that are not statistically significantly different from each other. The averages (standard errors) for different shades are: 83.9 (15.3) for clear shade; 79.0 (17.1) for light grey; 74.4 (22.8) for dark grey; and black cells are empty.

expression: $W = 51$ $p = 0.005$; reading: (n{aphasics} = 0); writing (n{aphasics} = 2): $W = 12, p = 0.554$

b) Middle aged (40–59), middle education (10–12 years), men (n{aphasics} = 4; n{normals} = 8): Auditory comprehension: $W = 32, p = 0.005$; oral expression: $W = 32$ $p = 0.005$; reading: (n{aphasics} = 3) $W = 24$ $p = 0.003$; writing (n{aphasics} = 1)

c) Middle aged (40–59), higher education (13+ years), men (n{aphasics} = 2; n{normals} = 10): Auditory comprehension: $W = 20, p = 0.015$; oral expression: $W = 20$ $p = 0.015$; reading: (n{aphasics} = 3) $W = 10$ $p = 0.035$; writing (n{aphasics} = 0).

3.3. Fluency measures

Qualitative analysis of free conversation (i.e., response to questions regarding occupation, history of events related to the accident, current hospitalization, and general autobiographical information) and picture description (the 'cookie theft'), both of which are subsections of the conversational and expository speech subtest, revealed different types of errors. We used as fluency measures the 'cookie theft' picture description and the spontaneous speech questions. These sections of BDAE-SF were scored from 1–100 according to the instructions (100 depicting fluent speech with complex grammatically correct sentences). Patients scored low in both fluency measures ('cookie theft' mean = 40, SD = 20.7; spontaneous speech mean = 58.75, SD = 23.57). In particular, patients presented syntactic errors (e.g. lack or incorrect use of passive voice, lack of anaphoric propositions, pronouns and clitics), elliptic speech (e.g., lack of nouns/verbs, inadequate sentence construction), word finding difficulties, stereotypic phrases and perseverations (e.g. one patient repeated: "working and drinking, working and drinking"), neologisms (e.g., one patient used the word "dapi" instead of the Greek word "doulapi," meaning cupboard). A translated example of a patient's speech output when asked to describe the "cookie theft" picture reads as follows: "Mom, how can I say this, in the kitchen, wiping the plate dry, her children, on a stool the boy and his little hand is up, how can I say this, to get the sweets to eat, he … probably secretly, he extends his hand to give her one, on the water, water, basin, how can I say this, the si … the sink upside down, and the water is coming out, the water is overflowing."

4. Discussion

In the current study we adapted the Boston Diagnostic Aphasia Examination – Short Form to the Greek language and culture, for use in screening for aphasia and language functioning assessment in acute and sub-acute stroke. We aimed to determine whether demographic variables such as age, gender, and education, would have an effect on performance. Further, we aimed to develop norms for the Greek population, and determine the validity of the test for discriminating between neurological patients and healthy controls.

Our results suggest that amongst the factors we examined, i.e., age, education and gender, it was only education that influenced consistently the scores in all 4 subtests of the battery. In detail, education was the only factor influencing reading and auditory comprehension and it had a main effect in both oral expression and writing. In addition, education interacted with age in both oral expression and writing and in writing only it interacted with gender as well. Amongst education groups, the higher and mid education group (10–12, and 13+, years of education) performed significantly higher than the low education group (1–9 years of education) in all subtests. Furthermore, in the oral expression subtest there was an additional difference between the mid and higher education group as well. Although we are not aware of any studies exploring the influences of demographic variables on the short form of the BDAE, the present findings that emphasize the important role of eduation in language tests is consistent with previous studies on the BDAE [1–4]. Additionally, the differentiation between the 3 eduation levels in the oral expression subtest shows the particular importance of education in oral expression. This finding corresponds very well with our previous finding on the influence of education in oral semantic fluency measures [14]. In the previous study, we also found that education had an incremental effect on semantic fluency, i.e. the lower education group performed worse than the mid-education group, and that group was also worse than the higher education one. Another point we would like to make is that the effect of education becomes more pronounced in old age. In all subtests, within the older population group, those with lower education (1–9 years) performed significantly worse than older people with mid and higher education. Education is, thus, a predictive factor of good language performance, especially in old age.

Many normal controls achieved a full score, as expected. This is a common finding and a common problem in aphasia tests (e.g. [4,15]). This ceiling effect does not invalidate the predictive value (R-square) of the best-fitted linear models we explored. It does imply, though, that an even higher predictive value can be achieved by a two-stage model, predicting first whether or not the individual has a full score, and, if not, then using a linear model. Such a model for the subtests is a subject for future work. Furthermore, the highly predictive effects of education and age of the linear model show that the test is sensitive to language performance across the education and age span.

Most importantly for the purpose of this study, the test had good discriminant validity, as the performance of a small sample of neurological patients already diagnosed with aphasia after a left hemisphere stroke was found to be significantly different than that of the normative sample on most subtests of the test. Writing was the test with the least discriminant validity because most patients had severe motor deficits and could not perform this subtest. To circumvent this generic but quite prevalent problem in acute stroke, we suggest that instead of the actual writing, patients could be asked to spell the words orally. Here, we would also like to make a note that in the cases where a single patient should have been compared to this control group we did not perform Crawford and Garthwaite's [16] very useful method for such comparisons because this method assumes a normal distribution of the control sample, something that was not true in most subtests. (In [16] the authors provide a very useful statistical method that can be applied when one needs to compare a single subject, often a patient in neuropsychology, with a modestly sized matched control sample.) In general, this short version adapted to the Greek culture and language seems to be appropriate for use with stroke patients.

A limitation of this test is that is does not allow for detailed assessment of syntactic, morphosyntactic or morphophonological problems as already found for Greek patients with aphasia [11–13]. Assessment of spontaneous speech is only qualitative, and the measure does not assess degree of severity of deficits or broader functional limitations. Furthermore, our analysis is limited to the group of patients available at the time since their profile of aphasia may change with time. Therefore more research is needed to validate the full battery in chronic stroke when plasticity mechanisms are at work and provide more variable profiles. Alternatively, it comprises a sensitive screening tool that is quick to administer in medical settings for the purpose of diagnosing and further referring patients with aphasia.

The adaptation and validation of the BDAE-SF presented in this study serves as a lesson for the issues, decisions and most importantly the challenges that the clinical researcher faces when adapting a standardized aphasia test in a different language and culture. Besides learning about the effects of education in different language functions and documenting the discriminant validity of this test, the present endeavor shows that when adaptations use principles that respect each language and cultural properties the test preserves its discriminative power to detect language attrition.

Acknowledgements

We would like to thank all the patients and control subjects who participated in this study. We would also like to thank Anna Emanouil, Kristi Passalidou, and Georgia Nasiopoulou, students at the Master's program in Cognitive Psychology of the Department of Psychology at the University of Thessaloniki, who participated in early control data collection and preliminary analysis for research course credit, as well as Eleni Peristeri for patient data collection and analysis. We are grateful to Dr Constantine Frangakis, Professor of Biostatistics at Johns Hopkins University, for his help with the statistical analysis. No conflicts of interest and no sources of financial support exist for this study.

References

[1] H. Goodglass, E. Kaplan and B. Baressi, *The assessment of aphasia and related disorders* (3rd ed.), M.A. Boston, ed., Lippincott, Williams, & Wilkins, 2000.

[2] H. Goodglass, E. Kaplan and B. Baressi, *Boston Diagnostic Aphasia Examination: Short form record booklet* (3rd ed.), M.A. Boston, Lippincott, Williams, & Wilkins, 2001.

[3] D.M. Jacobs, M. Sano, S. Albert, P. Schofield, G. Dooneief and Y. Stern, Cross-cultural neuropsychological assessment: A comparison of randomly selected, demographically matched cohorts of English- and Spanish-speaking adults, *Journal of Clinical and Experimental Neuropsychology* **19**(3) (1997), 331–339.

[4] D.A. Pineda, M. Rosselli, A. Ardila, S.E. Mejia, M.G. Romero and C. Perez, The Boston Diagnostic Aphasia Examination – Spanish Version: The influence of demographic variables, *Journal of the International Neuropsychological Society* **6**(7) (2000), 802–814.

[5] M. Radanovic, L.L. Mansur and M. Scaff, Normative data for the Brazilian population in the Boston Diagnostic Aphasia Examination: influence of schooling, *Brazilian Journal of Medical and Biological Research* **37** (2004), 1731–1738.

[6] M. Radanovic and L.L. Mansur, Performance of a Brazilian population sample in the Boston Diagnostic Aphasia Examination. A pilot study, *Brazilian Journal of Medical and Biological Research* **35** (2002), 305–317.

[7]   A. Patricacou, E. Psalida, T. Pring and L. Dipper, The Boston Naming Test in Greek: Normative data and the effects of age and education on naming, *Aphasiology* **21**(12) (2007), 1157–1170.

[8]   I. Papathanasiou, V. Pliogkas, P. Salavoura, E. Tsigaras and S. Malefaki, The validation of the aphasia screening test in Greek speaking population. In International Aphasia Rehabilitation Conference: International Aphasia Rehabilitation Conference (2006: 12th: Sheffield. UK: 4–6 June, 2006).

[9]   V. Nell, *Cross-Cultural Neuropsychological Assessment: Theory and Practice*, N.J. Mahwah, Lawrence Erlbaum Associates, Inc, 2000.

[10] M.H. Kosmidis, C.H. Vlahou, P. Panagiotaki and G. Kiosseoglou, The Verbal Fluency Task in the Greek population: Normative data and clustering and switching strategies, *Journal of the International Neuropsychological Society* **10** (2004), 164–172.

[11] K. Tsapkini, G. Jarema and E. Kehayia, (2001). Manifestations of morphological impairments in Greek aphasia: A case study, *Journal of Neurolinguistics* **14** (2001), 281–229.

[12] K. Tsapkini, G. Jarema and E. Kehayia, A morphological processing deficit in verbs but not in nouns: a case study in a highly inflected language, *Journal of Neurolinguistics* **15** (2002), 265–288.

[13] S. Varlokosta, N. Valeonti, M. Kakavoulia, M. Lazaridou, A. Economou and A. Protopappas, The breakdown of functional categories in Greek aphasia: Evidence from agreement, tense, and aspect, *Aphasiology* **20** (2006), 723–743.

[14] M.H. Kosmidis, K. Tsapkini, V. Folia, C. Vlahou and G. Kioseoglou, Semantic and phonological processing in illiteracy, *Journal of the International Neuropsychological Society* **10** (2004), 818–827.

[15] A. Ardila, A note of caution: Normative neuropsychological test per formance: Effects of age, education, gender and ethnicity: A comment on Saykin et al. (1995), *Applied Neuropsychology* **5** (1998), 51–53.

[16] J.R. Crawford and P.H. Garthwaite, Investigation of the single case in neuropsychology: Confidence limits on the abnormality of test scores and test score differences, *Neuropsychologia* **40** (2002), 1196–1208.

6

Test-retest reliability of fMRI during nonverbal semantic decisions in moderate-severe nonfluent aphasia patients

Jacquie Kurland[a,b,*], Margaret A. Naeser[a,b], Errol H. Baker[a], Karl Doron[a], Paula I. Martin[a], Heidi E. Seekins[a], Andrew Bogdan[a], Perry Renshaw[c] and Deborah Yurgelun-Todd[c]

[a]*Harold Goodglass Boston University Aphasia Research Center, Department of Neurology, Boston University School of Medicine and the Veterans Affairs Boston Healthcare System, USA*
[b]*University of Colorado at Boulder, Departments of Speech, Language and Hearing Sciences and Neuroscience, USA*
[c]*Brain Imaging Center, McLean Hospital, Belmont, MA and Harvard Medical School, USA*

Abstract. Cortical reorganization in poststroke aphasia is not well understood. Few studies have investigated neural mechanisms underlying language recovery in severe aphasia patients, who are typically viewed as having a poor prognosis for language recovery. Although test-retest reliability is routinely demonstrated during collection of language data in single-subject aphasia research, this is rarely examined in fMRI studies investigating the underlying neural mechanisms in aphasia recovery.

The purpose of this study was to acquire fMRI test-retest data examining semantic decisions both within and between two aphasia patients. Functional MRI was utilized to image individuals with chronic, moderate-severe nonfluent aphasia during nonverbal, yes/no button-box semantic judgments of iconic sentences presented in the Computer-assisted Visual Communication (C-ViC) program. We investigated the critical issue of intra-subject reliability by exploring similarities and differences in regions of activation during participants' performance of identical tasks twice on the same day. Each participant demonstrated high intra-subject reliability, with response decrements typical of task familiarity. Differences between participants included greater left hemisphere perilesional activation in the individual with better response to C-ViC training. This study provides fMRI reliability in chronic nonfluent aphasia, and adds to evidence supporting differences in individual cortical reorganization in aphasia recovery.

Keywords: Nonfluent aphasia, fMRI reliability, nonverbal semantic decisions

1. Introduction

Cortical reorganization underlying poststroke language recovery, while not well understood, is now being actively studied with functional neuroimaging. Some studies link recovery with greater activation of right hemisphere (RH) language homologues [7,10,39]. These findings, however, have been challenged by studies suggesting that abnormal and/or over-activation of RH structures during language tasks may be, in part, a maladaptive process [1,29,30,35]. Other studies suggest that activation of residual left hemisphere (LH) perilesional areas may be critical to better, or more efficient, language recovery [5,14,15,30,40]. Some reasons underlying the different conclusions offered by these studies include heterogeneity of subjects, task selection, and differences in methodologies used to acquire data [6].

Recently, it has been suggested that important insights can be gained via the single-subject approach to studying aphasia recovery with functional imaging [30]. A well-established methodological issue in

*Corresponding author: Jacquie Kurland, M.S., Aphasia Research Center (12-A), V.A. Boston Healthcare System, 150 South Huntington Ave., Boston, MA 02130 USA. E-mail: kurlandj@bu.edu.

single-subject research is the need for test-retest reliability [20]. Test-retest reliability provides a measure of stability, repeatability, and consistency over time. Although test-retest reliability is routinely performed during collection of behavioral data, it is still fairly uncommon among published studies investigating the underlying neural mechanisms supporting those behaviors. This oversight may be due to the relatively high cost and low availability of functional neuroimaging time. Nonetheless, the issue of test-retest reliability in functional neuroimaging research remains important.

Previous functional neuroimaging and lesion studies investigating semantic processing in healthy normal controls and aphasia patients have suggested a broad network of regions to be necessary and/or sufficient in the performance of lexical-semantic tasks [10,11, 13,18,19,22–24,30,31,39]. This semantic network includes, but is not limited to, the following areas: superior, middle and inferior temporal gyri (BA 22, 21, 20), fusiform gyrus (T4 and BA 18, 19, 37), temporal pole (BA 38), SMA (BA 6), angular gyrus (BA 39), supramarginal gyrus (BA 40), prefrontal areas (BA 8, 9, 10, 46, 47), and posterior inferior frontal gyrus (BA 44, 45). These studies examined a wide variety of healthy and language impaired subjects (of varying type and severity of aphasia) during performance of variable receptive and expressive semantic tasks. No two studies suggest the exact same necessary and/or sufficient regions, but this is not surprising given differences in subjects, tasks and control conditions that differentially emphasize various aspects of the complex phenomenon of lexical-semantic processing.

We have utilized functional imaging to investigate the neural networks supporting language recovery in aphasia. The present study is part of a larger investigation into semantic decision-making in patients with chronic, severe nonfluent aphasia. These patients have been treated with the iconic, nonverbal Computer-assisted Visual Communication (C-ViC) program [16, 17]. To our knowledge, no other functional imaging studies with aphasia patients have reported results post-treatment with an alternative nonverbal communication system. Moreover, none of the studies investigating semantic processing in aphasia patients have reported test-retest reliability.

This study addresses the issue of test-retest reliability in two individuals with chronic, moderate-to-severe nonfluent aphasia during acquisition of blood oxygenation level dependent (BOLD) functional magnetic resonance imaging (fMRI). During fMRI, they performed a nonverbal, yes/no, button-box semantic judgment task

on C-ViC icon "sentences". We investigated the critical issue of intrasubject reliability by exploring similarities and differences in regions of activation during each participant's performance of two identical tasks on the same day. We also explored hemispheric lateralization and localization associated with different degrees of aphasia recovery in these two patients.

We hypothesized the following: 1) Patients with moderate-to-severe nonfluent aphasia can provide reliable fMRI data during performance of language tasks in the scanner; 2) During fMRI, these patients will activate RH regions homologous to LH regions previously associated with lexical-semantic functions. These patients may also activate undamaged LH regions as well as perilesional regions; 3) The patient with "best response" to C-ViC training [28] will demonstrate better performance (accuracy and response times), and will have a different pattern of fMRI activation than the patient with "moderate response", including more LH activity in the patient with "best response".

2. Methods

2.1. Participants

Each participant suffered a single left hemisphere stroke (Figs 1 and 2). Participant 1 (P1) is a right-handed, 69-year old man, former carpenter, 11 years poststroke onset, with severe nonfluent speech. Structural MRI scan revealed that both Broca's and Wernicke's cortical areas were spared. This patient primarily had a subcortical lesion centered over the putamen with lesion extension into two white matter areas near ventricle, compatible with nonfluent speech (arrows on MRI scan in Fig. 1): 1) medial subcallosal fasciculus (MScF), deep to Broca's area, adjacent to the left (L) frontal horn (affecting pathways from SMA and cingulate gyrus BA 24 to head of caudate); and 2) middle 1/3 periventricular white matter (M 1/3 PVWM), located deep to sensorimotor cortex, adjacent to the L body of lateral ventricle (affecting sensori-motor pathways deep to mouth, inter- and intra-hemispheric pathways including in part, limbic and motor thalamo-cortical pathways) [27]. Some cortical lesion was present in the supramarginal gyrus and part of the angular gyrus.

P2 is a right-handed, 59-year old man, former construction engineer, 10 years poststroke onset, with moderate-severe nonfluent speech. Structural MRI scan showed cortical lesion in all of Broca's area and portion of Wernicke's area. Subcortical white mat-

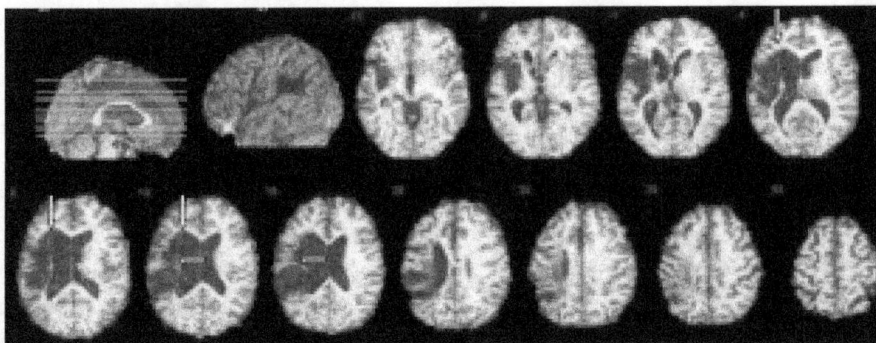

Fig. 1. Structural T1-weighted, three-dimensional spoiled gradient echo (3D SPGR) MRI scan for P1 (severe nonfluent, "moderate" response to C-ViC training). Both Broca's and Wernicke's cortical areas were largely spared. Subcortical lesion was centered over the putamen with lesion extension into two white matter areas near ventricle, compatible with nonfluent speech: 1) medial subcallosal fasciculus (MScF), deep to Broca's area, adjacent to the left (L) frontal horn (vertical arrows); and 2) middle 1/3 periventricular white matter (M 1/3 PVWM), located deep to sensorimotor cortex, adjacent to the L body of lateral ventricle (horizontal arrows). Some cortical lesion was present in the supramarginal gyrus and part of the angular gyrus.

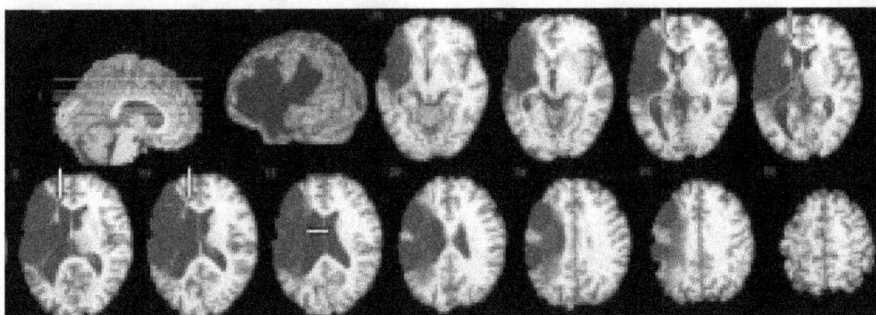

Fig. 2. Structural T1-weighted, 3D SPGR MRI scan for P2 (moderate-severe nonfluent, "best" response to C-ViC training). Cortical lesion was present in all of Broca's area and portions of Wernicke's area. Subcortical white matter lesion was present in both white matter areas near ventricle, compatible with nonfluent speech: 1) MScF (vertical arrows); and 2) M 1/3 PVWM (horizontal arrows). Cortical lesion was present in lower sensorimotor cortex (mouth region) with sparing in the upper regions; lesion was also present in the supramarginal gyrus and part of the angular gyrus.

ter lesion was present in both white matter areas near ventricle, compatible with nonfluent speech (arrows on MRI scan in Fig. 2): 1) MScF; and 2) M 1/3 PVWM. Cortical lesion was present in lower sensorimotor cortex (mouth region) with sparing in the upper regions; lesion was also present in supramarginal gyrus and part of the angular gyrus.

Longitudinal scores in auditory comprehension, repetition and naming on the Boston Diagnostic Aphasia Exam (BDAE) [12] demonstrate chronic nonfluent aphasia (Table 1). P1 at 6.5 Yr. poststroke had severe nonfluent speech (0-1 word phrase length). When P2 entered C-ViC training at 2 Yr. poststroke, he had severe nonfluent speech (0–1 word phrase length). By 10 Yr. poststroke, P2 had moderate nonfluent speech (2–3 word phrase length). Neither patient was classified as having global aphasia because each had relatively preserved auditory comprehension (70th percentile). The study was approved by the Institutional Review Boards

at all hospitals where the authors are affiliated, and signed informed consent was obtained.

2.2. fMRI experimental design

Functional MRI measurements were collected while participants made yes/no button-box semantic decisions regarding appropriateness of icon "sentences" presented in Computer-assisted Visual Communication (C-ViC) [35]. C-ViC is an icon-based alternative communication system designed for patients with severe aphasia including limited oral, gestural, or written expressive output. Both participants had received at least 9 months of training in the C-ViC program with one of the authors (EB) within four years of undergoing this fMRI experiment. Both attended several weeks of C-ViC refresher training with EB during the month prior to this fMRI study. In response to previous C-ViC training, P1 had been classified as having "moderate response", whereas P2 had been classified as having

Table 1
Boston Diagnostic Aphasia Exam (BDAE) test scores for participants

Patient data			Fluency	Auditory comprehension				Repetition	Naming
Patient	MPO when tested	Date when tested	Max. No. words per phrase	AC: Mean of 3 %iles	Word discrim	Commands	Complex ideational material	Single word repetition	Visual confr'n. naming
	Maximum score:		7		72	15	12	10	114
1/ severe	4.5 Yr.	4/97[a]	0-1	72.3	66	14	6	–	–
nonfluent	6.5 Yr.	2/99[b]	0-1	69.3	68	11	7	1	8
speech									
2/ mod-severe	10 Mo.	7/94[c]	0-1	38.3	46	9	3	8	28
nonfluent	4 Yr.	3/97[d]	2	62.1	62.5	8	9	8	59
speech	10 Yr.	5/03[e]	2-3	74.3	65	13	9	9	(12/20)

[a]2 Yr. post-C-ViC training
[b]4.5 Yr. prior to fMRI study
[c]immediately pre-C-ViC training
[d]2 Yr. post-C-ViC training
[e]6 Mo. prior to fMRI study

"best response" [28]. While both individuals could utilize C-ViC to respond to questions posed by others, only P2 used C-ViC to initiate communication, and did so generally with better syntactic and semantic ability than did P1.

The C-ViC subject-verb-object icon "sentences" were either acceptable (e.g., "woman cut pizza") or unacceptable due to semantic unrelatedness (SUR) of the verb and object (e.g., "man build cheese"). See Fig. 3.

During fMRI sessions, participants viewed two runs of alternating blocks of rest (passively viewing "nonnameable" black and white patterns, 7.5 sec. per pattern) and the semantic decision task (7.5 sec. per icon sentence). Patients had been trained to press the left button to accept the icon sentence (if it "makes sense"), and the right button to reject it. Each run lasted 2.5 minutes, and each block of rest or semantic decision task lasted 30 seconds and consisted of four 7.5-second trials. After approximately 25 minutes of other MR imaging, and while the participant was still in the same position in the MRI scanner, the identical session with two runs of S-V-O sentences judged earlier, was repeated for test-retest fMRI reliability.

2.3. Data acquisition

Functional MRI images were acquired using a 1.5 T GE Signa scanner. Scout images were acquired in the sagittal plane in order to define the anterior commissure-posterior commissure (AC-PC) line. Functional images were acquired in the same plane (parallel to AC-PC) using a T2*-weighted gradient echo, EPI sequence with TR = 3000 ms, TE = 40 ms, FOV = 24 × 24 cm, 64 × 64 matrix size with an in-plane resolution of 3.75 mm and 30 slices of

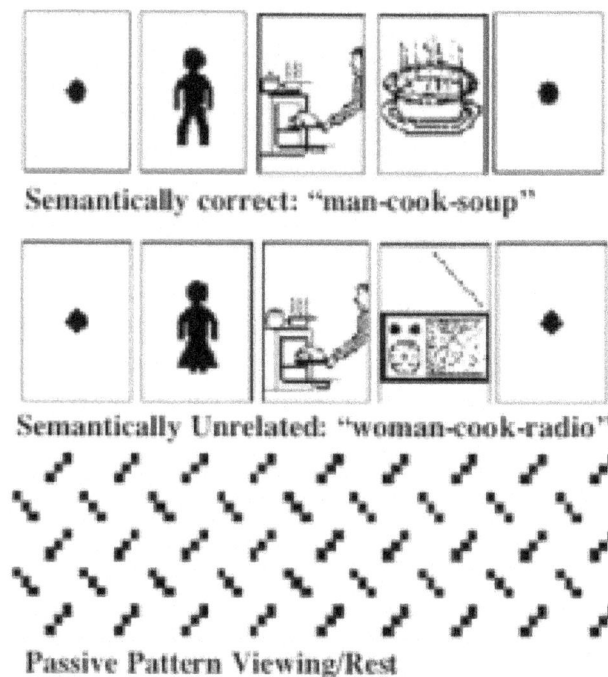

Fig. 3. C-ViC subject-verb-object (S-V-O) icon "sentences" were judged to be acceptable (e.g., "man cook soup") or they were judged to be unacceptable, due to semantic unrelatedness (SUR) of the verb and object (e.g., "woman cook radio"). During the passive pattern viewing/rest condition, one of six different black and white "non-nameable" patterns was viewed.

5 mm thickness with no gap. A high-resolution three-dimensional spoiled gradient echo (3D SPGR) image was acquired at the end of the scanning session, TR = 35 ms, TE = 5 ms, FOV = 24 × 24 cm, 256 × 256 matrix size with an in-plane resolution of 0.94 mm and 124 slices of 1.5 mm thickness with no gap.

During each of the two, 2.5-minute fMRI runs, each condition lasted 30 seconds (4 stimuli at 7.5 seconds each), during which 10 scans were acquired. The resting (pattern) condition alternated with the yes/no button-box task condition, for a total of 50 volumes (30 pattern, 20 task for each run). After less than half an hour of performing other tasks in the scanner, with rest between tasks, these two 2.5-minute fMRI runs (TEST session) were repeated (RETEST session).

2.4. Data analysis

Data were analyzed with MatLab 6.5 (MathWorks, Natick, MA) and SPM2 (Wellcome Department of Cognitive Neurology, London, UK) on a Dell Workstation Precision 360. Functional runs begin with 12 s, 4 images, of dummy scans to establish longitudinal magnetization. Images were realigned using the first (post-dummy) functional image as a reference. The mean realigned EPI image was coregistered to the 3D SPGR using mutual coregistration information with these orientation shifts applied to the realigned EPI time series. The 3D SPGR was normalized to the MNI T1 template and resampled to $2 \times 2 \times 2$ mm matrix size. These warping parameters were then applied to the EPI time series. Functional data were smoothed with a 6 mm^3 FWHM isotropic Gaussian kernel. Each voxel was regressed against a box-car reference waveform convolved with a canonical hemodynamic response function and subsequent T-tests were performed [uncorrected $p < 0.001$; corrected Family Wise Error (FWE) $p < 0.05$] to determine task-related functional activation patterns contrasting semantic decisions with pattern viewing/rest. The FWE adjustment protects against family-wise false positives using a Gaussian field correction for spatially extended data that is analogous to the Bonferroni correction for discrete data. This procedure controls the FWE rate at or below alpha (0.05), which represents the chance of one or more false positives anywhere (not limited to supra-threshold voxels). Significantly activated voxels were transformed from MNI space to the standard stereotaxic space of Talairach and Tournoux [38] using MEDx 3.42 medical imaging processing software [3]. Graphic imaging was performed using MRIcro software [34].

3. Results

3.1. Behavioral results

Figure 4 reports accuracy and response times (RTs, for accurate responses only) for each participant. Percent accuracy was stable across test-retest in each par-

ticipant. Errors were not identical for either participant across sessions. P1 ("moderate response" to C-ViC training), correctly judged 12/16 (75%) icon sentences in the first session (TEST) and also 12/16 (75%) in the second session (RETEST). His errors (3/4 each session) predominantly consisted of accepting semantically unrelated icon sentences, i.e., judging them to be correct. For example, he judged the sentence, "man build cheese" to be semantically acceptable.

P2 ("best response" to C-ViC training), correctly identified 12/14 (86%) during the TEST session and 13/15 (87%) during the RETEST session. Although 16 stimuli were presented in each session (8 per run), some response data are missing due to excessively long reaction time (>7500 msec). In addition, not all fMRI data could be analyzed for P2, due to head motion artifact (>0.5 mm in any direction). Among the data that could be analyzed during the TEST session, he scored 5/7 (71%); during the RETEST session he also scored 5/7 (71%). Errors were mixed, i.e., both judging semantically acceptable sentences to be inaccurate, and accepting SUR sentences.

Paired t-tests between each participant's own TEST and RETEST scores showed each subject was faster on RETEST (P1: mean difference = 407 msec, $t = 2.08$, $df = 11$, $p = 0.062$; P2: mean difference = 1480 msec, $t = 3.68$, $df = 4$, $p = 0.021$). See Fig. 4. There was no significant difference between the RTs of the two participants.

3.2. Functional MRI results

Figure 5 shows activated regions superimposed on each participant's reconstructed images during TEST and RETEST. Significant activation is shown at $p < 0.001$ uncorrected, for display purposes. Table 2 reports selected regions showing significantly higher BOLD activations during semantic decisions than during passive viewing/rest. These regions were selected from previously published functional neuroimaging studies investigating semantic processing, as reviewed above. Significant clusters in Table 2 are corrected for multiple comparisons using $p < 0.05$ Family-Wise Error correction. Some clusters demonstrated significance at the less conservative, $p < 0.05$ False Discovery Rate, especially during RETEST, and are noted as such (by asterisk).

In general, regions which were strongly activated during TEST were also activated during RETEST, but with less spatial extent and intensity of activation (lower p levels) on RETEST. Normal subjects have also

Semantic Judgments: Accuracy and RTs (for accurate responses)

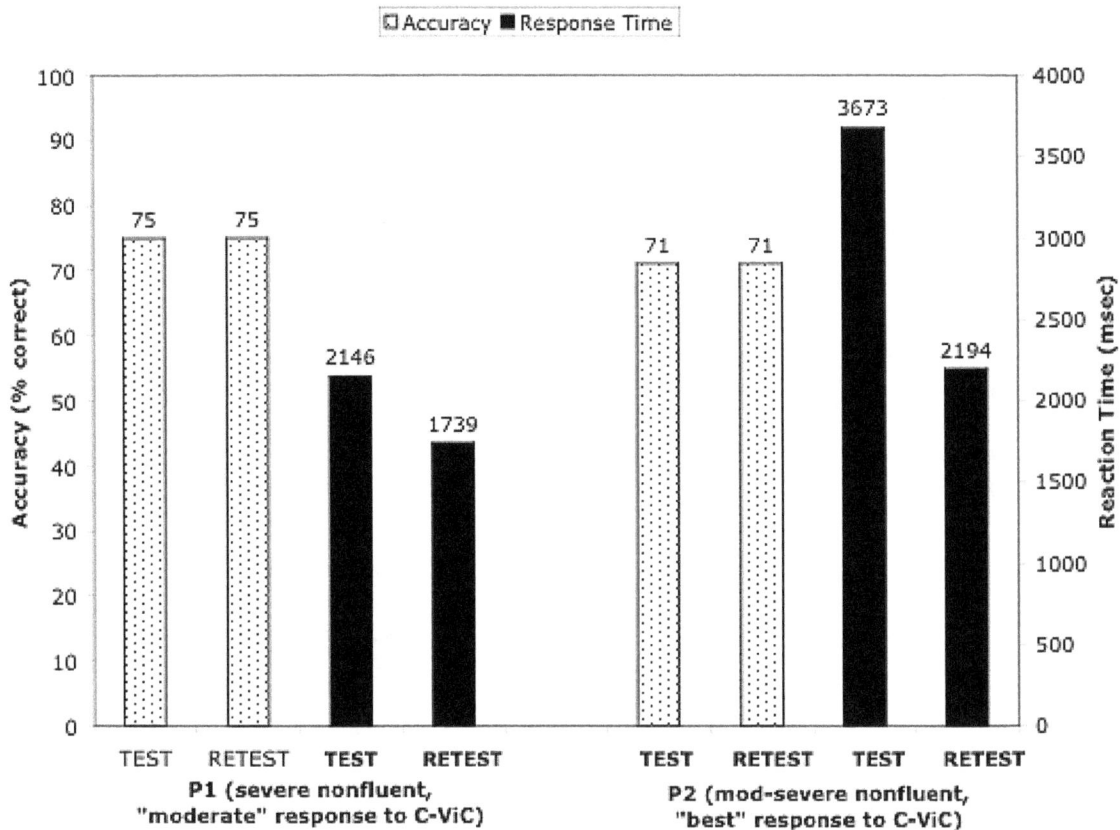

Fig. 4. Accuracy and response times (for accurate responses) for P1 and P2 during TEST and RETEST. Both participants showed no change in accuracy between TEST and RETEST runs, although errors were not identical between sessions. Both decreased RTs: P1 marginally significant ($t = 2.08$, $df = 11$, $p = 0.062$, mean difference $= 407$ msec); P2 significant decrease in RT ($t = 3.68$, $df = 4$, $p = 0.021$, mean difference $= 1480$ msec).

demonstrated this phenomenon of 'repetition suppression', i.e., decreased neuronal activation on delayed, identical tasks [4]. Results for each patient are reviewed separately below.

P1. Severe Nonfluent ("moderate" response to C-ViC training)

During the first session (TEST), P1 predominantly activated RH language homologues commonly activated in the LH during semantic tasks with normals. In P1, this included in part, R IFG (BA 47, 44), R MFG (BA 46, 10, 6), and R temporal areas (BA 37, 38). The RH regions with the highest levels of activation on TEST were also significantly activated on RETEST, but on RETEST, they demonstrated less spatial extent and intensity (Fig. 5 and Table 2). A notable exception to this was observed in the L temporal fusiform gyrus (TFG, BA 37) on TEST, $z = 7.1$; but on RETEST, adjacent voxels were highly activated in L TFG (BA 19), $z > 8$. Regions that were weakly activated during TEST, such as L MTG (BA 21) and R BA 44 did not reach significance during RETEST. Even though

P1's lesion spares both Broca's and Wernicke's cortical areas, he failed to activate either of these LH cortical regions during either TEST or RETEST.

P2. Moderate-Severe Nonfluent ("best" response to C-ViC training)

During TEST, P2 also predominantly activated RH language homologues commonly activated in the LH in normals during semantic tasks. In P2, this included in part, R IFG (BA 47), R MFG (BA 46, 10, 6), R SMA (BA 6), R TFG (BA 37), and R angular gyrus (BA 39). These significantly activated regions on TEST also were significantly activated on RETEST, although with less spatial extent and intensity. See Table 2. In spite of his large perisylvian cortical lesion, P2 also weakly activated L supramarginal gyrus (BA 40), but only during TEST. Overall, Table 2 shows that P2 had significant activation in more LH areas on TEST and/or RETEST (frontal, temporal and parietal) than P1 (frontal and temporal, only).

Table 2
Activation foci in selected Brodmann areas relevant for semantic tasks: Semantic decisions vs. rest

Area[2]	P1: TEST[3]	P1: RETEST	P2: TEST	P2: RETEST
Left frontal				
L SFG (8)	–	–	–6,18,52 (4.9)	–
L SFG (6) (**=SMA)	–	–	–	–10,9,58 (5.1)**
L MedFG (8)	–	–	–4,28,46 (6.6)	–8,26,48 (5.2)
	–	–	0,26,47 (6.5)	–
L MedFG (10)	–	–6,56,–6 (5.0)	–	–
Left temporal				
L TFG (36)	–38,–38,–25 (7.5)	–	–	–
L TFG (37)	–44,–61,–14 (7.1)	–	–28,–51,–18 (7.3)	–42,–61,–7 (4.8)
	–	–	–36,–45,–13 (6.7)	–36,–63,–19 (4.6)
L TFG (19)	–	–46,–70,–10 (>8)	–	–
L MTG (21)	–61,–39,–8 (5.8)	–	–	–
L MTG (39)	–	–	–	–48,–60,8 (4.5)
L STG (39)	–	–	–	–32,–55,32 (4.1)*
Left parietal				
L SupraMarg (40)	–	–	–42,–41,37 (3.5)*	–
Right frontal				
R IFG (9)	44,4,31 (7.2)	48,7,25 (6.3)	–	50,19,27 (4.64)*
R IFG (44)	44,16,5 (4.3)*	–	–	–
R IFG (45)	–	–	–	51,24,10 (3.6)*
R IFG (47)	40,15,–6 (5.2)	–	28,27,–8 (5.6)	28,27,–6 (4.8)
	–	–	38,26,–15 (4.9)	46,18,1 (3.2)*
R MFG (46)	40,34,22 (5.6)	–	44,19,21 (7.7)	42,18,19 (5.1)
	–	–	–	50,32,9 (3.7)*
R MFG (10)	38,48,–4 (6.4)	–	38,39,13 (6.6)	40,39,13 (4.1)*
	34,46,–4 (6.3)	–	24,54,–11 (6.4)	–
R MFG (6)	30,–11,45 (>8)	32,–11,45 (7.1)	42,14,49 (>8)	38,12,47 (>8)
	–	42,–3,53 (7.1)	26,3,62 (5.0)	–
R MedFG (6)	8,–19,51 (6.9)	8,–19,51 (6.3)	2,29,35 (5.6)	–
R MedFG (10)	–	4,58,–4 (5.6)	–	–
	–	4,60,3 (5.0)	–	–
R Cing (32)	–	6,6,47 (5.6)	–	8,34,26 (4.3)*
R SFG (6) (**=SMA)	–	24,–8,67 (5.8)	2,16,54 (6.5)**	6,18,54 (6.3)**
R MFG (9)	44,27,26 (6.0)	48,27,34 (5.7)	59,21,28 (4.9)	36,17,36 (4.2)*
Right temporal				
R TFG (37)	38,–59,–16 (>8)	38,–59,–16 (7.8)	34,–59,–11 (5.8)	36,–51,–15 (5.6)
	42,–61,–7 (7.6)	–	–	–
R STG (38)	50,15,–7 (4.3)*	–	–	–
Right parietal				
R AngG (39)	–	–	34,–55,34 (5.5)	32,–55,36 (4.4)*
	–	–	–	34,–57,32 (4.4)*

[1]$P < 0.001$ uncorrected; Family-Wise Error Rate < 0.05 corrected ; (* = False Discovery Rate <0.05 corrected)
[2]Numbers in parentheses refer to Brodmann areas. MedFG = Medial Frontal Gyrus; TFG = Temporal Fusiform Gyrus; MTG = Middle Temporal Gyrus; MFG = Middle Frontal Gyrus; SFG = Superior Frontal Gyrus; ** = SMA; SMA = Supplementary Motor Area; SupraMarg = supramarginal gyrus; AngG = angular gyrus; Cing = Cingulate
[3]Numbers refer to stereotaxic coordinates x, y, z from Talairach & Tournoux (1988) converted from MNI space (Brett, 2003); numbers in parentheses refer to Z scores

4. Conclusion

This study demonstrates that fMRI can be performed with chronic, moderate-to-severe nonfluent aphasia patients and that reasonably reliable test-retest results can be obtained in this patient group. Intrasubject reliability in fMRI responses was established in two participants during identical semantic judgment tasks, with expected repetition suppression [4]. Reliability is an important finding given the enormous clinical potential for utilizing fMRI in future applications, e.g., in patient selection for appropriate treatment, monitoring of rehabilitation, and verification of treatment efficacy.

The finding of repetition suppression has also been described by Raichle and colleagues [33], and Blasi and colleagues [2] as a response decrement that is modu-

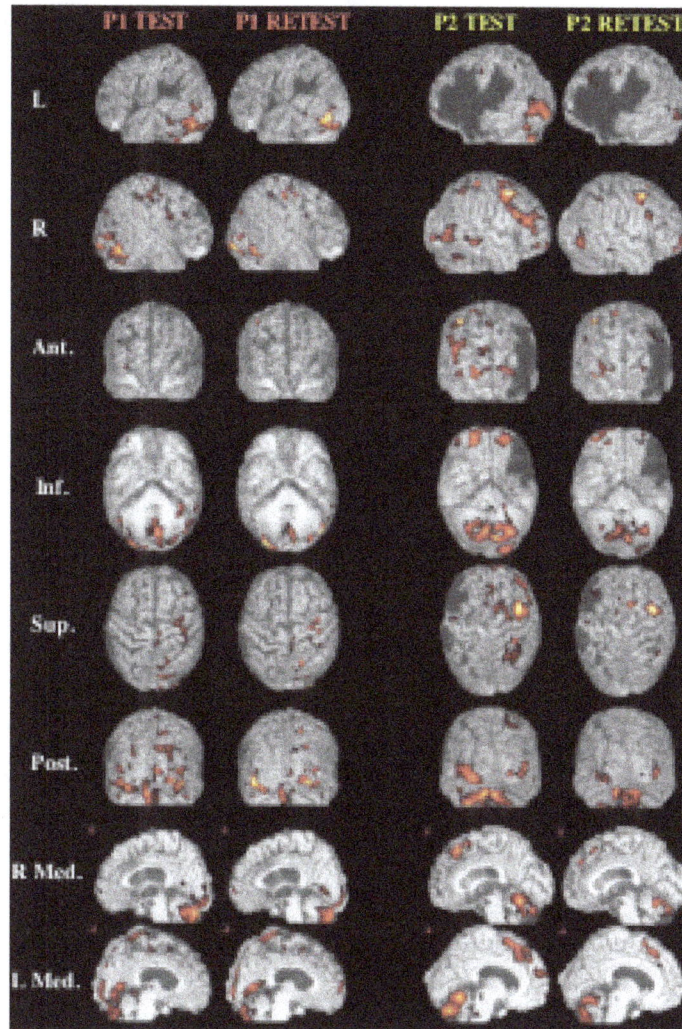

Fig. 5. Cortical activation maps for P1 (severe nonfluent) and P2 (moderate-severe nonfluent) during TEST and RETEST, superimposed on each participant's reconstructed images. Areas activated ($p < 0.001$ uncorrected, for display) during the nonverbal semantic decision task compared to a passive viewing/rest condition.

lated by practice, learning, or familiarity with the task. Raichle demonstrated decreased activations in L prefrontal cortex during a semantic task (verb generation) in normal, healthy subjects. Blasi reported similar physiological modulations of activity in R frontal cortex (dorsal IFG) in patients with L IFG damage during learning of a word stem completion task. Their results suggested that compensatory pathways in the RH may be capable of plasticity through learning.

Recently, Fridriksson and Morrow [9] examined changes in cortical activation as a result of manipulating task difficulty on a picture-word verification task. They found greater activation in the difficult condition, compared to the easy condition, for participants with aphasia and healthy, age-matched controls. Their findings, as well as those of Blasi [2], highlight the significant role of both task familiarity and task difficulty in modulating cortical activations. Their results suggest

that in order to verify treatment-induced brain plasticity, these factors may need to be calibrated pre- and post-treatment.

Participants in the current study were already familiar with the task stimuli, which had comprised part of their training in C-ViC. They nonetheless both demonstrated considerable fMRI response decrements between TEST and RETEST. This decrement in both spatial extent and intensity of cortical activation was also associated with decrements in response time, although accuracy in both participants remained stable. Future investigations would benefit from using more stimuli, including some novel stimuli, as well as a mixed block/event-related paradigm, in which post-hoc analyses might reveal differences between accurate and inaccurate, easy and difficult, or fast and slow trials.

In addition to establishing intrasubject test-retest reliability in fMRI, this study also supports evidence of individual differences for LH and RH involvement in long-term aphasia recovery. P1 ("moderate response" to C-ViC training), whose predominantly subcortical lesion spares many of the LH cortical areas previously associated with semantic processing, nonetheless demonstrates a strongly RH-lateralized pattern of activation. Although his lesion does not extend into Broca's or Wernicke's cortical areas, neither of these regions (nor most of the spared LH perisylvian cortex, with the exception of L TFG and L MTG) was recruited in performance of this semantic judgment task. This failure to recruit classical cortical language areas that appear undamaged by structural MRI may be due to disconnection or diaschisis resulting from the subcortical white matter damage, or may reflect microscopic infarcts, or some combination of these factors [21,26]. As Nadeau and Crosson [26] have suggested, separating the direct effects of white matter lesions from the effects of associated vascular events (e.g., sustained cortical hypoperfusion), has not generally been possible. Future investigations utilizing converging evidence from structural and functional MRI, diffusion tensor imaging, and perfusion MRI, in conjunction with detailed behavioral data, may further address this question.

As one might expect, neither patient significantly activated identical clusters on TEST and RETEST. However, each patient activated similar parts of his own network for lexical-semantic processing on RETEST. For example, both P1 and P2 activated parts of RH homologous regions on TEST and RETEST analogous to LH regions activated on lexical-semantic tasks in normals: IFG, MFG and TFG. P2, however, the patient with "best" response to C-ViC training, was also able to activate more of these LH regions than P1, on TEST and/or RETEST, including L supramarginal gyrus.

P2 demonstrated a strongly RH-lateralized pattern of activation. Compared to P1, however, P2 showed more activation in LH frontal, temporal and parietal areas, despite large LH lesion that destroyed most of the LH cortical regions critical to semantic processing. It is tempting to characterize the differences in LH activation between our two subjects as supporting previous treatment studies. For example, new LH activation has been associated with better language outcome in aphasia patients post- speech/language therapy intervention [8,18,25,36]. Leger et al. [18], for example, studied an aphasic patient pre- and post- speech therapy on a confrontation naming (and control rhyming) task. Their patient demonstrated greater perilesional activity (including L Broca's area and the L supramarginal gyrus) as performance on the task improved. As their

study suggests, it may be the case that restoration of LH language-related networks is critical for efficient or effective recovery in poststroke aphasia.

In the current study, we observed greater LH perilesional activation in the patient with more extensive long-term recovery during a nonverbal semantic judgment task. Unfortunately, one methodological weakness of our design was the lack of a true baseline task to which these two patients' pattern-viewing and semantic-processing could be compared. Not having normalized each subjects' data to this common baseline, evidence of greater LH activation must be interpreted with caution. Future investigations exploring the question of relative degrees of hemispheric recruitment in aphasia recovery should include a true resting/baseline condition.

In summary, the three hypotheses tested in the present, small study were generally supported by the results – i.e., 1) chronic aphasia patients with moderate-to-severe nonfluent speech can provide reliable fMRI data during performance of a nonverbal semantic decision task in the scanner; 2) during fMRI, our two patients activated RH regions homologous to LH regions previously associated with lexical-semantic functions in normals; and they each activated some L perilesional regions and undamaged LH regions; and 3) the patient with "best response" to C-ViC training had a different pattern of fMRI activation than the patient with "moderate response", possibly including more LH activity in the patient with "best response". Additional fMRI studies with a larger number of aphasia patients where the language tasks include a baseline condition and are calibrated to account for the modulatory effects of practice, familiarity, and task difficulty are recommended. Future investigations would also benefit from analyses which might provide converging evidence of the significance of BOLD signal activation in these patients, including lesion volume analysis, perfusion, and diffusion weighted imaging.

Acknowledgements

Research supported by grants from the Medical Research Service, Department of Veterans Affairs, Washington, D.C., and R01 DC05672 (to M.A.N.); and P30 DC05207 to the BU Aphasia Research Center from the National Institute on Deafness and Other Communication Disorders, Bethesda, MD. The authors would like to acknowledge the assistance of the MRI staff at McLean Hospital; Ashley Young, Patricia Pimentel, Anne Smith, RT and Eileen Connolly, RT.

References

[1] P. Belin, Ph. Van Eeckhout, M. Zilbovicius, Ph. Remy, C.Francois, S. Guillaume, F. Chain, G. Rancurel and Y. Samson, Recovery from nonfluent aphasia after melodic intonation therapy: A PET study, *Neurology* **47** (1996), 1504–1511.

[2] V. Blasi, A.C. Young, A.P. Tansy, S.E. Petersen, A.Z. Snyder and M. Corbetta, Word retrieval learning modulates right frontal cortex in patients with left frontal damage, *Neuron* **35** (2002), 159–170.

[3] M. Brett, *The MNI brain and the Talairach atlas*, [On-line], 2003, Available: http://www.mrc-cbu.cam.ac.uk/Imaging/mnispace.html.

[4] C. Buchel and K. Friston, Extracting brain connectivity, in: *Functional MRI: An introduction to methods*, P. Jezzard, P.M. Matthews and S.M. Smith, eds, Oxford: New York, 2001, pp. 295–308.

[5] Y. Cao, E.M. Vikinngstad, K.P. George, A.F. Johnson and K.M.A. Welch, Cortical language activation in stroke patients recovering from aphasia with functional MRI, *Stroke* **30** (1999), 2331–2340.

[6] S.F. Cappa and G. Vallar, The role of the left and right hemispheres in recovery from aphasia, *Aphasiology* **6** (1992), 359–372.

[7] S.F. Cappa, D. Perani, F. Grassi, S. Bressi, M. Alberoni, M. Franceschi, V. Bettinardi, S. Todde and F. Fazio, A PET follow-up of recovery after stroke in acute aphasics, *Brain and Language* **56** (1997), 55–67.

[8] K. Cornelissen, M. Laine, A. Tarkiainen, T. Jarvensivu, N. Marin and R. Salmelin, Adult brain plasticity elicited by anomia treatment, *J of Cognitive Neuroscience* **15** (2003), 444–461.

[9] J. Fridriksson and L. Morrow, *Cortical activation and language task difficulty in aphasia*, Poster presented at 34th Annual Clinical Aphasiology Conference, May, 2004, Park City, UT.

[10] B.T. Gold and A. Kertesz, Right hemisphere semantic processing of visual words in an aphasic patient: An fMRI study, *Brain and Language* **73** (2000), 456–465.

[11] B.T. Gold and R.L. Buckner, Common prefrontal regions coactivate with dissociable posterior regions during controlled semantic and phonological tasks, *Neuron* **35** (2002), 803–812.

[12] H. Goodglass and E. Kaplan, *The Assessment of Aphasia and Related Disorders*, Second Edition. Philadelphia: Lea & Febiger, 1983.

[13] T.J. Grabowski, H. Damasio and A.R. Damasio, Premotor and prefrontal correlates of category-related lexical retrieval, *Neuroimage* **7** (1998), 232–243.

[14] W.D. Heiss, J. Kessler, A. Thiel, M. Ghaemi and H. Karbe, Differential capacity of left and right hemispheric areas for compensation of post-stroke aphasia, *Annals of Neurology* **45** (1999), 430–438.

[15] H. Karbe, A. Thiel, Weber-Luxenburger, J. Kessler, K. Herholz and W.D. Heiss, Reorganization of the cerebral cortex in poststroke aphasia studied with positron emission tomography, *Neurology* **50** (1998), A321.

[16] J. Kurland, E.H. Baker, M.A. Naeser, P.I. Martin, K. Doron, A. Bogdan, H. Seekins, P. Renshaw and D. Yurgelun-Todd, *fMRI in severe aphasia: Semantic yes/no decisions on icon sentences in C-ViC*, Poster presented at 32nd annual meeting of the International Neuropsychological Society, February, 2004, Baltimore, MD.

[17] J. Kurland, E.H. Baker, M.A. Naeser, K. Doron, P.I. Martin, H. Seekins, A. Bogdan, P. Renshaw and D. Yurgelun-Todd, *Non-verbal semantic decisions in severe*, global aphasia: An fMRI investigation with test/re-test reliability, Poster presented at 34th Annual Clinical Aphasiology Conference, May, 2004, Park City, UT.

[18] A. Leger, J-F. Demonet, S. Ruff, B. Aithamon, B. Touyeras, M. Puel, K. Boulanouar and D. Cardebat, Neural substrates of spoken language rehabilitation in an aphasic patient: An fMRI study, *NeuroImage* **17** (2002), 174–183.

[19] A. Martin, C.L. Wiggs, L.G. Ungerleider and J.V. Haxby, Neural correlates of category-specific knowledge, *Nature* **379** (1996), 649–652.

[20] L.V. McReynolds and C.K. Thompson, Flexibility of single-subject experimental designs, Part I: Review of the basics of single-subject designs, *Journal of Speech and Hearing Disorders* **51** (1986), 194–203.

[21] E.J. Metter, J.C. Mazziotta, H.H. Itabashi, N.J. Mankovich, M.E. Phelps and D.E. Kuhl, Comparison of glucose metabolism, x-ray CT, and postmortem data in a patient with multiple cerebral infarcts, *Neurology* **35** (1985), 1695–1701.

[22] R.A. Muller, N. Kleinhans and E. Courchesne, Linguistic theory and neuroimaging evidence: An fMRI study of Broca's area in lexical semantics, *Neuropsychologia* **41** (2003), 1199–1207.

[23] C.J. Mummery, K. Patterson, J.R. Hodges and C.J. Price, Functional neuroanatomy of the semantic system: Divisible by what? *Journal of Cognitive Neuroscience* **10** (1998), 766–777.

[24] S. Murtha, H. Chertkow, M. Beauregard and A. Evans, The neural substrate of picture naming, *Journal of Cognitive Neuroscience* **11** (1999), 399–423.

[25] M. Musso, C. Weiller, S. Kiebel, S.P. Muller, P. Bulau and M. Rijntjes, Training-induced brain plasticity in aphasia, *Brain* **122** (1999), 1781–1790.

[26] S.E. Nadeau and B. Crosson, Subcortical aphasia, *Brain and Language* **58** (1997), 355–402.

[27] M.A. Naeser, C.L. Palumbo, N. Helm-Estabrooks, D. Stiassny-Eder and M.L. Albert, Severe non-fluency in aphasia: Role of the medial subcallosal fasciculus plus other white matter pathways in recovery of spontaneous speech, *Brain* **112** (1989), 1–38.

[28] M.A. Naeser, E.H. Baker, C.L. Palumbo, M. Nicholas, M.P. Alexander, R. Samaraweera, M.N. Prete, S.M. Hodge and T. Weissman, Lesion site patterns in severe, nonverbal aphasia to predict outcome with a computer-assisted treatment program, *Archives of Neurology* **55** (1998), 1438–1448.

[29] M.A. Naeser, P.I. Martin, E.H. Baker, S.M. Hodge, S.E. Sczerzenie, M. Nicholas, C.L. Palumbo, H. Goodglass, A. Wingfield, R. Samaraweera, G. Harris, A. Baird, P. Renshaw and D. Yurgelun-Todd, Overt propositional speech in chronic nonfluent aphasia studied with the dynamic susceptibility contrast fMRI method, *Neuroimage* **22** (2004), 29–41.

[30] D. Perani, S.F. Cappa, M. Tettamanti, M. Rosa, P. Scifo, A. Miozzo, A. Basso and F. Fazio, A fMRI study of word retrieval in aphasia, *Brain and Language* **85** (2003), 357–368.

[31] J. Postler, R. De Bleser, J. Cholewa, V. Glauche, F. Hamzei and C. Weiller, Neuroimaging the semantic system(s), *Aphasiology* **17** (2003), 799–814.

[32] C.J. Price, E.A. Warburton, C.J. Moore, R.S.J. Frackowiak and K.J. Friston, Dynamic diaschisis: Anatomically remote and context-sensitive human brain lesions, *J Cogn Neurosci* **13** (2001), 419–429.

[33] M.E. Raichle, J.A. Fiez, T.O. Videen, A.K. MacLeod, J.V. Pardo and P.T. Fox, Practice-related changes in human brain

functional anatomy during non-motor learning, *Cerebral Cortex* **4** (1994), 8–26.

[34] C. Rorden and M. Brett, Stereotaxic display of brain lesions, *Behavioural Neurology* **12** (2000), 191–200.

[35] H.J. Rosen, S.E. Petersen, M.R. Linenweber, A.Z. Snyder, D.A. White, L. Chapman, A.W. Dromerick, J.A. Fiez and M. Corbetta, Neural correlates of recovery from aphasia after damage to left inferior frontal cortex, *Neurology* **55** (2000), 1883–1894.

[36] S.L. Small, D.K. Flores and D.C. Noll, Different neural circuits subserve reading before and after therapy for acquired dyslexia, *Brain and Language* **62** (1998), 298–308.

[37] R.D. Steele, M. Weinrich, R.T. Wertz, M.K. Kleczewska and G.S. Carlson, Computer-based visual communication in aphasia, *Neuropsychologia* **27** (1989), 409–426.

[38] J. Talairach and P. Tournoux, *Co-planar stereotaxic atlas of the human brain: 3-dimensional proportional system – an approach to cerebral imaging*, New York: Thieme, 1988.

[39] K.R. Thulborn, P.A. Carpenter and M.A. Just, Plasticity of language-related brain function during recovery from stroke, *Stroke* **30** (1999), 749–754.

[40] E. Warburton, C.J. Price, K. Swinburn and R.J. Wise, Mechanisms of recovery from aphasia: Evidence from positron emission tomography studies, *Journal of Neurology, Neurosurgery and Psychiatry* **66** (1999), 155–161.

[41] R. Zahn, E. Drews, K. Specht, S. Kemeny, W. Reith, K. Willmes, M. Schwarz and W. Huber, Recovery of semantic word processing in global aphasia: A functional MRI study, *Cognitive Brain Research* **18** (2004), 322–336.

7

Action and object word writing in a case of bilingual aphasia

Maria Kambanaros[a,*], Lambros Messinis[b] and Emmanouil Anyfantis[c]

[a]*Cyprus Acquisition Team, Department of English Studies, University of Cyprus, Nicosia, Cyprus*
[b]*Department of Neurology, Neuropsychology Section, University of Patras Medical School, Patras, Greece*
[c]*Department of Speech and Language Therapy, Technological Educational Institute Patras, Patras, Greece*

Abstract. We report the spoken and written naming of a bilingual speaker with aphasia in two languages that differ in morphological complexity, orthographic transparency and script Greek and English. AA presented with difficulties in spoken picture naming together with preserved written picture naming for action words in Greek. In English, AA showed similar performance across both tasks for action and object words, i.e. difficulties retrieving action and object names for both spoken and written naming. Our findings support the hypothesis that cognitive processes used for spoken and written naming are independent components of the language system and can be selectively impaired after brain injury. In the case of bilingual speakers, such processes impact on both languages. We conclude grammatical category is an organizing principle in bilingual dysgraphia.

Keywords: Lexical access, dysgraphia, Orthographic Autonomy Hypothesis (OAH), Greek

1. Introduction

Verbs and nouns are universal categories across languages. Verbs express states and events, that is, what happens to things, including actions, whereas nouns refer to entities such as people, animals, objects, and concepts. In Indo-European languages, verbs are usually marked for tense, aspect, mood, and number, while nouns are marked for case, gender, number, and definiteness (among other features). On the basis of their unique core linguistic function, the term verb can be used interchangeably with *action* (*name*) and correspondingly the term noun with *object* (*name*).

Studies of patients with brain damage report differences in processing actions and objects across languages [4]. Dissociations between action and object naming have also been reported in bilingual brain-impaired individuals in both languages spoken [11,12, 21,24]. Such findings can be taken as evidence for the claim that words are organized in the language system according to semantic and grammatical categories, and (perhaps more controversially) that verbs and nouns are linked to specific cortical regions [2,28]. Brain damage can selectively impair verb and noun processing at many levels in the language system: the conceptual level, the semantic-syntactic level, including lemma retrieval, the phonological level, including lexeme retrieval, and the level of articulation (see [22] and references within). The question of whether patterns of dissociation emerge across modalities of processing in bilingual speakers is our focus in the present study.

A small group of studies has reported an effect of word class on written picture naming of actions and objects in individuals with aphasia. Caramazza and colleagues [14–19,33,34] investigated written lexical access for action and object names in monolingual speakers with aphasia and compared their performance to spoken word production. In these cases, the writing performance of patients was typically spared relative to spoken word production [34]. However, a selective deficit for actions can be restricted to writing in some subjects and to speech in others [3] or a selective deficit for objects in speech only [17]. Most intriguingly, the

*Corresponding author: Maria Kambanaros, Cyprus Acquisition Team, Department of English Studies, University of Cyprus, 75 Kallipoleos, P.O. Box 20537, 1678 Nicosia, Cyprus. E-mail: kambanaros@gmail.com.

same patient may have difficulty with verbs in spoken but not written word production and with nouns in written but not spoken word production [34]. Such results suggest there are modality-specific (spoken or written) input and output components available for writing verbs and nouns in the brain [17].

Few studies have investigated the written production of verbs and nouns (i.e. actions and objects) in bilingual speakers with aphasia. Hernández et al. [12] described spoken and written output of a bilingual speaker with word-finding difficulties due to degenerative neuropathology. Before the onset of the illness, the patient (JPG) was highly proficient in Catalan and Spanish. When he was presented with the same set of action and object pictures, selected to elicit noun and verb production during spoken and written output, he performed better on object than action words in both modalities. A dissociation between action and object naming in written and spoken word output supports the hypothesis that the grammatical category of verbs and nouns is shared for cognitive and neural mechanisms across languages in a bilingual speakers [28]. However, the evidence to date is limited to participants who speak languages from the same linguistic family.

Our aim in the present report is to investigate the written and oral naming of actions and objects in a bilingual speaker with aphasia in two languages from different linguistic families: (Standard Modern) Greek and English. Unlike Spanish and Catalan, these languages differ in a number of features including morphological complexity, orthographic transparency and the type of script that is used for reading and writing. The key linguistic differences between Greek and English are summarized in Table 1. Unlike English, which is characterized as a word-based language, Greek is a stem-based language with a relatively complex morphology [13]. As in some English words, morpho-phonological word forms are inflected according to *grammatical category*, for instance '*skoup-izi*' is a verb [translation '*he/she sweeps*'] and '*skoup-a*' is a noun [translation '*broom*']. Nouns and verbs are differentiated by suffixes and marked for person and gender. Each stem in Greek is bound and presented for correct output after the correct inflectional suffix is attached to the stem at the morphological level. The Greek gender system with masculine, feminine and neuter gender is relatively complex. Nouns inflect gender at a morphological level. However, nouns are not only assigned gender on the basis of word meaning, but also on the basis of more general morphological rules. For instance, nouns ending with the nominative singu-

lar suffix –as ('*o papas*' [translation '*the priest*']) and with the accusative singular –a ('*ton papa*') are masculine, whereas nouns ending with the nominative singular –as ('*to kreas*' [translation '*the meat*']) and the accusative singular –as ('*to kreas*') are neuter. Gender agreement is also marked in Greek throughout the whole noun phrase, including determiners and adjectives. Information about the grammatical category and morpho-syntactic features of a Greek word, such as person, tense and mood for verbs or gender and case for nouns, are prominent aspects in the language as they must be accurately projected, marked and expressed during single word production. Thus, grammatical information can be assumed *prima facie* to be a constraint on selection and retrieval of appropriate phonological or orthographic representations (or lexeme) for output via language-specific processes necessary for morpho-phonological and morpho-orthographic encoding.

All cognitive models of lexical retrieval assume that spoken and written word production share conceptual representations but, post-semantically, to have different output mechanisms [2]. To retrieve a picture name, the speaker must first identify an action or object (e.g. a picture of scissors) and recognize the concept. This is considered a *pre-semantic* stage of processing. Next, a name is retrieved after the concept is distinguished the visually and semantically similar items. This is called the *lexical-semantic* stage. It is at this stage that morphosyntactic information first becomes available; e.g. in English and Greek, *scissors* is a single noun and in Greek it comes with neuter gender. Finally, the phonological or orthographic form of the word *scissors* is delivered. For spoken naming, the corresponding representation of the sound of the word is stored in the phonological output lexicon and instructions are given to the sensori-motor system to coordinate and produce speech sounds. For written naming, a corresponding orthographic form is retrieved from the orthographic output lexicon, which activates graphemic patterns for written output including allograph selection, retrieval of graphic motor patterns and motoric execution [5].

One theoretical issue in the study of lexical retrieval during written word production is the question of whether the sound of a word must be activated prior to retrieval of orthographic information. The Obligatory Phonological Mediation Hypothesis (OPMH) assumes the mapping of a lexical-semantic structure to an orthographic word form in the orthographic output lexicon first *requires* access to the phonological output lexicon. By contrast, the Orthographic Autonomy Hypothesis (OAH) assumes that orthographic representa-

Table 1
Key differences between the orthographic and phonological systems of Greek and English

Language system	Greek	English
Orthographic system		
Orthography	Transparent	Non-transparent
Letter inventory	More characters/letters than corresponding sounds	Fewer characters/letters than corresponding sounds
Orthographic principle	Phonemic basis	Largely morphophonemic basis
Alphabetic script	Mapping Greek letters to Greek phonemes	Mapping Roman letters to English phonemes
Phonological system		
Vowel inventory size and complexity	Unmarked five-vowel system with vowels evenly distributed in the periphery of the vowel space.	Complex and highly marked vowel system with over 20 vowels (depending on dialect) comprising of both monophthongs that mark length and diphthongs.
Prosody	Trochaic but syllable-timed	Trochaic but stress-timed

Table 2
Self – rated estimates of proficiency in his different languages across linguistic domains and of language use (percentage)

Estimates of proficiency					Language use background (percentage)				
	Understanding	Speaking	Reading	Writing		Home life	Tertiary education	Socializing	Reading	TV/ Radio
L1 (Greek)	7.0	7.0	7.0	7.0	L1 (Greek)	75%	100%	75%	75%	12.5%
L2 (English)	6.0	7.0	5.0	6.0	L2 (English)	12.5%	–	12.5%	25%	75%
L3 (Arabic)	5.0	5.0	–	–	L3 (Arabic)	12.5%	–	12.5%	–	12.5%

Key: 5 = good abilities, 6 = very good abilities, 7 = excellent (native-like) abilities.

tions are directly retrieved without any phonological mediation [33]. These theoretical views make different predictions about the effect of grammatical class on written word output. According to the OPMH, grammatical class effects in written word production should be accompanied by an effect of grammatical class on spoken word production. However, the OAH makes no such prediction allowing for dissociable effects. Any dissociation between action and object naming in written and spoken word output is strong evidence against the OPMH. If such dissociations can be found in a bilingual speaker, this would be evidence that grammatical category is an organizing principle of the language system shared across languages as argued by Miozzo et al. [28, see also 17]. We report such evidence below.

2. Case report

AA is a 25-year-old right-handed male student who has a left parieto-occipital lesion verified by neuroimaging (CT) as a result of cerebral hemorrhage on 19 February 2006, while sleeping. An angiography conducted on 21 February 2006 revealed an arteriovenous malformation (AVM). AA has a right hemi paresis involving the arm and leg. He was right-handed before the stroke but now writes only with his left hand. AA was born in Athens, Greece, and raised as a simultaneous bilingual speaking Greek, English and Arabic from infancy. However, he was educated in Greek only with some years of English language instruction during schooling in Greece. AA's mother is Greek, his father Palestinian and the home language is English. He has two younger brothers. AA was asked to rate his abilities in each language prior to and post stroke and the results of these ratings are presented in Table 2. His family members verified the responses. AA was asked to quantify his current domain of language use. This information is presented in Table 2. AA considers Greek his predominant language and English his second language. Hence we classified Greek as L1 and English L2. AA had no premorbid writing disorder and vision and his hearing were normal. At the time of testing he was in the third year of a 4-year bachelor degree (Building Renovation and Restoration at the Technological Educational Institute Patras), and he read and wrote in Greek on a daily basis. This course contains three English language modules of graded difficulty, which AA completed prior to his stroke. A (bilingual) language questionnaire [26] administered in Greek was used to assess his language background. Information included the age of language acquisition, domains of language use and estimated proficiency in each language [30].

2.1. Neuropsychological evaluation

During collection of demographic information and checklist completion, AA was able to provide personal information such as age, nationality, education and family history of neurological and psychiatric conditions. He was co-operative with testing. AA's understanding of task instructions was good. Premorbid intellectual ability was estimated using subtests (Vocabulary and Matrix Reasoning) taken from the Wechsler Abbreviated Scale of Intelligence (WASI) [27,35] giving a Full Scale IQ score of 95 (37th percentile). His score on the Greek adapted version of the Mini Mental State Examination (MMSE) [6] was 29/30 (absence of dementia). AA's verbal and visual memory was assessed with the CNS Vital Signs memory test, which is translated into Greek [9]. In this test participants must learn 15 words and 15 geometric figures and recognize them from distractors. This task has immediate and delayed recognition/recall trials. AA obtained a standard score (age and education adjusted) of 110 on the verbal immediate recall trial (75th percentile rank for his age and education level) and 97 on the verbal delay recall trial (42nd percentile rank for his age and education level) indicating an average overall verbal memory performance, but difficulties in recalling previously learned information. On visual memory testing, his standard score (age and education adjusted) was 107 on the immediate recall trial (68th percentile rank for his age and education level) and 87 on the visual delay recall trial (19th percentile rank for his age and education level). This is in the low average range, especially recall of visual information after a delay. Executive functions were assessed with the CNS Vital Signs STROOP Test [9]. This is a measure of goal directed behaviour and flexibility required for self-correction. His score was in the impaired range between 1st and 13th percentile age and education adjusted. The CNS Vital Signs Symbol Digit Coding Test [9] was also administered to assess psychomotor speed and visual-motor coordination. Performance was poor (1st percentile age and education adjusted) showing slowed information processing when perceiving, attending and responding to visual information. We assessed his mood with the Beck Depression Inventory – Fast Screen (BDI-FS) [1] and the Beck Anxiety Inventory (BAI) [1]. AA scored 5/21 on the BDI-FS and 14/63 on the BAI, showing no significant depression but some mild anxiety.

2.2. Language assessment

Language testing was carried out in a quiet treatment room at the Speech and Language Clinic of the Technological Educational Institute (TEI) Patras. AA was tested over three-months. He was administered (a) the Boston Diagnostic Aphasia Examination (BDAE) in English [8] and Greek [29] to determine aphasia type and severity; (b) Greek Object and Action Test (GOAT) [21] of spoken and written retrieval of action and object names; and (c) phonological and orthographic processing subtests of the Athina Diagnostic Test of Learning Difficulties [31].[1] To test spelling, AA was given (i) nonwords in Greek and English to test sub-lexical/phonological spelling ability and (ii) homophones and cognate words to test lexical-semantic/non-phonological processing. A Greek-English speaker (the first author) administered all tasks. According to the BDAE, AA presented with anomic aphasia characterized by fluent, well-articulated speech but mild to moderate anomia (word-finding difficulties) [7] in Greek (L1) and English (L2). His auditory comprehension across language tasks was within normal limits in both languages. As writing impairments are our focus, writing subtests from the BDAE were administered. There was no evidence of motor writing impairments and we note that AA had trained himself to write with his non-paretic (left) hand. He showed a good writing style with well-formed letters and legible cursive writing. As a full-time university student, AA reported spending many hours per day writing (by hand) in Greek and also in English. In both scripts, on all tasks, AA wrote in lower case letters only. Writing was assessed on the following tasks in Greek and English: a) mechanics of writing (automatic writing: name and address) including recall of written symbols (serial writing-alphabet and numbers; primer-level dictation-writing individual numbers, letters, primer words to dictation; b) written word finding (spelling to dictation and written confrontation naming); and c) written formulation (narrative writing). These results are summarized in Table 3.

2.3. Tests of hypotheses

Previous studies of bilingual speakers have reported effects of grammatical class on spoken and written word

---

[1]The Athina Diagnostic Test of Learning Difficulties is partly based on the Illinois Test of Psycholinguistic Abilities and is standardized on healthy Greek speakers.

Table 3
AA's results on the writing subtests of the BDAE in L1 and L2

Subtest	Greek (L1)	English (L2)
Automatic writing (name and address)	Judged to be similar to pre-morbid writing	Judged to be similar to pre-morbid writing
Recall of alphabet	24/24 correct	8/26 correct
Recall of numbers	21/21 correct	21/21 correct
Writing letters	No impairment	No impairment
Writing numbers	No impairment	No impairment
Copying	No impairment	1 letter substitution (dog ⇒ bog)
Written word finding	10/10	2/10
Written picture description "Cookie Theft"	Organized coherent account: 31 words, 1 spelling error	Organized coherent account: 24 words, 7 spelling errors, 1 grammatical error

naming with better performance for actions than objects in both languages [11]. According to the obligatory phonological mediation hypothesis (OPMH), effects of grammatical class on written word naming must be accompanied by the same effect on spoken word naming. Our first goal was to assess whether AA was impaired on lexical retrieval tasks. We did this with subtests from the Greek Object and Action Test (GOAT) [21] administered to assess spoken and written naming of actions and objects. The GOAT has 84 items: 42 action and 42 object colored photographs measuring 10 × 14 cm in size. No items were cognates in Greek and English [30]. Pictured actions were mono-transitive verbs. Actions included instrumental verbs (sweeping) and non-instrumental verbs (climbing). Objects were all inanimate nouns. There were no significant differences in mean word frequency, age of acquisition (AoA) or stimulus length between nouns and verbs in Greek (see Appendix 1) and no differences in written frequency in English between nouns (mean 89.31 per million) and verbs (mean 69.95 per million) on GOAT subtests [35]. Responses were recorded via audiotape. Error coding was based on a standard system [24].

2.4. Spoken and written naming

AA was shown photographs individually and asked to describe the picture using one word either in Greek or English, according to language tested. Each language was tested at least one week apart and all subtests presented in random order. Oral and written naming was tested separately.

AA was able to produce the correct spoken name in Greek for 19/42 (45.2%) actions and 17/42 (40.5%) objects and in English for 12/42 (28.5%) actions and 12/42 (28.5%) objects. Chi-square analysis found a significant difference in spoken naming between Greek and English $\chi^2 = 21.42$ $p < 0.001$, with better performance in Greek compared to English for actions $\chi^2 =$

8.67, $p = 0.003$ and objects $\chi^2 = 27.42$, $p < 0.001$. Within languages, there were no significant differences in action and object naming. In Greek, "Don't know" responses were dominant for actions 13/23 (56.5%) and objects 7/25 (28%) although semantic errors 8/25 (32%) and code-switching errors 5/25 (20%) were observed. In English, "Don't know" responses were dominant for actions 16/25 (64%) followed by semantic errors 7/23 (30.4%) and omissions 6/25 (24%) whereas for objects, omissions were dominant 24/29 (83%).

AA was able to produce the correct written name in Greek for 34/42 (81.0%) actions and 28/42 (66.6%) objects and in English for 8/42 (19.0%) actions and 8/42 (19.0)% objects. Chi-square analysis found a significant difference in written naming between Greek and English $\chi^2 = 3.42$, $p < 0.001$, with better performance in Greek compared to English for actions $\chi^2 = 5.25$, $p = 0.022$ and objects $\chi^2 = 42.85$, $p < 0.001$. There was a significant difference in written performance for actions compared to objects in Greek $\chi^2 = 5.95$, $p < 0.001$, with better performance for actions. There was no significant difference in action and object written naming in English. In Greek, the predominant error type was letter substitutions when writing actions (7/7) and objects (13/14). Greek errors involved substitution of a single vowel in either word initial (3/7) or word medial position (4/7) for action and word final (8/13), initial (3/13), and both initial and final positions in the same word (2/13), for object words. Moreover, all written naming errors for actions and objects were phonologically plausible alternatives in Greek. In English, errors with action and object names were mostly omissions and performance for both word types was close to the floor.

3. Discussion

We observed differential effects of word class on spoken and written word retrieval: an effect of grammatical class on written word production but not spoken word production in Greek and no effect of word class on spoken or written word retrieval in English. Our findings contrast with previous studies of bilingual speakers reporting effects of grammatical class on spoken word *and* written word naming with superior performance on nouns compared to actions in each language.

AA was better at writing action than object names in his native language (Greek) only. According to the obligatory phonological mediation hypothesis (OPMH), effects of grammatical class on written word naming must be accompanied by the same effect on spoken word naming. We therefore reject the OPMH as an explanation for written word naming in bilingual speakers. In addition to the effect of grammatical class on writing in Greek, AA was more impaired at spoken (43% correct) than written naming (73% correct) in Greek with no differences between spoken (28.5%) and written naming in English (19%). We assume there was damage at the level of the phonological output lexicon and the orthographic output lexicon in Greek and English (see Fig. 1) given AA has normal comprehension in both languages. Semantic errors in spoken naming were observed in both languages when the target was unavailable [2,19]. However, semantic errors were absent in writing. Writing errors were more likely to reflect knowledge of phonology to orthography correspondences in both Greek and English. We take this dissociation in error types as evidence of selective damage to phonological and orthographic output lexica.

The orthographic autonomy hypothesis [33] can explain the effect of selective damage to the orthographic output lexicon and the effect of grammatical class on written word output in Greek. According to this account, separate input and output components are available for writing verbs and nouns in the orthographic output lexicon [18] as in the phonological output lexicon [14]. AA's writing of action names – although not perfect – was significantly better than writing object names. The dominant writing error for objects was letter substitutions i.e. phonological-orthographic errors, involving the vowel "i" [ι] (iota) in word final position replaced by the vowel "i" [η] (ita); iota is the most common ending for singular neuter nouns, while ita is the most common ending for singular feminine nouns in Greek. Writing errors on (neuter) object words in Greek could be called morphological as AA assigned feminine gender to neuter nouns. However, we can reject this account for two reasons: first, he retrieved the gender of every noun correctly (100%) on

the spoken naming task when asked to provide gender by the examiner, and second, he was able to write other neuter nouns ending with *iota*, e.g. spoon, sponge, fishing rod. Furthermore, all other errors for objects in Greek involved letter substitutions or phonological-orthographic replacements of similar-sounding vowels (e.g., αναπτύρας instead of αναπτήρας "lighter"). As Greek has a transparent orthography, one explanation for performance on written picture naming of Greek neuter nouns is that spelling proceeded via a sublexical route (phoneme to grapheme conversion), delivering phonologically plausible alternatives lacking word-specific orthographic knowledge. There are alternative spellings of the vowel "i" and other vowels in Greek [32]. Word-specific knowledge is required to write words containing (vowel) orthographic ambiguity. Moreover, it is likely that access to morphological rules for neuter noun declensions was partly available to AA (after stroke), which would explain his mixed written picture naming performance mainly on (neuter) nouns.

Errors in action word written naming also show phonological-orthographic substitutions of word-medial or final vowels (e.g., κλειδόνει for κλειδώνει "locking", τριπάει for τρυπάει "drilling") that are also phonologically plausible alternatives. We contend that AA's action word writing (close to ceiling) involves an orthographic lexicon for spelling (orthographic ambiguous) action words and b) contribution from sublexical language-specific phonological to orthographic conversion procedures for action words. There was also evidence that AA relied on a sublexical route to spell object names in Greek. He produced written errors on vowel phonemes that are represented by many spellings in Greek. Considering that the orthography of Greek words is based not only on the phonological but also on the etymological information of a word, it would be expected that AA developed a visual orthographic representation that allows him to write all known words, but particularly words with phonemes that are ambiguous, i.e. can be spelled with more than one grapheme. Relying on a phonological transcription strategy will not automatically give a correct spelling for Greek words. It is not clear why damage to the orthographic output lexicon would have a greater effect on writing object names compared to action names but some explanations can be excluded. There were no significant differences in mean word frequencies, age of acquisition or stimulus length between objects and actions in Greek. It is important to note that regularity of spelling in action and object names was not controlled, but this is irrelevant to explaining writing performance according to the OAH. The OAH assumes that writing picture names does not require access to phonological representations, which are necessary to spell from dictation and thus could lead to differential effects on the spelling of regular and irregular words. According to the OAH, damage to the orthographic output mechanism for writing objects must be more impaired for AA due to greater loss of word specific orthographic knowledge or due to greater damage to morpho-syntactic properties for the retrieval of nouns from the lexical system.

There was evidence of impairment to the lexical retrieval of nouns in spoken production. However, AA's performance on spoken word naming of objects (40.5%) was worse than written word naming of the same objects (66.6%) a pattern that was magnified for spoken word naming of actions (42.5%) compared to written word naming of actions (81%). Therefore, it is not likely that impaired writing of object names simply reflects AA's impairment in lexical retrieval only. We contend that effects of grammatical class on object naming in Greek reflect a loss of specific orthographic knowledge about linguistic features of Greek nouns. We noted above a tendency for AA to assign feminine gender when writing neuter nouns although he could retrieve the gender of every noun correctly on the spoken naming task. This suggests that AA has a specific problem with retrieval of knowledge about noun gender at the orthographic level. Of interest, preserved knowledge of orthography allowed AA to produce better written word naming than spoken word naming of both actions and objects, although superior written word naming always has a benefit from preserved knowledge of spoken as well as orthographic information (and this is not true in spoken picture naming).

AA demonstrated deficits across spoken and written production in English (L2) with differences in performance reflecting premorbid familiarity with written English. The absence of any effects of grammatical class in L2 when compared to the effect on written word naming in L1 does not challenge the OAH provided the hypothesis is able to assume selective damage across both languages of a bilingual speaker (as well as between word class and modality of output). An advantage for nouns over verbs in L1 and L2 written picture naming was reported for a bilingual Spanish-Catalan speaker, JPG [12]. The effect of word class was reported for spoken picture naming in both languages. In general, JPG's performance was qualitatively very similar across languages and tasks, but the magnitude of the effect was larger in Catalan (L2).

Dissociations between actions and objects in written and spoken word naming support the claim that grammatical category is an organizing principle of the language system. However, we predicted equivalent impairments across both languages of a bilingual speaker following Miozzo et al. [28]. The absence of any effect of grammatical class in L2 is not necessarily a problem for the grammatical processing hypothesis in bilingual aphasia. Effect of word class on spoken and written picture naming in English may be difficult to detect given that performance was so near to floor. However, this does not explain why action naming in L1 is better than action naming in L2 or effects of language on performance across tasks. One possibility is that these effects reflect impairment to cognition such as attention, executive function and memory. AA's recall of visual information after a delay was poor and executive functions was impaired, with slow information processing given visual information. Slow processing and impairment to delayed visual memory may have more impact on writing verbs and nouns in English than in Greek since there are more irregular words in English requiring retrieval of word specific orthographic knowledge. This is likely to affect performance on picture naming tasks because phonological input is limited. We contend that it is important to consider cognitive impairments when explaining grammatical class effects on performance in any language.

To conclude, the results support the view that word class is a constraint on lexical retrieval. The results can be explained by the OAH because effects of grammatical class were restricted to lexical retrieval of word specific orthographic knowledge in Greek. Differences in morphological and orthographic features between languages explain effects of word class on writing in bilingual dysgraphia. For most writers, word patterns of English are picked up during the acquisition of reading and writing skills and most are learned through familiarity with the alphabetic symbols and their pronunciations or by memorizing of whole-word forms.

Appendix

Picture characteristics of the GOAT based on psycholinguistic variables: lemma frequency, syllable length, age-of-acquisition (mean years;months), word imageability (0 = not imageable, 7 = highly imageable) and picture complexity (0 = high complexity, 7 = low complexity).

Picture type	Lemma frequency	Syllable length	Age-of-acquisition	Imageability	Picture complexity
Objects	40.91	2.88 (0.80)	2.98 (0.76)	6.49 (0.49)	6.49 (0.28)
Actions	40.11	2.95 (0.73)	2.82 (0.58)	6.42 (0.16)	6.16 (0.67)

Key: ( ) = standard deviations.

References

[1] A. Beck and R.A. Steer, *Beck Anxiety Inventory*: Manual, Harcourt Assessment: The Psychological Corporation, 1993.

[2] A. Caramazza, How many levels of processing are there in lexical Access? *Cognitive Neuropsychology* **14** (1997), 177–208.

[3] A. Caramazza and A. Hillis, Lexical organization of nouns and verbs in the brain, *Nature* **349** (1991), 788–790.

[4] J. Druks, Verbs and nouns: A review of the literature, *Journal of Neurolinguistics* **15** (2002), 289–315.

[5] A.W. Ellis and A.W. Young, *Human Cognitive Neuropsychology*, Psychology Press, Hove, East Sussex, 1988.

[6] N.K. Fountoulakis, M. Tsolaki, H. Chantzi and A. Kazis, Mini mental state examination (MMSE): A validation study in Greece, *American Journal of Alzheimer's Disease and Other Dementias* **15** (2000), 342–345.

[7] H. Goodglass, *Understanding Aphasia*, Academic Press, San Diego, 1993.

[8] H. Goodglass and E. Kaplan, *The Assessment of Aphasia and Related Disorders*, (2nd ed.), Lea and Febiger, Philadelphia, 1983.

[9] T.C. Gualtieri and G.L. Johnson, Reliability and validity of a computerized neurocognitive test battery, CNS Vital Signs, *Archives of Clinical Neuropsychology* **21** (2006), 623–643.

[10] M.N. Hatzigeorgiou, S. Gavrilidou, G. Piperidis, A. Carayannis, A. Papakostopoulou, Spiliotopoulou et al., Design and implementation of the online ILSP corpus, *Proceedings of the Second International Conference of Language Resources and Evaluation (LREC)* **3** (2000), 1737–1740.

[11] M. Hernández, A. Costa, N. Sebastián-Gallés, M. Juncadella and R. Reñe, The organization of nouns and verbs in bilingual speakers: A case of bilingual grammatical category-specific deficit, *Journal of Neurolinguistics* **20** (2007), 285–305.

[12] M. Hernández, A. Caño, A. Costa, N. Sebastián-Gallés, M. Juncadella and J. Gascón-Bayarri, Grammatical category-specific deficits in bilingual aphasia, *Brain and Language* **107** (2008), 68–80.

[13] P.P.D. Holton, P. Mackridge and I. Philippaki-Warburton, *Greek: A Comprehensive Grammar of the Modern Language*, Routledge, London, 1997.

[14] A. Hillis and A. Caramazza, Mechanisms for accessing lexical representations for output: Evidence from a category-specific semantic deficit, *Brain and Language* **40** (1991), 106–144.

[15] A. Hillis and A. Caramazza, Category–specific naming and comprehension impairment: a double dissociation, *Brain* **114** (1991), 2081–2094.

[16] A. Hillis and A. Caramazza, The compositionality of lexical semantic representations: Clues from semantic errors in object naming, *Memory* **3** (1995), 333–358.

[17] A. Hillis and A. Caramazza, Representation of grammatical categories of words in the brain, *Journal of Cognitive Neuroscience* **7** (1995), 457–458.

[18] A.E. Hillis, B.C. Rapp and A. Caramazza, When a rose is a rose in speech but a tulip in writing, *Cortex* **35** (1999), 337–356.

[19] A. Hillis, E. Tuffiash and A. Caramazza, Modality-specific deterioration in naming verbs in nonfluent primary progressive aphasia, *Journal of Cognitive Neuroscience* **14** (2002), 1099–1108.

[20] C.I. Iribarren, G. Jarema and R.A. Lecours, Two different dysgraphic syndromes in a regular orthography, Spanish, *Brain and Language* **77** (2001), 166–175.

[21] M. Kambanaros, *Verb and noun processing in late bilingual individuals with anomic aphasia*, Doctoral dissertation, Flinders University, Adelaide, 2003.

[22] M. Kambanaros, Grammatical word class distinctions in bilingual aphasia, in: *Aphasia: Symptoms, Diagnosis, and Treatment*, Grigore Ibanescu and Serafim Pescariu, eds, Nova Science Publishers, NY. 2009.

[23] M. Kambanaros, The relationship between single-word naming and connected speech in bilingual aphasia: Evidence from bilingual Greek–English-speaking individuals, *Aphasiology* **24** (2010), 1–21.

[24] M. Kambanaros and W. van Steenbrugge, Noun and verb processing in Greek–English bilingual individuals with anomic aphasia and the effect of instrumentality and verb–noun name relation, *Brain and Language* **97** (2006), 162–177.

[25] H. Kucera and W.N. Francis, Computational analysis of present- day American English, Brown University Press, Rhode Island, 1970.

[26] P. Li, S. Sepanski and X. Zhao, Language history questionnaire: A web-based interface for bilingual research, *Behaviour Research Methods* **38** (2006), 202–210.

[27] L. Messinis, A. Biris and P. Papathanasopoulos, Wechsler abbreviated scale of intelligence (WAIS) [Greek adaptation and preliminary normative data]. Unpublished data, Neuropsychological laboratory, Department of Neurology, University of Patras Medical School, Greece, 2009.

[28] M. Miozzo, A, Costa, M. Hernández and B. Rapp, Lexical processing in the bilingual brain: Evidence from grammatical/morphological deficits, *Aphasiology* **24** (2010), 262–287.

[29] I. Papathanasiou, D. Papadimitriou, B. Gavrilou and A. Mixou, Psychometric data on the BDAE in a healthy adult population: the role of age and gender (English translation of Greek title), *Psychology* **15** (2008), 398–410.

[30] M. Paradis, A Neurolinguistic Theory of Bilingualism. John Benjamins Publishing Company, Amsterdam/Philadelphia, 2004.

[31] J. Paraskevopoulos, A. Kalantzi-Azizi and N. Gianitsas, 'Athina' test for diagnosis of learning disabilities (in Greek), Helleneka Grammata, ed,. Faculty of Philosophy, University of Athens, 1999.

[32] D.C. Porpodas, Literacy acquisition in Greek: Research review of the role of phonological and cognitive factors, in: *Handbook of Orthography and Literacy*, Erlbaum, Malwah, NJ, 2006, pp. 189–199.

[33] B. Rapp, L. Benzing and A. Caramazza, The autonomy of lexical orthography, *Cognitive Neuropsychology* **14** (1997), 71–104.

[34] B. Rapp and A. Caramazza, Selective difficulties with spoken nouns and written verbs: A single case study, *Journal of Neurolinguistics* **15** (2002), 373–402.

[35] D. Wechsler, *Wechsler Abbreviated Scale of Intelligence* (WAIS): Manual, The Psychological Corporation, New York, 1999.

8

Right hemisphere involvement in nonfluent primary progressive aphasia

Claudia Repetto[a,*], Rosa Manenti[b], Maria Cotelli[a], Marco Calabria[c], Orazio Zanetti[a], Barbara Borroni[d], Alessandro Padovani[d] and Carlo Miniussi[a,e]

[a]IRCCS S. Giovanni di Dio Fatebenefratelli, Brescia, Italy
[b]Department of Neuroscience, Vita Salute University and San Raffaele Scientific Institute, Milan, Italy
[c]Department of General Psychology, University of Padua, Italy
[d]Department of Neurology, University of Brescia, Italy
[e]Department of Biomedical Sciences and Biotechnologies, University of Brescia, Italy

Abstract. We described a 56-years-old man with a diagnosis of "non-fluent primary progressive aphasia" (NfPPA). An accurate neuropsychological, neurological and neuroimaging evaluation was performed in order to assess clinical and behavioural features of the patient.

From a neuropsychological point of view, the patient showed a typical cognitive profile of subjects affected by NfPPA: a prominent language deficit, associated with impairments in several cognitive domains after three years from the onset of the symptomatology. The most intriguing feature is that SPECT revealed hypoperfusion in the right frontal cortex, albeit the patient is right-handed. This unexpected finding shows that NfPPA may arise not only from cortical abnormalities in the language-dominant left hemisphere, but also from right hemisphere involvement in a right hander (crossed aphasia).

Keywords: Non-fluent primary progressive aphasia, language disorder, lateralization, frontotemporal dementia

1. Introduction

Primary Progressive Aphasia (PPA) is a neurodegenerative disease characterized by a) insidious onset, but progressive impairment of word finding, object naming, syntax, or word comprehension manifested during conversation or assessed with the use of standard neuropsychological tests of language; b) all major limitation in activities of daily living can be attributed to the language impairment for at least two years after onset; c) premorbid language function is known to be intact; d) prominent apathy, disinhibition, loss of memory of recent events, visuospatial impairment, visual-recognition deficits, and absence of sensory-motor dysfunction during the initial two years of illness, d) acalculia and ideomotor apraxia can be present even in the first two years of illness; e) other cognitive functions may be affected after the first two years of illness, but language remains the most impaired function throughout the course of the illness and deteriorates faster than other affected functions; f) specific cause of aphasia, such as stroke or tumor, as ascertained by neuroimaging, are absent [14,16].

PPA is observed in different forms: non-fluent PPA (NfPPA), characterized by effortful articulation, agrammatism, phonemic paraphasias, various degrees of anomia but relatively preserved comprehension; semantic dementia (SD), or fluent-PPA, in which prominent loss of the meaning of words and objects, gram-

*Corresponding author: Claudia Repetto, Neuroscience Unit, IRCCS S. Giovanni di Dio Fatebenefratelli, Via Pilastroni 4, Brescia, Italy. E-mail: claudia.repetto@cognitiveneuroscience.it.

matically correct speech, and preserved syntactic comprehension are present. A third variant, which differs from both NfPPA and SD is called "logopenic", and is characterized by a speech slowed in rate but without articulatory difficulties, syntactically simple but correct, halted by frequent word-finding pauses, in the absence of (syntactic or semantic) comprehension deficits [7].

Some reviews of demographic and clinical features of patients with diagnosis of NfPPA revealed that they are largely more males than females (66% vs 34%), and that the onset of the illness is shown between the age of 50 and 69, with the modal value at 64 years [23]. When the MRI shows abnormal findings, there are either in the left hemisphere or bilateral (for a review: Westbury, 1997 [23]).

We present here a new case of non-fluent primary progressive aphasia, characterized by right hemisphere involvement. The observation can be interpreted referring to the hypothesis of crossed aphasia (CAD), as originally defined by Bramwell [2]. He introduced this term to denote, in a broad sense, any aphasic syndrome resulting from a cerebral lesion ipsilateral to the dominant hand.

2. Case report

G.G. is a 56-years-old, right handed (50% dexterity,[1] following Biggs [3] evaluation), man. He used to work as a business manager and has had 13 years of education. His clinical history is unremarkable. Family history is positive for neurodegenerative diseases (grandfather and father with diagnosis of Alzheimer Disease).

By the age of 53th, the patient presented difficulties in word-finding, as he referred at his first neurological consultation in 2004. This consultation showed a normal neurological examination, but MRI revealed aspecific and puntiform signal hyperintensity in the right frontal lobe and SPECT showed hypoperfusion in the right frontal cortex.

He was autonomous in his daily activities except for the ones requiring oral and written language production. Formal neuropsychological evaluation at that time revealed an isolated deficit on verbal fluency. The great difficulties in language expression, associated to an almost preserved comprehension, made the patient deeply depressed.

We reported G.G.'s neurological and neuropsychological evaluation, assessed three years after the onset of the symptomatology, investigating with particular care his language abilities.

2.1. Neurological evaluation

Neurological examination revealed the cranial nerves to be intact. The muscle tone was normal in the upper and lower limbs. Gait and reflexes were normal. Tremors at the distal extremities were evident.

2.2. General neuropsychology

Neuropsychological testing was administered by an experienced examiner in a quiet environment at the hospital.

Approximately 60 to 90 minutes were needed to administer tests. Language impairment prevented from long-term verbal memory evaluation that requires production of complex sentences (story recall [18]).

The examination included screening test for dementia (Mini-Mental State Examination, MMSE [6]), test of nonverbal reasoning (Raven's Coloured Progressive Matrices, CPM), auditory language comprehension (Token Test), verbal fluency with phonemic and semantic cues, verbal and spatial short-term memory (Digit Span forward and Spatial Span), spatial long-term memory (Rey Recall), constructional abilities (Rey's complex copy), upper limbs [4] and buccofacial apraxia [21], visuospatial abilities (VOSP – The Visual Object and Space Perception battery subtests of incomplete letter detection, object decision and number location detection [22], Judgement of lines orientation - H form [1]), and attention (Trail Making Test).

Table 1 reports GG's performance in these tasks.

In sum, G.G. showed deficits in all these cognitive domains, with the exception of short-term verbal memory, letter, object and number position detection, and buccofacial praxic abilities. In addition, language comprehension and non-verbal reasoning were at a borderline level.

2.3. Language assessment

G.G.'s spontaneous speech was non-fluent, with anomic pauses, phonetic substitutions and articulatory disturbances; oral language was made up of short sentences, of no more than 2–3 words; syntax was simple.

A formal language evaluation with Aachener Aphasia Test (Italian version [9]) and BADA [15] showed

---

[1] The degree of dexterity ranges from 0 to 100%, whereas left-handedness assumes negative values.

Table 1
General neuropsychology (July 2006)

TEST	Original scores	Adjusted scores	Cut-off
MMSE (0–30)	27	25.99	24
Raven (CPM 0–36)	18	18	18
Rey Recall (0–36)*	4	2.25	9.47
Digit span	5	4.75	3.75
Spatial span*	3	2.75	3.75
Token test (0–36)	30.5	28.5	26.5
Fluency (phonological cue)*	2	0	17
Fluency (semantic cue)*	0	0	25
Rey copy (0–36)*	20	19.75	28.88
Trail making test A*	97	91	93
Trail making test B*	392	376	282
Trail making test B-A*	295	285	186
De Renzi right arm (0–72)*	52		62
De Renzi left arm (0–72)*	54		62
Buccofacial apraxia (0–20)	19	18.75	17–18
VOSP:			
Incomplete letters	18		16
Object decision	20		14
Number location	8		7
Benton lines*	11	14	17

*Score below cut-off.

difficulties repeating single words and sentences, associated with disorder of comprehension and verbs naming. Writing on composition was well performed, whereas hand writing, for both words and non-words was pathological and a qualitative analysis of his calligraphy showed an evident micrography.

Oral and written naming of verb appeared impaired. The nature of errors referred to the selection of wrong stem (i.e. "vote" rather than "put in envelope") or anomia (the pantomime of the gesture substitutes the verbs).

In comprehension BADA subtest, the patient demonstrated difficulties in tasks that require a judgment about sentence morphosyntactic features: subject – verb, noun – adjective and article – noun agreement, verb conjugation, location of constituents.

3. Discussion

In this report we described a case of NfPPA, a clinical syndrome due to a neurodegenerative process that affects primarily language functions. From the first clinical description of Mesulam [13], during recent years renewed interest has been developed in this form of aphasia that belongs to the spectrum of frontotemporal dementias (FTD).

The heritability of PPA is not well known. Krefft et al. [8] reported the first case of familial PPA, in which all members affected (three siblings of four) met criteria of PPA: genetic analysis revealed a probable autosomal inheritance (dominant or recessive).

Most studies in literature focused on neuropsychological and neuropathological characterisation of different forms of PPA, with particular concern of anatomical localization of brain damage. Despite the large data corpus, there is not a general consensus about brain areas involved in NfPPA, mainly for what concerns the lateralization of cerebral damage. Left brain involvement, consistently with the usual localization of language function, is well documented in several studies; among these the following imaging data may be mentioned: atrophy of the pars opercularis and triangularis of the left inferior frontal gyrus and grey matter loss in the left precentral gyrus of the insula [7]; cortical atrophy in inferior, orbital, insular, and dorsolateral regions of the left frontal lobe [11]; focal abnormality of the left insular region and frontal operculum extending onto the inferior frontal gyrus, with the epicentre of this hypometabolic cluster being in the anterior insula [17].

Bilateral anomalies were found in several cases, varying from 43% with MRI to 31% with PET or SPECT in Westbury's review [20,23].

The opposite pattern, with right side damage, is reported in left-handed patients by Mesulam [12] and Drezga [5].

Up to date and excluding our observation, only one case of right-handed subject showing right hypoperfusion at SPECT scan is reported in literature [19].

Table 2
Language assessment (July 2006)

Aachener Aphasie Test				
	Score	PT	Gravity	Performance
Repetition	116/150	51	5	Pathological
Written language	82/90	64	8	Normal
Objects naming	118/120	80	9	Normal
Comprehension	105/120	60	7	Pathological
B.A.D.A		Cut-off		
Non-words repetition	31/35	33		Pathological
Non-words reading	42/45	43		Pathological
Non-words writing	25/25	23		Normal
Oral lexical decision	78/80	78		Borderline
Visual lexical decision	77/80	76		Normal
Words repetition	32/45	43		Pathological
Words reading	77/92	90		Pathological
Words writing	41/46	44		Pathological
Oral objects comprehension	39/40	38		Normal
Visual objects comprehension	40/40	38		Normal
Oral verbs comprehension	19/20	18		Normal
Visual verbs comprehension	18/20	18		Borderline
Oral objects naming	29/30	28		Normal
Oral verbs naming	25/28	26		Pathological
Written objects naming	22/22	20		Normal
Written verbs naming	17/22	20		Pathological
Naming based in definition	15/16	14		Normal
Oral morphosyntactic comprehension	44/48	46		Pathological
Visual morphosyntactic comprehension	17/24	22		Pathological
Sentences repetition	12/20	18		Pathological
Oral syntactic comprehension	55/60	58		Pathological
Visual syntactic comprehension	38/45	43		Pathological

In this paper authors described a 65-years woman who presented gradual decrease in fluency with intact cognitive functions: her brain SPECT revealed ^{99m}Tc-HMPAO uptake reduction into the right frontal, perisylvian and temporal lobe regions.

This unusual finding is explained by authors referring to the hypothesis that women brain has greater bilateral representations of language. This is not true for our male patient.

Our data show that NfPPA may arise not only from cortical abnormalities in the language-dominant left hemisphere but also from right hemisphere involvement: this observation could be explained also referring to the hypothesis of crossed aphasia. Recently, Mariën et al. [10], reviewing a corpus of 152 case reports of CAD following cerebrovascular lesions, proposed a set of criteria allowing a classification of CAD into unreliable, possible and reliable.

If we extend these criteria to other possible etiologies (i.e. neurodegenerative disease), we can find that G.G. could be classified as "reliable CAD": in fact he met all the five points requested to assign this label (evidence of aphasia; evidence of natural right handedness; lesions restricted to right hemisphere; absence of familial left

handedness and no history of early brain damage or seizures).

In conclusion, G.G.' cognitive profile seems comparable with a clinical picture of NfPPA, with the peculiarity of right-hemisphere involvement suggesting the presence of CAD.

References

[1] A.L. Benton, A.B. Sivan, K.d. Hamsher et al., *Contribution to neuropsychological assessment*. A clinical manual, Oxford University Press, New York, 1994.

[2] B. Bramwell, On "crossed" aphasia and the factors wich go to determine whether the "leading" or "driving"speech-centers shall be located in the left or right hemisphere of the brain, with notes on a case of "crossed" aphasia (aphasia with right-sided hemiplegia in a left handed man), *Lancet* (1899), 1473–1479.

[3] G.G. Briggs and R.D. Nebes, Patterns of hand preference in a student population, *Cortex* **3** (1975), 230–238.

[4] E. De Renzi, F. Motti and P. Nichelli, Imitating gestures. A quantitative approach to ideomotor apraxia, *Arch Neurol* **1** (1980), 6–10.

[5] A. Drzezga, T. Grimmer, H. Siebner, S. Minoshima, M. Schwaiger and A. Kurz, Prominent hypometabolism of the right temporoparietal and frontal cortex in two left-handed patients with primary progressive aphasia, *J Neurol* **9** (2002), 1263–1267.

[6] M.F. Folstein, S.E. Folstein and P.R. McHugh, "Mini-mental state". A practical method for grading the cognitive state of patients for the clinician, *J Psychiatr Res* **3** (1975), 189–198.

[7] M.L. Gorno-Tempini, N.F. Dronkers, K.P. Rankin, J.M. Ogar, L. Phengrasamy, H.J. Rosen, J.K. Johnson, M.W. Weiner and B.L. Miller, Cognition and anatomy in three variants of primary progressive aphasia, *Ann Neurol* **3** (2004), 335–346.

[8] T.A. Krefft, N.R. Graff-Radford, D.W. Dickson, M. Baker and R.J. Castellani, Familial primary progressive aphasia, *Alzheimer Dis Assoc Disord* **2** (2003), 106–112.

[9] C. Luzzatti, K. Willmes and R. De Bleser, *Aachener Aphasie-Test,* Versione Italiana, Organizzazioni Speciali, Firenze, 1992.

[10] P. Marien, B. Paghera, P.P. De Deyn and L.A. Vignolo, Adult crossed aphasia in dextrals revisited, *Cortex* **1** (2004), 41–74.

[11] C. McMillan, J. Gee, P. Moore, K. Dennis, C. DeVita and M. Grossman, Confrontation naming and morphometric analyses of structural MRI in frontotemporal dementia, *Dement Geriatr Cogn Disord* **4** (2004), 320–323.

[12] M. Mesulam, S. Weintraub, T. Parrish and D. Gitelman, Primary progressive aphasia: reversed asymmetry of atrophy and right hemisphere language dominance, *Neurology* **3** (2005), 556–557.

[13] M.M. Mesulam, Slowly progressive aphasia without generalized dementia, *Ann Neurol* **6** (1982), 592–598.

[14] M.M. Mesulam, Primary progressive aphasia, *Ann Neurol* **4** (2001), 425–432.

[15] G. Miceli, A. Laudanna, C. Burani and R. Capasso, Batteria per l'Analisi dei Deficit Afasici B.A.D.A., CEPSAG Università Cattolica del Sacro Cuore, Roma, Italy, 1994.

[16] D. Neary, J.S. Snowden, L. Gustafson, U. Passant, D. Stuss, S. Black, M. Freedman, A. Kertesz, P.H. Robert, M. Albert, K. Boone, B.L. Miller, J. Cummings and D.F. Benson, Frontotemporal lobar degeneration: a consensus on clinical diagnostic criteria, *Neurology* **6** (1998), 1546–1554.

[17] P.J. Nestor, N.L. Graham, T.D. Fryer, G.B. Williams, K. Patterson and J.R. Hodges, Progressive non-fluent aphasia is associated with hypometabolism centred on the left anterior insula, *Brain* **Pt 11** (2003), 2406–2418.

[18] G. Novelli, C. Papagno, E. Capitani, M. Laiacona, S.F. Cappa and G. Vallar, Tre test clinici di memoria a lungo termine. Taratura su soggetti normali, *Archivio di Psicologia Neurologia e Psichiatria* **2** (1986), 278–296.

[19] E.C. San Pedro, G. Deutsch, H.G. Liu and J.M. Mountz, Frontotemporal decreases in rCBF correlate with degree of dysnomia in primary progressive aphasia, *J Nucl Med* **2** (2000), 228–233.

[20] M.H. Soriani-Lefevre, D. Hannequin, S. Bakchine, J.F. Menard, A. Manrique, A. Hitzel, P.O. Kotzki, V. Boudousq and P. Vera, Evidence of bilateral temporal lobe involvement in primary progressive aphasia: a SPECT study, *J Nucl Med* **7** (2003), 1013–1022.

[21] H. Spinnler and P. Tognoni, Standardizzazione eTaratura Italiana di Test Neuropsicologici, *The Italian Journal of Neurological Sciences* (1987), 8–119.

[22] E.K. Warrington and M. James, *Visual Object and Space Perception Battery,* Thames Valley Test, Bury St. Edmunds, UK, 1991.

[23] C. Westbury and D. Bub, Primary progressive aphasia: a review of 112 cases, *Brain Lang* **3** (1997), 381–406.

9

Spelling intervention in post-stroke aphasia and primary progressive aphasia

Kyrana Tsapkini[a],* and Argye E. Hillis[a,b,c]

[a]*Departments of Neurology, Johns Hopkins Medicine, Baltimore, MD, USA*
[b]*Physical Medicine and Rehabilitation, Johns Hopkins Medicine, Baltimore, MD, USA*
[c]*Department of Cognitive Science, Johns Hopkins University, Baltimore, MD, USA*

Abstract. Spelling – a core language skill – is commonly affected in neurological diseases such as stroke and Primary Progressive Aphasia (PPA). We present two case studies of the same spelling therapy (learning of phoneme-to-grapheme correspondences with help from key words) in two participants: one who had a stroke and one with PPA (logopenic variant). Our study highlights similarities and differences in the time course of each indivdual's therapy. The study evaluates the effectiveness and generalization of treatment in each case, i.e. whether the treatment affected the trained items and/or untrained items, and whether or not the treatment gains were maintained after the end of therapy. Both participants were able to learn associations between phonemes and graphemes as well as between phonemes and words. Reliable generalization to untrained words was shown only for the participant with post-stroke aphasia, but we were not able to test generalization to untrained words in the individual with PPA. The same spelling therapy followed a different time course in each case. The participant with post-stroke aphasia showed a lasting effect of improved spelling, but we were unable to assess maintenance of improvement in the participant with PPA. We discuss these differences in light of the underlying nature of each disease.

Keywords: Spelling, intervention, PPA, stroke, post-stroke aphasia

1. Introduction

Primary Progressive Aphasia (PPA) is a neurodegenerative disease characterized by language impairment at its onset. Although other cognitive functions are affected in the course of PPA, language deficits remain the most characteristic and frequent symptom. Furthermore, it has been shown that spelling is one of the earliest affected language skills [1]. There is currently no available pharmacological treatment for these patients; however, a few studies document behavioral interventions, mostly of naming [2-5,5-12) and only one of spelling [13]. Several variants of PPA have recently been identified: logopenic, semantic, and nonfluent/agrammatic [14]. These are associated with dis-tinct brain pathologies and different regions of brain atrophy. Different variants of PPA show atrophy in brain areas associated with performance in distinct language tasks such as grammatical processing, semantic processing, and fluency [15,16]. However, the unique features (language characteristics and areas of atrophy) that differentiate PPA variants at early-to-middle stages tend to lose their distinctiveness later on [16]. Many patients become nonverbal, but may retain some ability to write and type. Because they may depend on writing to communicate, recognizable spelling is crucial for basic communication. As for all people in today's society, use of e-mail, computers, and other texting that depends on spelling is crucial for basic activities. Spelling is not only one of the first language functions affected in all three variants of PPA but also has prognostic value for the evolution of the disease. Different variants of PPA have distinct spelling deficits. A recent study from our laboratory has identified early spelling patterns that predict the variant of PPA into which the patient is like-

*Corresponding author: Kyrana Tsapkini, PhD, Department of Neurology, Johns Hopkins Medical Institutions, 600 N. Wolfe Street, Meyer 6-113, Baltimore, MD 21237, USA.
E-mail: tsapkini@jhmi.edu.

ly to evolve, when only naming and spelling are affected (such that the patient does not yet meet criteria for any one variant). Our study further determined which cognitive processes underlying spelling are affected in each of the PPA variants [1,17].

In brief, there are three main cognitive processes involved in spelling of familiar words to dictation: recognition of the spoken word (access to the stored phonological representation of the word), access to the meaning of the word (access to the lexical-semantic representation of the word) and access to the correct spelling of the word (the stored orthographic lexical representation). In the case of unfamiliar words or pseudowords (non-existing, word-like utterances), the mechanism recruited is a sublexical letter-to-sound conversion (phoneme-to-grapheme correspondence mechanism). Spelling of all words and nonwords requires temporary storage of the sequence of letters in working memory–a storage system called the 'graphemic buffer' – while the individual letters are being written or spelled out loud. All of these mechanisms have been described in a series of case studies mainly of stroke patients [18–26].

In stroke and PPA any of these mechanisms (as well as combinations of them) may be disrupted, and therapeutic interventions have been shown to improve patients' communication. One of the most affected spelling processes in stroke is the phoneme-to-grapheme (PG) conversion mechanism: the mechanism that applies letter-sound associations during spelling and provides a way to write unfamiliar words. Successful remediation for this mechanism as described in relevant cognitive neuropsychological models has been shown to have beneficial effects for patients post-stroke [27–29]. Few studies treat spelling disorders and in particular treat the PG mechanism. Possible reasons include; (a) most literate subjects write lexically by directly accessing the orthographic lexicon, and (b) the PG mechanism is more useful in languages with transparent orthographies – one-to-one PG correspondences, like Italian but not English. Luzzatti et al. [29] include a comprehensive list of all studies treating the sublexical level [27,30–32] in spelling, but the results lack homogeneity, ranging from no effects to improvement involving either treated-only or both treated and untreated items. We review three studies using treatment of the PG conversion mechanism with generalizable and sustainable results [27–29]. Hillis [27] first used this approach to remediate spelling in a stroke patient who was not able to spell unfamiliar words or syllables to dictation. The patient was mute and was taught

PG conversion in order to use to text-to-speech synthesizer. She learned correspondence between phonemes and graphemes using a cuing hierarchy involving key words and maintained this system 12 months after the end of treatment. She could successfully spell monosyllabic words, but for longer words or sentences she relied on her impaired system of orthographic access resulting in frequent semantic errors. Luzzatti et al. [29] described the rehabilitation of dysgraphia in two Italian patients after stroke. Emphasis was given to phonological analysis of the auditory string to be written. After treatment, patients could spell at normal levels on most subsets of therapy items as well as in spontaneous writing and written naming tasks. Therapy gains were maintained 6-18 months post-treatment. Greenwald [28] documented treatment of severe global agraphia after stroke. Spelling performance on both regular and irregular words improved after treatment of sublexical spelling (PG conversion rules); however, regular words improved more than irregular words. With treatment, the patient's global agraphia evolved to surface dysgraphia but follow-up results were not mentioned.

There are few treatment studies in PPA [33] and these studies have focused on treatment of word retrieval with encouraging results for trained items, primarily in the semantic variant of PPA [4–7,11]. There are also a few studies of word retrieval treatment in non-fluent/agrammatic variant PPA [7–10], with no evidence of lasting effects. The logopenic variant of PPA (lvPPA) has received minimal attention. Only a few studies have documented treatment of language functions in lvPPA: two studies with naming interventions [2,3] and one with a spelling intervention [13]. In PPA, any of the aforementioned spelling mechanisms may be disrupted [1]. Phoneme-to-grapheme conversion (PGC), for example, has been shown to be disrupted mostly in patients with the logopenic variant PPA and nonfluent variant PPA, and spared in patients with semantic variant PPA. In general, there is a remarkable paucity of studies of spelling and even more so of treatment of spelling deficits in PPA.

We are aware of only one study of a spelling intervention in PPA. Rapp and Glucroft [13] documented a lexical (word-level) spelling intervention for a PPA patient (logopenic variant, although not mentioned explicitly), which examined the effectiveness of a non-intensive spelling therapy using a spell-study-spell procedure. They found that a spelling intervention can provide immediate and short-term benefits for dysgraphia in PPA, without, however, generalization to untrained items. Also, at 12 month follow-up, all word sets (trained, repeated, homework, and control) had declined even in comparison to pre-intervention baseline.

In our study we provided spelling therapy to an individual with logopenic variant PPA and compared results to results of the same therapy provided to an individual with post-stroke aphasia. Both participants experienced difficulties with spelling (dysgraphia) and in particular with PGC. Consistent with the severity of his initial aphasia, the one who had post-stroke aphasia had extensive left hemisphere damage. As far as we know, this is the first time such a therapy has been used in PPA. The aims of the present study were to: (1) report on the effectiveness of spelling therapy using letter-to-sound associations (PGC) in PPA; (2) directly compare the effectiveness of the spelling therapy used between PPA and severe damage from chronic stroke; (3) consider the similarities and differences in the course and pattern of spelling therapy results between the two types of dysgraphias (acquired, recovering vs. progressive) to evaluate possible compensatory mechanisms that could be recruited in each case.

2. Methods

2.1. Participants

WCR, was a 62-year-old right-handed man, with an MA in history who presented with a large, left-sided, middle-cerebral artery stroke 3 years before testing. The stroke affected most of left hemisphere, sparing only occipito-temporal and medial frontal areas but not sparing their connections to lateral frontal and parietal areas. Initial MRI revealed a large, left middle cerebral artery stroke and an incidental finding of a completely occluded right carotid artery. Initially, he was globally aphasic, but had improved mainly through rehabilitation and probably physiological reinstitution at least in the first year. Three years post-stroke, WCR lived independently, taking care of his own bills, and all of his own needs. His aphasia type was unclassifiable; he was classified by the Western Aphasia Battery (WAB) as anomic [34], but he had "asyntactic" auditory comprehension on sentence comprehension tasks. He was administered the WAB and supplemental tests of sentence comprehension and working memory (see Table 1). His scores in a sentence-picture matching task were at 85% correct for active sentences, 80% for passive, 65% for cleft subject (e.g., "It was the man that kicked the girl."), 55% for cleft object (e.g.,"It was the niece that the father kicked.), 48% for semantically

reversible (e.g., "The dog chased the boy."), and 95% for irreversible sentences (e.g., "The girl kicked the ball."). In an enactment task (in which he had to enact the sentence with paper dolls), he was 100% correct with active sentences, 35% with passive, 95% with cleft subject, 50% with cleft object, 55% with reversible and 90% with irreversible sentences. Notable sub-scores on the WAB (see Table 1 for a summary of results) are: 90% correct in sentence repetition, 100% correct in object naming, 100% correct in sentence completion and 100% correct in responsive speech (naming to definition). His spontaneous speech was generally fluent and well articulated, but he had hesitations for word finding and frequent circumlocutions. He followed and participated in conversations without difficulty.

FSE, was a 62-year-old right-handed woman with a BA degree who was an elementary teacher but retired 10 years before testing. Six years before treatment she started having difficulties forming sentences and finding words. She was first diagnosed with logopenic variant PPA three years prior to therapy on the basis of history, neurological examination, imaging, and neurocognitive assessment completed at Johns Hopkins. When she first presented, her speech was fluent and well-articulated but with frequent hesitations for word finding and many circumlocutions. MRI showed left greater than right temporoparietal atrophy. During the course of the disease her speech became full of stereotypic phrases and hesitations for word finding. She had difficulty formulating and repeating sentences. She could repeat the partial meaning of sentences but not the exact words. She made phonemic and semantic paraphasias. Her performance on the WAB and other neuropsychological tests is summarized in Table 1.

2.1.1. Spelling impairments of the two participants

WCR: The participant was tested before intervention on Johns Hopkins Dysgraphia Battery when he presented to the clinic, 3 years post-stroke. As shown in Table 2, his performance on words and pseudowords was very impaired (11% accurate on words and 0% on nonwords). The following information refers to his performance on words: Nouns were somewhat better preserved than verbs, but the difference was not significant (21% vs. 7% accurate). There was not a significant concreteness effect, although abstract words were slightly less accurate than concrete words (5% vs. 19% accuracy on abstract vs. concrete words). He did not show any frequency or regularity effect either (22% and 19% accurate on high vs. low frequency words and 33% vs. 36% on high vs. low regularity words).

Table 1

Performance of patients WCR and FSE in the Western Aphasia Battery (WAB) and other neuropsychological tests

Tests from the WAB	WCR (8/14/2009)	FSE (6/10/2009)
Overall aphasia quotient:	85	68
Aphasia type:	anomic (but asyntactic)	conduction
Spontaneous speech total:	15/20, 75% Correct	15/20, 75% Correct
– Information content:	10/10, 100% Correct	10/10, 100% Correct
– Fluency, grammatical competence:	5/10, 50% Correct	5/10, 50% Correct
Auditory verbal comprehension	86% correct	88% correct
– Yes/no questions:	54/60, 90% Correct	51/60, 85% Correct
– Auditory word recognition:	55/60, 92% correct	60/60, 100% correct
– Sequential commands:	60/80, 75% correct	64/80, 80% correct
Repetition total:	90/100, 90% correct	56/100, 56% correct
Naming and word finding		
– Object naming:	60/60, 100% correct	27/60, 45% correct
– Word fluency:	8/20, 40th percentile	3/20, 15th percentile
– Sentence completion:	10/10, 100% correct	8/10, 80% correct
Responsive speech:	10/10, 100% correct	8/10, 80% correct
Trail Making Test	Part A: 128 sec	Part A: 42,
	Part B: not completed	Part B: 16
Digit Span	Forward: 4	Forward: 3
	Backward: 3	Backward: 2
Word Span	Forward: 3	Forward: 2
	Backward: 2	Backward: 2

He only showed a significant word-length effect (43% correct on 4-letter vs. 7% on 5-letter vs. 14% on 6-letter vs. 7% on 7-letter and 0% on 8-letter words correct). His errors were mostly phonologically implausible nonwords (e,g., child -> chies; strange -> staging; happen -> happist; brother -> browets). WCR had a pronounced length effect that characterizes patients with impairment at the level of graphemic buffer, a working memory system that temporarily holds information about identity and sequence of letters while the word and nonword is written. In combination with his 0% accuracy on nonwords, his pattern of performance was congruent with impairments both at the level of the graphemic buffer and at the level of sublexical mechanisms for phoneme-grapheme conversion. We decided to treat his sublexical route – the phoneme-grapheme conversion mechanism – as a first step, to give him some rules he could rely on to transcribe from the auditory to the written word. Treatment of the graphemic buffer impairment was planned at a later stage.

FSE: Before treatment, on the Johns Hopkins Dysgraphia Battery, FSE spelled words and pseudowords with approximately equal accuracy (65.5 vs. 61.8% accuracy). The following information refers to her performance on words: There was no effect of grammatical class (68% correct in nouns and verbs, 61% in adjectives and 65% in function words). She did, however, show a concreteness effect (90.5% correct for concrete and 52% for abstract words). There was also a significant frequency effect (88% correct for high frequency words and 72% for low frequency ones). There was no significant difference between high/low regularity words (80.0 vs. 83.8% correct). There was no significant effect of word length; she correctly spelled 85.7% of 4-letter vs. 92.9% of 8-letter words (ns different by chi square). Only 15.2% of her errors were phonologically plausible errors (rooster-> rouster; pigeon-> picheon). Most of her errors were phonologically similar word errors (bright-> bride, brick; chain-> chant) or mixed phonological and semantically similar words including morphological errors (absence-> absent; speak-> speech; begin-> begun; jury-> juror). These types of errors have been proposed to occur as a result of an interaction between information from the semantic system and partial information from the impaired phoneme-to-grapheme conversion (PGC) mechanism, which each access lexical representations semantically or phonologically related to the target. According to this "summation hypothesis", lexical representations that are both semantically and phonologically related to the target will be activated nearly as much as the target is activated. When the target lexical orthographic representation is unavailable (due to damage at that level), the semantically and phonologically related representation might be activated for output instead [35]. Thus, we hypothesized that FSE was impaired both (1) in accessing orthographic lexical representations for output, and (2) in phoneme-to-grapheme conversion (PGC). We decided to treat the latter mechanism, as improvement might also improve access to orthographic lexical representations.

2.2. Treatment

For the spelling therapy, 30 English sounds were selected representing most common word-initial English phonemes (speech sounds) and were divided into 3 sets using a counterbalanced design with respect to the frequency of the initial phoneme. Then a set of 30 English words starting with these sounds were selected to be used as prompts to help the patients relate each sound to a grapheme (abstract letter identity or sequence of letter identities). The sequence of events in the therapy sessions was as follows: The participant was asked to write the letter or combination of letters corresponding to a particular phoneme, e.g., 'sh'. If the participant was correct, then s/he was reinforced, and asked to write a word that starts with this sound. However, if the participant could not write the correct letter, s/he was asked to think of a word that starts with this sound or, if needed, was provided with such a word (prompt); then s/he was asked to write the word and then instructed explicitly to associate that particular phoneme to the particular word and initial grapheme. Each session consisted of teaching the correct phoneme-grapheme correspondence of 10 initial word phonemes using 10 common English words. When the patient reached criterion for two consecutive sessions and a minimum of 3 sessions per set (80% correct, i.e., 8/10 of phoneme-grapheme or phoneme-word correspondences) for each set, s/he would continue to the second set and then to the third set. For each set, trial accuracy and response times for the letter and the word responses were recorded. The 3 sets were matched for several linguistic variables so that they were equivalent in difficulty. Baseline evaluation before each therapy session required that the participant would choose – from a series of possible initial letters or letter sequences of English (30 choices) written in front of him or her – the letter, or letter sequence, that corresponded to the phoneme the examiner provided each time. The same measurement was used as an independent evaluation of the therapeutic outcome after therapy. Participants received approximately one therapy session per week, with the duration of one to two hours each. Both liked to talk quite a bit during the session, accounting for the variability in the duration of the sessions.

2.3. Assessment

Follow-up assessment probed all three sets of trained phoneme-grapheme and phoneme-word correspondences to identify whether or not the participant had retained knowledge of the trained items. We also looked at generalization effects, that is, effects of training to untrained items. We trained all possible initial phoneme-grapheme correspondences of English in 3 sets (30 items), and compared trained to untrained items directly. Differences in baseline measures in pre- and post-therapy accuracy for phoneme-grapheme correspondences for each participant were evaluated using chi-square or Fisher's exact tests. We also compared the improvement of each participant in trained items using a chi-square test to evaluate whether either of them improved more than the other. Additionally, we evaluated pre- and post-therapy accuracy for graphemes and for words for the trained items for each participant using Fisher's exact tests. Finally, we did follow-up assessments when possible (for WCR only).

3. Results

Both participants completed all three sets of 10 phoneme-grapheme correspondences that comprised the spelling therapy; that is, they were able to learn the new associations and benefit from the intervention. However, each of them showed a different pattern of performance in the course of training. First, they completed the training in different lengths of time. WCR, the one with post-stroke aphasia, completed the training in 25 sessions; FSE, the one with PPA completed the training in 11 sessions. Furthermore, they showed a different pattern in learning of phoneme-grapheme and phoneme-word associations. Results are presented below in detail.

1. We first addressed the question of whether the participants showed generalization of treatment by comparing the percentage of trained vs. untrained items before and after the first set of the therapeutic intervention. Given that there are only 30 initial phoneme-grapheme correspondences in English and we trained 10 of them in each set we looked for generalization to untrained items before and after the first set. We used chi-square or Fisher's exact test to evaluate whether there was significant improvement in phoneme-grapheme correspondence (see Figs 1a and 1b for results in each set). We also evaluated generalization of treatment to other

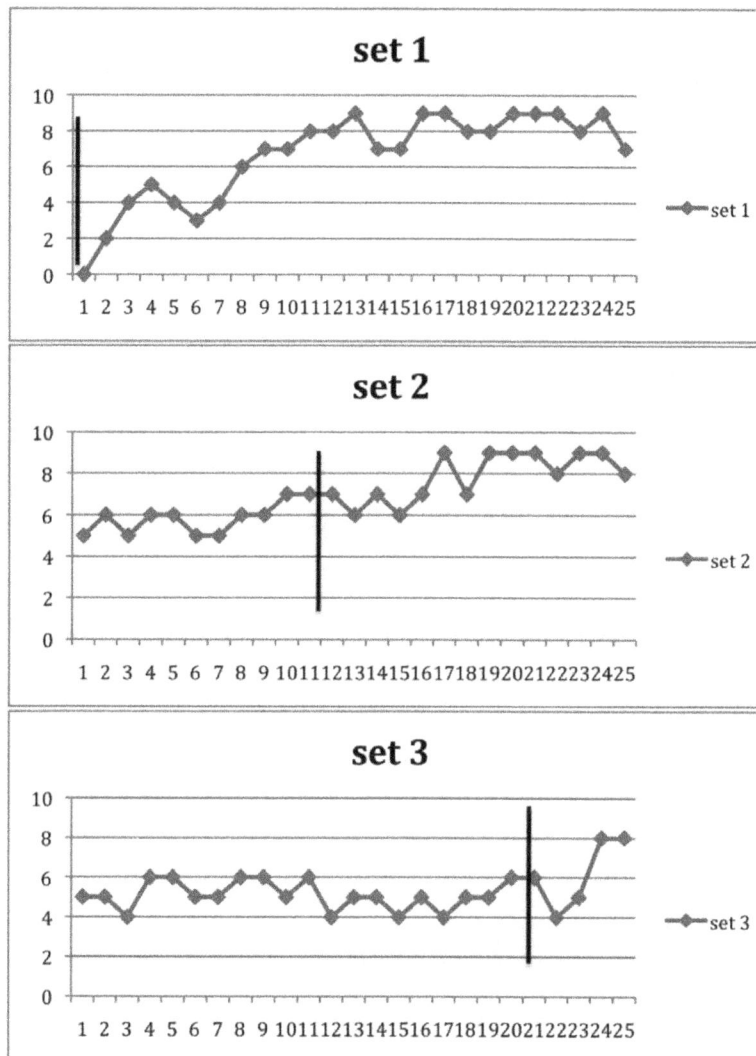

Fig. 1a. Effect of training in trained and untrained items of all 3 sets for patient FSE. Each dot corresponds to correct items per session for letter-phoneme correspondences. Horizontal axis corresponds to the number of therapy sessions and vertical axis corresponds to the level of success (out of 10 items per set). Vertical bars show when training began for each set.

spelling tasks before and after treatment (spelling to dictation, pointing to named letters) for WCR.

For FSE, we found that there was not a significant difference in the trained or untrained phoneme-grapheme correspondences between the beginning and the end of set 1 because she was not severely impaired at baseline: (Fisher's exact for trained: $p = 0.3$; Fisher's exact for untrained: $p = 1$). However, she improved with each set as it was trained (Fig. 1a). Also, there was an almost significant difference between the trained phoneme-word associations (Fisher's exact: $p = 0.057$, see Fig. 2). Therefore, in the first set she showed no significant improvement in trained items nor generalization to untrained items in phoneme-grapheme correspondences but she did show an improvement in her phoneme-word correspondences. Furthermore she reached criterion more

quickly for the consecutive training sets indicating that there had been at least some overall generalization to untrained phonemes. Unfortunately it was not possible to test her thoroughly post-intervention in spelling of unpracticed words and nonwords – such as the ones included in the JHU Dysgraphia battery – in order to demonstrate functional generalization. Generalization to other untrained tasks such as pointing to named letters, was, however, demonstrated by a significant improvement in her performance before and after intervention (Fisher's exact $p = 0.021$).

For stroke patient WCR there was a significant difference in trained but not in untrained phoneme-grapheme correspondences after the first set (Fisher's exact for trained: $p = 0.0007$; Fisher's exact for untrained: $p = 0.65$). Therefore, in the first set he showed no generalization to untrained phonemes. There was also no

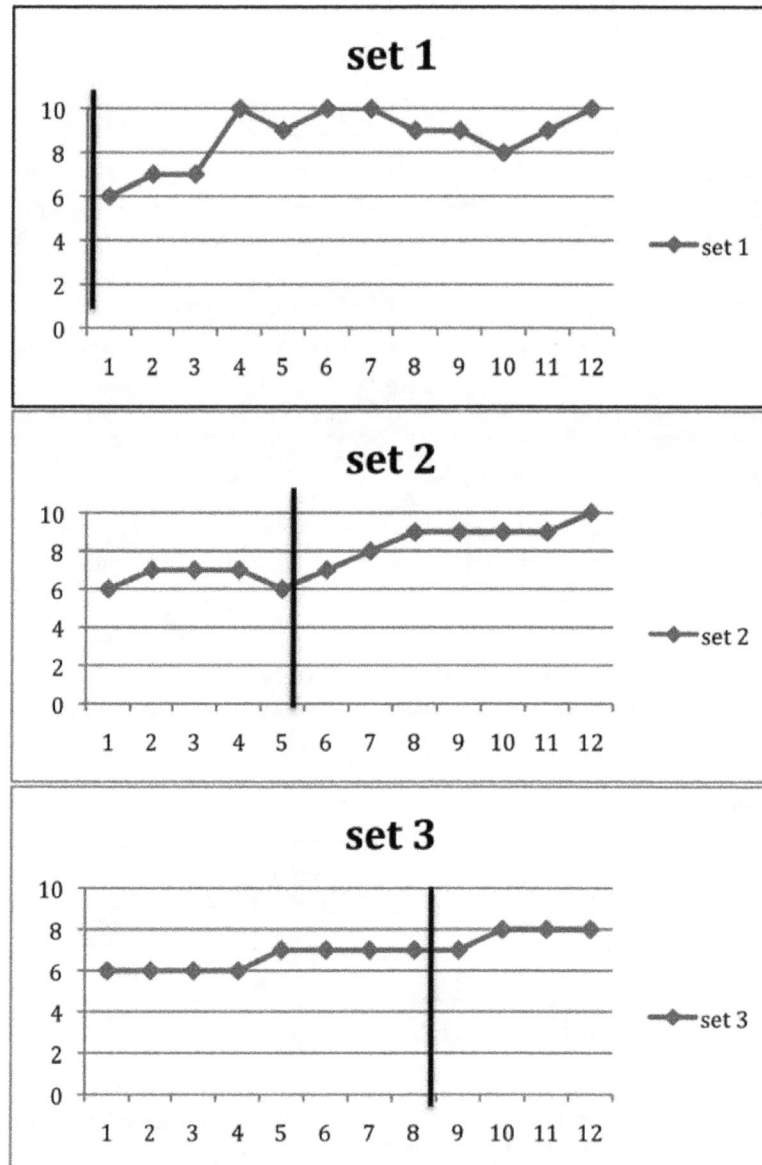

Fig. 1b. Effect of training in trained and untrained items of all 3 sets for patient WCR. Each dot corresponds to correct items per session for letter-phoneme correspondences. Horizontal axis corresponds to the number of therapy sessions and vertical axis corresponds to the level of success (out of 10 items per set). Vertical bars show when training began for each set.

difference between the trained phoneme-word associations before and after the first set (Fisher's exact: $p = 0.17$). WCR, like FSE, also reached criterion more quickly for each successive test suggesting that he generalized his new skill to untrained items (Figure 1b). However, generalization to untrained items and tasks was demonstrated by dramatically increased accuracy of spelling words to dictation in the JHU Dysgraphia battery (see Table 2) as well as pointing to named letters (chi-square $(1, N = 60) = 7$, $p < 0.001$). For example, WCR's performance in open class words improved significantly from 11 to 27% (chi-square $(1, N = 168) = 6.5$, $p < 0.01$). Pertinent to the therapy, his spelling of high probability words (words with reg-

ular phoneme-to-grapheme correspondence) improved significantly from 33 to 73% (chi-square $(1, N = 60) = 8.1$, $p < 0.001$); whereas his spelling of low probability (words with irregular phoneme-to-grapheme correspondence) improved, but not significantly (from 36 to 49%, chi-square $(1, N = 80) = 2.1$, $p < 0.1$, ns). His performance in nonwords included in the JHU battery did not improve significantly. A possible reason is that these nonwords are more than 4-letter, usually 2-syllable pronounceable nonwords that can be spelled with a minimum of 5–7 letters. This presented a further problem for WCR who also had a graphemic buffer impairment as manifested in the difference of his performance between 4-letter and longer words (see Table 2);

Table 2
WCR's performance in the JHU battery before and after spelling intervention

JHU Dysgraphia Battery	Before treatment	After treatment
Part of speech		
Open class words	9/84, 11%	23/84, 27%
Nouns	6/28, 21%	12/28, 43%
Verbs	2/28, 7%	5/28, 18%
Adjectives	1/28, 4%	6/28, 21%
Function words	1/20, 5%	1/20, 5%
Nonwords	0/34, 0%	1/34, 3%
Concreteness		
Concrete words	1/21, 5%	8/21, 38%
Abstract words	4/21, 19%	5/21, 24%
Word length		
4-letter	6/14, 43%	10/14, 71%
5-letter	1/14, 7%	3/14, 21%
6-letter	2/14, 14%	4/14, 29%
7-letter	1/14, 7%	1/14, 7%
8-letter	0/14, 0%	0/14, 0%
Probability (PG regularity)		
High probability	10/30, 33%	22/30, 73%
Low probability	29/80, 36%	39/80, 49%
Frequency		
High frequency	32/146, 22%	65/146, 45%
Low frequency	27/146, 19%	46/146, 32%

a difference maintained in the post-treatment evaluation as well. Overall, WCR showed clear indications of generalization of treatment to untrained items.

2. We also wanted to determine whether either of the patients improved more than the other. We compared the degree of improved performance (difference in correct phoneme-grapheme correspondences between the beginning and the end of therapy) for each patient to the utmost potential improvement for each patient: chi-square $(1, N = 51) = 0.003, p > 1$, showing that there was no difference in improvement between the two patients. Another indication that the patients were benefitting from therapy is that both of them reached criterion for the final set in fewer sessions than those of the first. Patient FSE completed the first set in 5 sessions, the second in 3 sessions and the third in 4 sessions. Patient WCR completed the first set in 11 sessions, the second in 9 sessions and the third in 5 sessions. (see Figs 2 and 3 for performance on letters and words in each set).

3. In order to evaluate whether either patient had improved more in any domain, that is, the phoneme-grapheme associations or phoneme-word associations, we also compared the difference between their initial and final performances in phoneme-grapheme and phoneme-word associations. WCR showed a dramatic improvement in phoneme-grapheme associations from 10/30 to 24/30 (chi-square $(1, N = 60) = 7, p < 0.001$) and a significant improvement in phoneme-word asso-

ciations (Fisher's exact $p = 0.02$) (see Fig. 3). FSE did show a significant difference in phoneme-grapheme associations learned in therapy (Fisher's exact $p = 0.021$): her performance improved from 20/30 to 28/30 correct. She also showed an improvement in phoneme-word associations learned in therapy (chi-square $(1, N = 60) = 8.4, p < 0.01$). (see Fig. 3). These results indicate that both participants were helped in both domains.

4. We were able to perform a 6-month follow-up session only for WCR who had post-stroke aphasia. WCR showed good maintenance of learned phoneme-grapheme conversion (see Table 3). Performance was not significantly different from that at the end of training for any measurement; for phoneme-grapheme associations: chi-square $(1, N = 60) = 0, p > 1$; for phoneme-word associations (Fisher's exact $p = 0.33$). Unfortunately, at the time of the scheduled follow-up appointment FSE's condition in other cognitive domains (recognition memory, attention, executive functions) had deteriorated to the point she had to be moved to a nursing home facility for people with dementia and could not be tested.

4. Discussion

We documented two case studies of spelling therapy (training of the phoneme-to-grapheme conversion system) in post-stroke aphasia and PPA. We compared the course and outcomes of therapy in these two participants to determine whether treatment of phoneme-to-grapheme conversion previously applied successfully in post-stroke aphasia [27–29] can be applied in the case of neurodegenerative diseases such as PPA. Only one study in the literature [13] shows that individuals with PPA may benefit from a spelling intervention at the word-level without, however, generalization to unpracticed items. Our study validates alternative approaches. The therapy of these two participants showed similarities but also differences. Both participants learned all three training sets of phoneme-grapheme associations and reached criterion in all of them in fewer sessions, showing that even in a degenerative disease learning is possible when the therapy is targeted. There were indications of possible generalization of treatment to other items and tasks for the PPA participant and reliable generalization to untrained items and tasks for the participant with post-stroke aphasia as shown in spelling to dictation on the JHU Dysgraphia battery and pointing to named letters. The participant with PPA required fewer

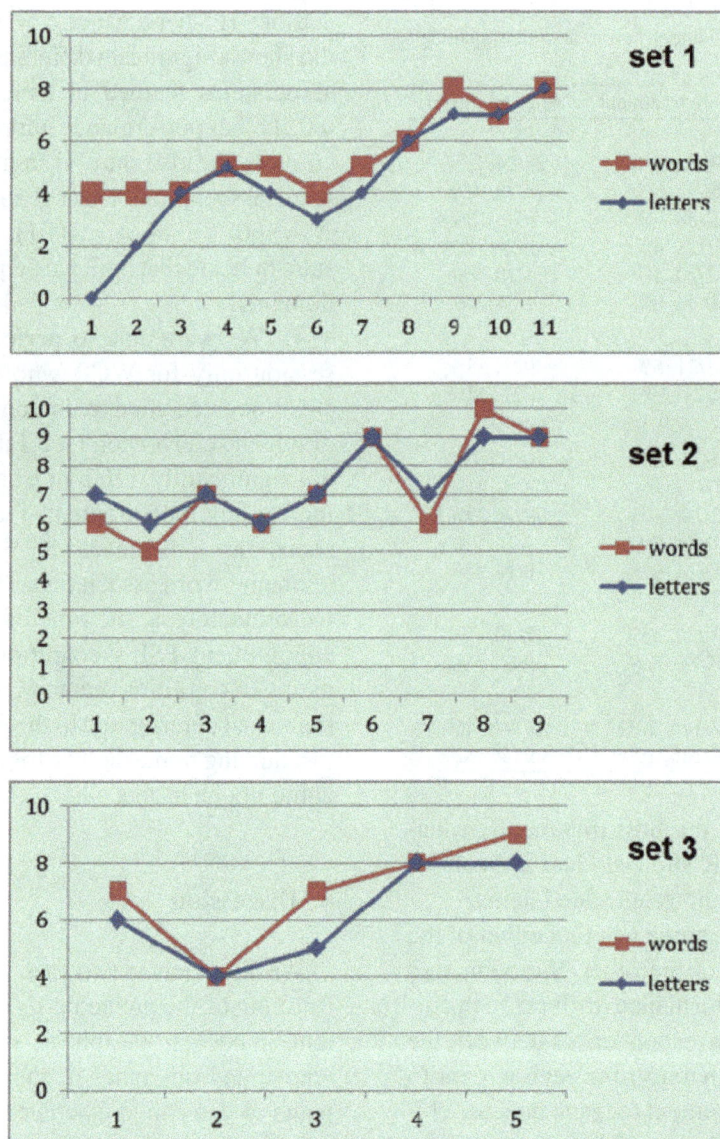

Fig. 2. Effect of training on trained items in each session for letter- and word-sound correspondences for patient FSE. Each dot corresponds to correct items per session for letter- and word- sound correspondences. Consecutive training sets are depicted in consecutive charts (set 1: 5 sessions, set 2: 3 sessions, set 3: 4 sessions).

sessions in consecutive sets and performed significantly better in pointing to named letters at the end of the therapy but functional generalization was not shown since her health did not allow comprehensive evaluation of untrained items at the end of treatment. There was no generalization to untrained phonemes after the first set of trained phonemes in either participant. Moreover, there was no difference in the effectiveness of therapy between the two participants, indicating that individuals with PPA are as trainable as those with stroke. This is a very encouraging result for a degenerative disease such as PPA, as decline can be rapid and dramatic.

Unfortunately, we were not able to evaluate long-term effects of treatment in the PPA patient. Follow-

up is often difficult in treatment studies of patients with neurodegenerative diseases. Other patients with logopenic variant PPA who had treatment of spelling and naming [3,13] had serious cognitive decline that did not allow follow-up investigations of therapy gains. Nevertheless, there is one therapy study of a logopenic PPA patient who received a naming/word retrieval intervention and showed generalization as well as retained therapy gains after 6 months [2]. Our stroke participant (WCR) retained the therapy gains at a 6-month follow-up, but during that time the PPA participant (FSE) had a major decline in her cognitive condition that did not allow further testing, indicating that 6-month follow-up may be a long time for some par-

Table 3
Follow-up evaluation of WCR on letter- and word-sound associations in all 3 trained sets after 6 months

set	letters			words		
	Baseline	End of therapy	Follow-up	Baseline	End of therapy	Follow-up
1	0/10	9/10	8/10	4/10	9/10	8/10
2	5/10	8/10	6/10	6/10	8/10	7/10
3	5/10	7/10	8/10	7/10	9/10	7/10

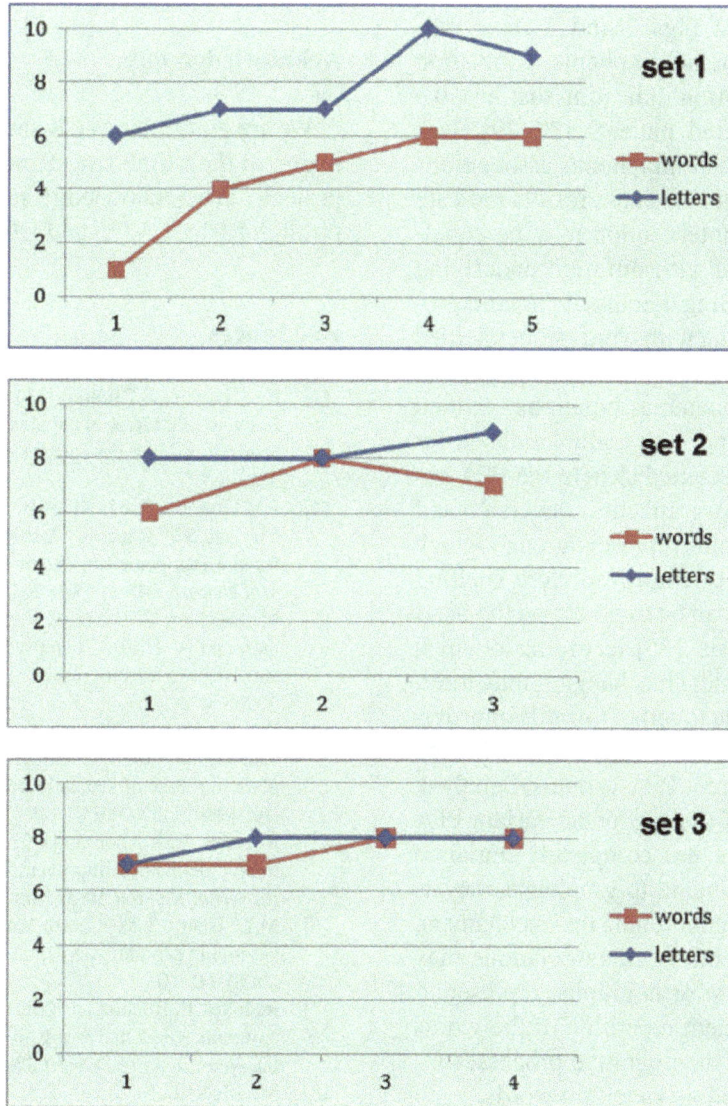

Fig. 3. Effect of training on trained items in each session for letter- and word-sound correspondences for patient WCR. Each dot corresponds to correct items per session for letter- and word- sound correspondences. Consecutive training sets are depicted in consecutive charts (set 1: 11 sessions, set 2: 9 sessions, set 3: 5 sessions).

ticipants with PPA. Therefore, future studies of PPA should consider shorter follow-up periods and perhaps repetition of the therapeutic procedures to improve retention.

The other difference between the two participants was that the one with stroke actually required more sessions to learn phoneme-grapheme associations than the one with PPA. This difference likely had more to

do with differences in the underlying cognitive impairment in spelling than the neurological etiology of the dysgraphia. That is, when the PG mechanism is partially preserved (as in the case of the participant with PPA), training can occur in a shorter period of time. Overall, the response to treatment in PPA was good, despite the fact that she did not show generalization of effects after training the first set of phoneme-grapheme and phoneme-word associations. However, even at that early stage, her trained phoneme-word associations showed a trend toward significant improvement, indicating that the therapeutic intervention improved other functions that were deficient, that is, word finding.

Even though WCR showed no statistically significant improvement in phoneme-word associations, examination of the graphs in Figs 2 and 3 show parallel improvement in phoneme-grapheme association and phoneme-word association indicating that he (like FSE and previously reported patients [27–29]) was also likely learning phoneme-grapheme associations via phoneme-word associations. These results indicate that the same therapeutic intervention may be equally effective for participants with different underlying deficits and etiologies. Spelling therapy of phoneme-to-grapheme conversion training with word-probes helped the participant with post-stroke aphasia strengthen and improve his phoneme-grapheme associations – which was a major weakness, along with a graphemic buffer deficit. The same therapy seemed to help the PPA patient to strengthen phoneme-grapheme conversion and improve access to orthographic representations – which were her major weaknesses. Improved word spelling with improvement in PGC can be expected on the basis of the 'summation hypothesis' [35] according to which lexical-semantic and sublexical mechanisms may interact in synergy and contribute together towards improvement of performance. In the only study that has looked at spelling patterns in different PPA variants, Sepelyak et al. [1] found that half of the logopenic variant PPA patients had a partially but not completely impaired sublexical mechanism (phoneme-to-grapheme conversion mechanism). Thus, strengthening this mechanism, particularly through phoneme-word associations may result in improved access to orthographic representations, perhaps via the frequent repetition of the words or the frequent practice of the cognitive processes involved in retrieving the spelling of taught words.

Improved word spelling by WCR despite his persistent graphemic buffer deficit may be explained by reliance on improved PGC to self-correct phonologically implausible errors in spelling. That is, even though he showed no generalization of training from trained phonemes to untrained phonemes in the first set when learning PGC, at the end of therapy, he clearly showed generalization of improvement in spelling to untrained tasks (word spelling to dictation) by applying PGC to untrained words. He maintained his ability to use PGC to compensate for his graphemic buffer deficit to spell short words six months later.

Although we were not able to follow the PPA participant long-term, it was encouraging that she showed improvement in spelling words despite having a condition in which language is generally declining. The long-term improvement in spelling by WCR, and his ability to apply the learned skill to an untrained task and untrained words, was also very encouraging.

Acknowledgments

We are grateful to WCR and FSE for the generous donation of their time and effort to the completion of this project. We acknowledge support from NIH/NIDCD through R01 DC5375 and DC03681 for this work.

References

[1] K. Sepelyak, J. Crinion, J. Molitoris, Z. Epstein-Peterson, M. Bann, C. Davis et al., Patterns of breakdown in spelling in primary progressive aphasia, *Cortex* **47**(3) (Mar 2011), 342–352.

[2] P.M. Beeson, R.M. King, B. Bonakdarpour, M.L. Henry, H. Cho and S.Z. Rapcsak, Positive effects of language treatment for the logopenic variant of primary progressive aphasia, *J Mol Neurosci* **45**(3) (Nov 2011), 724–736.

[3] M. Newhart, C. Davis, V. Kannan, J. Heidler-Gary, L. Cloutman and A. Hillis, Therapy for naming deficits in two variants of primary progressive aphasia, *Aphasiology* **23** (2009), 823–834.

[4] K.S. Graham, K. Patterson, K.H. Pratt and J.R. Hodges, Relearning and subsequent forgetting of semantic category exemplars in a case of semantic dementia, *Neuropsychology* **13**(3) (Jul 1999), 359–380.

[5] R. Jokel, E. Rochon and C. Leonard, Treating anomia in semantic dementia: improvement, maintenance, or both? *Neuropsychol Rehabil* **16**(3) (Jun 2006), 241–256.

[6] M.L. Henry, P.M. Beeson and S.Z. Rapcsak, Treatment for anomia in semantic dementia, *Semin Speech Lang* **29**(1) (Feb 2008), 60–70.

[7] R. Jokel, E. Rochon and N.D. Anderson, Errorless learning of computer-generated words in a patient with semantic dementia, *Neuropsychol Rehabil* **20**(1) (Jan 2010), 16–41.

[8] M. McNeil, S. Small, R.J. Masterson and T. Fossett, Behavioral and pharmacological treatment of lexical-semantic deficits in a single patient with primary progressive aphasia, *American Journal of Speech-Language Pathology* **4**(4) (1995), 76–87.

[9] S. Schneider, C. Thompson and B. Luring, Effects of verbal plus gestural matrix training on sentence production in a patient with primary progressive aphasia, *Aphasiology* **10**(3) (1996), 297–317.

[10] K. Marcotte and A.I. Ansaldo, The neural correlates of semantic feature analysis in chronic aphasia: discordant patterns according to the etiology, *Semin Speech Lang* **31**(1) (Feb 2010), 52–63.

[11] C.G. Heredia, K. Sage, M.A.L. Ralph and M.L. Berthier, Relearning and retention of verbal labels in a case of semantic dementia, *Aphasiology* **23**(2) (2009), 192–209.

[12] K. Dressel, W. Huber, L. Frings, D. Kümmerer, D. Saur, I. Mader et al., Model-oriented naming therapy in semantic dementia: A single-case fMRI study, *Aphasiology* **24**(12) (2010), 1537–1558.

[13] B. Rapp and B. Glucroft, The benefits and protective effects of behavioral treatment for dysgraphia in a case of primary progressive aphasia, *Aphasiology* **23**(2) (1 Feb 2009), 236–265.

[14] M.L. Gorno-Tempini, A.E. Hillis, S. Weintraub, A. Kertesz, M. Mendez, S.F. Cappa et al., Classification of primary progressive aphasia and its variants, *Neurology* **76**(11) (15 Mar 2011), 1006–1014.

[15] E. Rogalski, D. Cobia, T.M. Harrison, C. Wieneke, C.K. Thompson, S. Weintraub et al., Anatomy of language impairments in primary progressive aphasia, *J Neurosci* **31**(9) (2 Mar 2011), 3344–3350.

[16] E. Rogalski, D. Cobia, T.M. Harrison, C. Wieneke, S. Weintraub and M.M. Mesulam, Progression of language decline and cortical atrophy in subtypes of primary progressive aphasia, *Neurology* **76**(21) (24 May 2011), 1804–1810.

[17] A. Faria, J. Crinion, K. Tsapkini, M. Newhart, C. Davis, S. Cooley et al., Patterns of Dysgraphia in Primary Progressive Aphasia Compared to Post-Stroke Aphasia, *Behavioral Neurology* (in press).

[18] A. Caramazza, G. Miceli, G. Villa and C. Romani, The role of the Graphemic Buffer in spelling: evidence from a case of acquired dysgraphia, *Cognition* **26**(1) (Jun 1987), 59–85.

[19] A.E. Hillis and A. Caramazza, The graphemic buffer and attentional mechanisms, *Brain Lang* **36**(2) (Feb 1989), 208–235.

[20] A.E. Hillis and A. Caramazza, Mechanisms for accessing lexical representations for output: evidence from a category-specific semantic deficit, *Brain Lang* **40**(1) (Jan 1991), 106–144.

[21] J.R. Folk, B. Rapp and M. Goldrick, The interaction of lexical and sublexical information in spelling: What's the point? *Cogn Neuropsychol* **19**(7) (1 Oct 2002), 653–671.

[22] B. Rapp and A. Caramazza, Selective difficulties with spoken nouns and written verbs: A single case study, *Journal of Neurolinguistics* **15**(3) (05//May-Sep 2002), 373–402.

[23] G. Miceli, R. Capasso and A. Caramazza, The interaction of lexical and sublexical processes in reading, writing and repetition, *Neuropsychologia* **32**(3) (Mar 1994), 317–333.

[24] A.E. Hillis and A. Caramazza, Converging evidence for the interaction of semantic and sublexical phonological information in accessing lexical representations for spoken output, *Cognitive Neuropsychology* **12**(2) (1995), 187–227.

[25] K. Patterson, N. Graham and J.R. Hodges, The impact of semantic memory loss on phonological representations, *J Cogn Neurosci* **6**(1) (1994), 57–69.

[26] L. Posteraro, P. Zinelli and A. Mazzucchi, Selective impairment of the graphemic buffer in acquired dysgraphia: A case study, *Brain and Language* **35** (1988), 274–286.

[27] A. Hillis Trupe, Effectiveness of retraining phoneme-to-grapheme conversion, in: *Clinical Aphasiology Conference 1986 Minneapolis: BRK Publishers*, R. Brookshire, ed., 1986, pp. 163–171.

[28] M. Greenwald, Blocking Lexical Competitors in Severe Global Agraphia: A Treatment of Reading and Spelling, *Neurocase* **10**(2) (2004), 156–174.

[29] C. Luzzatti, C. Colombo, M. Frustaci and F. Vitolo, Rehabilitation of spelling along the sub-word-level routine, *Neuropsychological Rehab* **10**(3) (2000), 249–278.

[30] S. Carlomagno and V. Parlato, Writing rehabilitation in brain damaged adult patients: A cognitive approach, *Cognitive Approaches in Neuropsychological Rehabilitation* (1989), 175–209.

[31] S. Carlomagno, A. Iavarone and A. Colombo, Cognitive approaches to writing rehabilitation: From single case to group studies, *Cognitive Neuropsychology and Cognitive Rehabilitation* (1994), 485–502.

[32] A. Caramazza, A. Hillis, E.C. Leek and M. Miozzo, The organization of lexical knowledge in the brain: Evidence from category-and modality-specific deficits, *Mapping the Mind: Domain Specificity in Cognition and Culture* (1994), 68–84.

[33] M.M. Mesulam, Primary progressive aphasia: a 25-year retrospective, *Alzheimer Dis Assoc Disord* **21**(4) (Oct–Dec 2007), S8–S11.

[34] A. Kertesz, Western aphasia battery test manual, *Psychological Corp*, 1982.

[35] A.E. Hillis, B.C. Rapp and A. Caramazza, When a rose is a rose in speech but a tulip in writing, *Cortex* **35**(3) (Jun 1999), 337–356.

[36] Edmonds LA, Kiran S. Effect of semantic naming treatment on crosslinguistic generalization in bilingual aphasia. Journal of Speech, Language, and Hearing Research 2006; 49(4): 729.

[37] Thompson C, Shapiro L. Treating agrammatic aphasia within a linguistic framework: Treatment of Underlying Forms. Aphasiology 2005; 19(10–11): 1021-1036.

10

Degenerative jargon aphasia: Unusual progression of logopenic/phonological progressive aphasia?

Paolo Caffarra[a,b,*], Simona Gardini[a], Stefano Cappa[c], Francesca Dieci[b], Letizia Concari[a], Federica Barocco[a], Caterina Ghetti[d], Livia Ruffini[e] and Guido Dalla Rosa Prati[f]

[a]Department of Neuroscience, University of Parma, Parma, Italy
[b]Outpatient Clinic for the Diagnosis and Therapy of Cognitive Disorders, AUSL, Parma, Italy
[c]Department of Clinical Neuroscience, Vita-Salute San Raffaele Hospital, Milan, Italy
[d]Medical Physic Department, Azienda Ospedaliero-Universitaria, Parma, Italy
[e]Department of Nuclear Medicine, Azienda Ospedaliero-Universitaria, Parma, Italy
[f]Poliambulatorio Dalla Rosa Prati, Centro Diagnostico Europeo, Parma, Italy

Abstract. Primary progressive aphasia (PPA) corresponds to the gradual degeneration of language which can occur as nonfluent/agrammatic PPA, semantic variant PPA or logopenic variant PPA. We describe the clinical evolution of a patient with PPA presenting jargon aphasia as a late feature. At the onset of the disease (ten years ago) the patient showed anomia and executive deficits, followed later on by phonemic paraphasias and neologisms, deficits in verbal short-term memory, naming, verbal and semantic fluency. At recent follow-up the patient developed an unintelligible jargon with both semantic and neologistic errors, as well as with severe deficit of comprehension which precluded any further neuropsychological assessment. Compared to healthy controls, FDG-PET showed a hypometabolism in the left angular and middle temporal gyri, precuneus, caudate, posterior cingulate, middle frontal gyrus, and bilaterally in the superior temporal and inferior frontal gyri. The clinical and neuroimaging profile seems to support the hypothesis that the patient developed a late feature of logopenic variant PPA characterized by jargonaphasia and associated with superior temporal and parietal dysfunction.

Keywords: Primary progressive aphasia, logopenic aphasia, language, jargon

1. Introduction

Progressive language disorders without generalized dementia are defined primary progressive aphasia (PPA) [1]. PPA is usually associated with the degeneration of the language dominant network and the dysfunctional pattern shown with neuroimaging includes mainly left fronto-temporal and parietal regions [2].

Patients with PPA are commonly classified as having nonfluent or fluent speech production. Nonfluent speech output or nonfluent/agrammatic PPA may include or not apraxia of speech, while fluent output corresponds to semantic variant PPA or logopenic variant PPA [3]. The nonfluent/agrammatic PPA clinical picture corresponds to a deficit mainly in left frontal and insular regions. Semantic variant PPA presents with fluent grammatically correct speech, single words comprehension deficit and difficulty in objects meaning

*Address for correspondence: Paolo Caffarra M.D., Department of Neuroscience, University of Parma, Via Gramsci, 14, 43100 Parma, Italy.E-mail: paolo.caffarra@unipr.it.

recognition, caused by atrophy in bilateral anterior temporal regions. Logopenic variant PPA shows phonemic paraphasia, word-finding hesitation, slow speech and decreased verbal output with long word-finding pauses and preserved grammar and articulation, corresponding to left posterior temporal and parietal lobules degeneration. The inferior parietal lobule would be the site for phonological store portion of the phonological loop [4,5].

Patients with permanent and spontaneous jargon language appear to be more common in acute neurological disorders involving critical language networks, in particular Wernicke's aphasia, than in neurodegenerative disease. There are two case reports of jargonagraphia, a condition often, but not invariably, associated with jargonaphasia. LEA was a patient with severely reduced speech production and defective articulation, affected by what seems to be a severe, rapidly progressive form of fronto-temporal degeneration [6], who produced fluent, neologistic writte jargon. FM, a patient described by the Cambridge group in at least seven papers, appears to be a case of the semantic variant of PPA. He never developed a spoken jargon. After 7 years of follow up he produced fluent, "empty" speech with perseveration of a set of "general" words (special, set, etc.). In contrast, his written production was fluent, replete of written neologisms that followed the graphotactic rules of English [7]. Two patients with fluent jargonaphasia were present among the pathological series reported by Deramecourt and colleagues [8]. Both showed left temporo-parietal hypoperfusion on SPECT, and had a pathological diagnosis of Alzheimer's disease. Two detailed case reports of neologistic jargon in PPA have been published by Rohrer and colleagues [9]. The first case presented with word-finding difficulties, which progressed to neologistic jargonaphasia associated with semantic impairment. The imaging data were atypical for the semantic variant of PPA, as they showed progressive atrophy of the temporal lobes, without an anterior-posterior gradient, and of the parietal cortex. The second presented with non-fluent, agrammatic production, but in the next year started to produce profuse neologisms in speaking and reading. Auditory comprehension also deteriorated. Imaging finding revealed progressive perisylvian atrophy, with severe involvement of the inferior parietal lobule.

The present single case study aimed to describe the clinical evolution of a similar patient who developed neologistic jargon in the course of PPA, reporting both cognitive and neuroimaging correlates of this unusual clinical picture.

2. Case study

The patient is a 68-year-old right handed woman with 18 years of education, teacher of Italian literature, who, ten years ago, came to our observation for language impairment.

At the onset of the disease in 2001, the patient showed word-finding difficulties with prolonged anomic pauses. In addition, neuropsychological testing disclosed mild executive dysfunction, whereas, language comprehension, syntax, semantic, memory, praxic and visuo-perceptual abilities were in the normal range (see Table 1).

CT scan revealed mild frontal atrophy. Tc-HMPAO SPECT disclosed a reduced regional cerebral blood flow (rCBF) in right inferior frontal areas and in left temporo-parietal and occipital regions.

Cognitive follow-ups showed a worsening of linguistic abilities, due to the progressive occurrence of phonemic paraphasias and appearance of neologisms. Deficits in repetition, objects naming, verbal short-term memory, verbal learning, selective attention, phonemic and semantic fluencies were also observed. She had a stressful response to illness, with depressive symptoms and apathy, caused by a complete insight of disease.

After January 2004, due to the lack of family compliance, the patient's follow-up was interrupted. We have no additional clinical data until 2008. At this time, a neuropsychological assessment, cerebral MRI, ^{18}F-FDG PET, cerebrospinal fluid (CSF) analysis and APOE genotype survey were carried out. The cognitive assessment showed a severe impairment of speech production and repetition, characterized by a fluent but totally unintelligible language. Verbal comprehension, reading and writing were completely lost, while prosody and communicative gestures continued to be relatively appropriate to the context. The severe language impairment prevented any further neuropsychological assessment. Along with the language impairment, the patient developed a loss in daily functions (sparing eating and body movement), while depression and apathy were no longer present. The neurological examination was unremarkable. She developed stereotyped behaviour with the tendency to compulsive wandering and hoarding (pathological collection of objects, such as leaves or stones). Emotional response to both unpleasant (see images of dead at the television) and pleasant (see a baby) stimuli was preserved.

Some examples of her speech in different conversational situations are reported below. During the clinical interview she spontaneously manifested a jargon

Table 1
Neuropsychological testing of the patient in the disease course

Neuropsychological test	Cut-off normal range	May 2001	May 2002	July 2003	January 2004	October 2008
Mini Mental State Examination (MMSE)	⩾ 23.8	26	29	27	18	N.A.
Activity Daily Living (ADL)		6/6	6/6	6/6	6/6	2/6
Instrumental Activities of Daily Living (IADL)		8/8	8/8	7/8	7/8	0/8
Mental Deterioration Battery (MDB)						
Progressive Matrices (PM 47)	⩾ 18.96	26.2	24.45	32.55	28.45	N.A.
Verbal Fluency	⩾ 17.35	20.2	9.5*	9.5*	6.5*	N.A.
Sentence Construction	⩾ 8.72	10.4	2.75*	N.A.	N.A.	N.A.
Immediate Visual Memory	⩾ 13.85	19.6	22	18.75	18.75	N.A.
Rey Auditory Verbal Learning Test (RAVLT)						
Immediate	⩾ 28.53	42.8	29.65	30.65	20.65*	N.A.
Delayed	⩾ 4.69	10.6	8.85	4.85	6.3	N.A.
Constructional apraxia	⩾ 7.18	10.1	10.2	10.2	8.2	N.A.
Laiacona semantic memory test						
Visual naming	⩾ 61	–	73/80	68/80	–	–
Semantic questionnaire	⩾ 447	–	461/480	–	–	–
Semantic Fluency	⩾ 25	35	10.5*	13*	9*	N.A.
Boston naming test	⩾ 16	19	16*	15*	13*	N.A.
Digit Span	⩾ 3.75	4.5	4.5	3.5*	1.5*	N.A.
Visuo-Spatial Span – Corsi Test	⩾ 3.50	5	5.12	4.12	4.12	N.A.
Attentive Matrices	⩾ 31	–	–	18.12*	18.12*	N.A.
Object decision test – BORB subtest 10 Easy A	⩾ 24	28	28	–	–	–
Associative match task – BORB subtest 12	⩾ 22	29	29	–	–	–
Stroop test						
Interference time	⩽ 36.91	69.65*	76.7*	37.2*	59.7*	N.A.
Interference errors	⩽ 4.23	2.25	0	0	0.5	N.A.
Wisconsin Card Sorting Test						
Categories	⩾ 3	2*	2*	2*	1*	N.A.
Perseverations	⩽ 6.40	5.75*	13.75*	11.75*	11.75*	N.A.
Test for aphasia (Aachener Aphasie Test)						
Spontaneous speech						
Communicative Behavior	4	4	3	2	0	
Prosody	5	5	5	5	5	
Automatic language	5	5	4	4	3	
Semantic Structure	4	4	4	3	1	
Phonemic Structure	5	5	4	3	1	
Syntactic Structure	5	5	4	3	2	
Token test	⩽ 6	5	–	–	–	N.A.
Repetition	⩾ 144	144	129*	119*	114*	N.A.
Naming	⩾ 106	101*	104*	102*	89*	N.A.
Written language	⩾ 82	88	85	83	82	N.A.
Comprehension	⩾ 107	112	113	112	110	N.A.
Hospital Anxiety and Depression Scale						
Anxiety	⩽ 10	10	8	8	8	N.A.
Depression	⩽ 10	16*	8	8	13*	N.A.

Legend: N.A. Not Applicable due to illness severity; *pathological scores; – not administered.

like: *"I asked, I looked for, towards and so, co, here around, yes, there is people, it is a hundred"*; in response to the question "When were you born?", patient replies: *"Born? Pento, bande bande and go. That I don't say, to say, danno, I have some, so doctor"*; in response to "Goodbye", patient said: *"Goodbye, ah there will be. . . no, I saw a porsa, there is a land, I know that migenda vincite avò so so"*. An example of spontaneous speech was: *"rasapele ripata ripata, labela, debelito, eh, mitota bolu"*. (Underlined words are non-

existent Italian words). The language was totally unintelligible, with fluent jargon characterised by mainly non-existing words and real words put together in meaningless sequences as a mixed jargon [9,10].

The three-dimensional MRI showed an increased atrophy in the left temporo-parietal lobe, in the absence of vascular lesions.

A t-test comparison between the ^{18}F-FDG PET of the patient and those of a group of ten healthy controls (mean age 68.36, SD 8.59; mean education 9.55,

Table 2
Brain regions of decreased hypo-metabolism in the patient

Brain area	BA	L/R	Number of voxels in cluster	Cluster-level p-value (corrected)	Z value at local maximum	Talairach coordinates		
						x	y	z
Superior temporal gyrus	22	L	2903	0.000	5.11	−59	−44	15
	22	R	253		4.56	61	−55	19
	39	R	253		3.91	55	−61	18
Angular gyrus	39	L	2903	0.000	4.98	−46	−61	33
Middle Temporal gyrus	21	L	2903	0.000	4.47	−55	−56	5
Posterior cingulate	31	L	948	0.000	4.49	−6	−57	21
Precuneus	7	L	948	0.000	4.10	−4	−62	42
Inferior frontal gyrus	45	R	126	0.012	4.14	61	24	10
	44	R	126		3.74	53	16	14
	44	L	245		3.98	−51	7	20
Middle frontal gyrus	6	L	245	0.000	3.25	−51	4	37
Caudate		L	165	0.002	3.73	−16	5	16

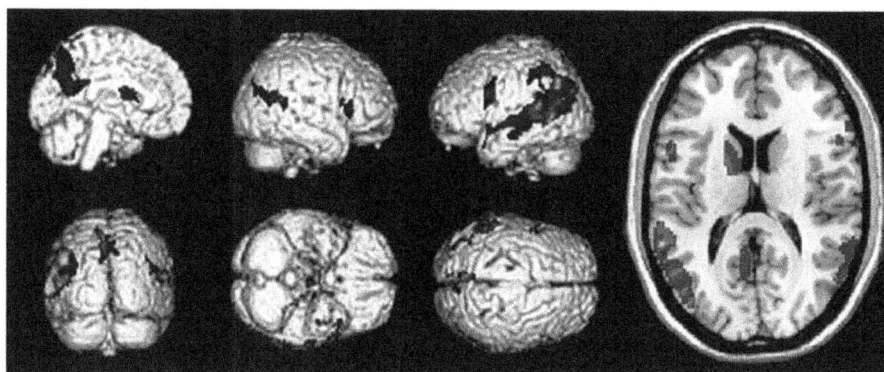

Fig. 1. Areas of hypometabolism revealed by FDG-PET in the patient compared to healthy controls.

SD 4.48) was computed using SPM5. Education was entered as covariate variable in the analysis. Areas of significant hypo-metabolism were found mainly in the left hemisphere in the angular (BA 39) and middle temporal (BA 21) gyri, precuneus (BA 7), posterior cingulate (BA 31), middle frontal gyrus (BA 6), caudate, and bilaterally in the superior temporal (BA 22) and inferior frontal (BA 44) gyri, ($p < 0.001$), (see Table 2 and Fig. 1).

The CSF analysis revealed a significant decrease of ß-amyloid (203, cut off > 600 pg/mL), a slight increase of total Tau protein (394, cut off < 300 pg/mL) and normal value of phosphorylated Tau (value 42, cut off < 60 pg/mL). APOE genotype was $\varepsilon3/\varepsilon3$.

3. Discussion

The language disorder profile of the patient at onset was characterised by anomic pauses, and progressed within ten years into a severe form of fluent, unintelligible speech including a severe deficit in repetition, corresponding to the characteristics of mixed, semantic and neologistic jargonaphasia, associated with severe comprehension deficits. The recent ^{18}F-FDG PET exam showed a significant hypo-metabolism in the same regions evidenced by at onset SPECT scan, but with an increase in damage extension in left fronto-temporo-parietal regions, extending also to the controlateral superior temporal and inferior frontal cortex (BA 44 and BA 22, respectively Broca's and Wernicke's areas).

From the neurolinguistic standpoint, the cause of jargon is a matter of debate. It is often considered as a consequence of defective monitoring of language production, due to defective auditory comprehension, associated with a severe impairment of phonological encoding [11]. Neologisms may be the production of a phonological sequence generator to fill "gaps" in lexical retrieval [12,13]. In vascular aphasia, jargon is typically observed in the context of Wernicke's aphasia, associated with damage in the posterior-superior temporal cortex. The results of some neuropathological studies, as well as of neuroimaging investigations, suggest that extension of damage towards the temporal and parietal cortex is responsible for jargon occurrence. More specifically, parietal vs. temporal extension may be associated with, respectively, semantic and neologistic jargon [14].

The prominent involvement of the temporo-parietal region observed in our patient, as well as in the cases reported by Demeracourt [8] and Rohrer [9], are in agreement with the data from vascular aphasia.

Why is progressive jargonaphasia rare, and how is it related to the three main clinical varieties of PPA? A prominent involvement of the left temporo-parietal regions is typical of the logopenic/phonological variety, which is often due to Alzheimer's disease. Jargonaphasia may thus represent a relatively unusual evolution of this syndrome. The evolution may be late, such as in the present case, or relatively early, as in Rohrer's case 1. The possibility that the responsible pathology may be AD is strengthened by the observation of the low CSF ß-amyloid level and high level of total Tau found in our patient. The patient was not ε4 carrier, and this is consistent with the atypical forms of AD [15].

The present clinical observation provides further evidence for the heterogeneity of clinical presentations of PPA, which reflects underlying differences in the topographical pattern of pathological involvement. This variability may be particularly extensive in the case of the logopenic/phonological variant, frequently associated with atypical patterns of AD neuropathology.

Acknowledgments

The authors thank the patient and the patient's family for the cooperation. This study was supported by a grant from the Fondazione Cassa di Risparmio of Parma and Piacenza to PC.

References

[1] M.M. Mesulam, Primary progressive aphasia, *Ann Neurol* **49** (2001), 425–432.

[2] D.G. Clark, A. Charuvastra, B.L. Miller et al., Fluent versus non fluent primary progressive aphasia: A comparison of clinical and functional neuroimaging features, *Brain Lang* **94** (2005), 54–60.

[3] M.L. Gorno-Tempini, N.F. Dronkers, K.P. Rankin et al., Cognition and Anatomy in Three Variants of Primary Progressive Aphasia, *Ann Neurol* **55** (2004), 335–346.

[4] M.L. Gorno-Tempini, S.M. Brambati, V. Ginex et al., The logopenic/phonological variant of primary progressive aphasia, *Neurology* **71** (2008), 1227–1234.

[5] M.L. Gorno-Tempini, A.E. Hillis, S. Weintraub et al., Classification of primary progressive aphasia and its variants, *Neurology* **76** (2011), 1006–1014.

[6] P. Ostberg, N. Bogdanovic, S.E. Fernaeus et al., Jargonagraphia in a case of frontotemporal dementia, *Brain Lang* **79** (2001), 333–339.

[7] N.L. Graham, K. Patterson and J.R. Hodges, The emergence of jargon in progressive fluent dysgraphia: The widening gap between target and response, *Cogn Neuropsychol* **18** (2001), 343–361.

[8] V. Deramecourt, F. Lebert, B. Debachy et al., Prediction of pathology in primary progressive language and speech disorders, *Neurology* **74** (2010), 42–49.

[9] J.D. Rohrer, M.N. Rossor and J.D. Warren, Neologistic jargon aphasia and agraphia in primary progressive aphasia, *J Neurol Sci* **277** (2009), 155–159.

[10] B. Butterworth, Jargon aphasia: processes and strategies, in: S. Newman and R. Epstein, eds, Current perspectives in dysphasia. Edinburgh, UK: Churchill Livingstone, 1985, pp. 61–96.

[11] A. Kertesz and D.F. Benson, Neologistic jargon: a clinicopathological study, *Cortex* **6** (1970), 362–386.

[12] H.W. Buckingham and A. Kertesz, Neologistic jargon aplasia. Amsterdam: Swets and Zeitlinger, 1976.

[13] B. Butterworth, Hesitation and the Production of Verbal Paraphasias and Neologisms in Jargon Aphasia, *Brain Lang* **8** (1979), 133–161.

[14] A. Kertesz, Neuropsychological evaluation of language, *J Clin Neurophysiol* **11** (1994), 205–215.

[15] W.M. van der Flier, Y.A. Pijnenburg, N.C. Fox et al., Early-onset versus late-onset Alzheimer's disease: the case of the missing APOE ε4 allele, *Lancet Neurol* **10** (2011), 280–288.

Patterns of dysgraphia in primary progressive aphasia compared to post-stroke aphasia

Andreia V. Faria[a], Jenny Crinion[c], Kyrana Tsapkini[b], Melissa Newhart[b], Cameron Davis[b], Shannon Cooley[e], Susumu Mori[a] and Argye E. Hillis[b,d,f,*]

[a]*Department of Radiology, Johns Hopkins University School of Medicine, Baltimore, MD, USA*
[b]*Department of Neurology, Johns Hopkins University School of Medicine, Baltimore, MD, USA*
[c]*University College London, London, UK*
[d]*Department of Physical Medicine and Rehabilitation, Johns Hopkins University School of Medicine, Baltimore, MD, USA*
[e]*Johns Hopkins University, Baltimore, MD, USA*
[f]*Department of Cognitive Science, Johns Hopkins University, Baltimore, MD, USA*

Abstract. We report patterns of dysgraphia in participants with primary progressive aphasia that can be explained by assuming disruption of one or more cognitive processes or representations in the complex process of spelling. These patterns are compared to those described in participants with focal lesions (stroke). Using structural imaging techniques, we found that damage to the left extrasylvian regions, including the uncinate, inferior fronto-occipital fasciculus, and sagittal stratum (including geniculostriate pathway and inferior longitudinal fasciculus), as well as other deep white and grey matter structures, was significantly associated with impairments in access to orthographic word forms and semantics (with reliance on phonology-to-orthography to produce a plausible spelling in the spelling to dictation task). These results contribute not only to our understanding of the patterns of dysgraphia following acquired brain damage but also the neural substrates underlying spelling.

Keywords: Dysgraphia, primary progressive aphasia, phonology, orthography, MRI

1. Introduction

Patterns of impairment in spelling have revealed distinct cognitive processes underlying normal spelling. For example, some patients after focal brain lesions are selectively unable to spell irregular words (e.g. spell leopard as lepperd), but are able to spell regular words and pseudowords (e.g. glimp). Others are able to spell both regular and irregular words, but cannot come up with a plausible spelling of an unfamiliar proper name or pseudoword. These patients provide evidence for relatively distinct mechanisms of sublexical phonology-to-orthography conversion and access to orthographic word forms (learned spellings of words). Other patients show modality-specific output impairments (impaired written spelling with intact oral

spelling), indicating that the problem is in accessing a letter shape or motor plan. Still others have a very generalized impairment in oral and written spelling of words and pseudowords that is dependent on the number of letters in the stimulus, which can be explained by an impairment in working memory or a "buffer" system for holding the sequence of abstract letter identities while the word is written or spelled aloud.

Most of these patterns have been described in chronic stroke patients with large lesions. It has been difficult to localize the lesions associated with distinct components of the spelling process, although Rapcsak and colleagues have found that chronic left perisylvian lesions (supramarginal gyrus, superior temporal gyrus, posterior inferior frontal gyrus, and precentral gyrus) are associated with impaired phonology-to-orthography; while extra-striate lesions are associated with impairments in other components that result in reliance on phonology-to-orthography (and "regular" or sublexical spelling) [1]. Some fMRI studies of spelling

*Corresponding author: Argye E. Hillis, MD, Meyer 6-113, Johns Hopkins Hospital, Baltimore, MD, 21287, USA.
E-mail: argye@JHMI.edu.

have supported these hypotheses [2]. In a large study of acute stroke, we did not find distinct regions associated with pseudoword and word spelling; however, few participants in that study showed a dissociation between word and pseudoword spelling, so there was insufficient power to detect distinct regions associated with one or the other [3]. In a separate series, we did find that lesions of posterior inferior frontal cortex were associated with impaired sublexical phonology-to-orthography conversion in some participants [4,5].

In this paper we report patterns of dysgraphia very similar to the patterns that have been reported in chronic unilateral stroke, but in participants with primary progressive aphasia (PPA), a neurodegenerative disease that disproportionately affects language for at least two years before the onset of other cognitive symptoms [6]. These data are of interest, because they demonstrate that these patterns of spelling impairment observed in both patient populations cannot be accounted for by rehabilitation alone. As PPA affects somewhat distinct areas of brain that are not typically affected by vascular lesions, they also provide the opportunity to look for unique patterns, not seen after unilateral focal stroke. Using structural imaging techniques, we found that PPA participants who relied on phonology-to-orthography conversion for successful spelling could be distinguished from those who were disproportionately impaired in phonology-to-orthography conversion. Damage to the left extrasylvian regions was significantly associated with impairments in access to orthographic word forms and semantics (with reliance on phonology-to-orthography to produce a plausible spelling in the spelling to dictation task) including the uncinate, inferior fronto-occipital fasciculus, and sagittal stratum (including geniculostriate pathway and inferior longitudinal fasciculus), as well as other deep white and grey matter structures. These imaging data directly complement the imaging obtained from chronic stroke participants and furthers our understanding of the role of the left perisylvian regions involved in spelling.

2. Methods

2.1. Participants

We enrolled a series of 30 participants with PPA who were seen in the senior author's outpatient clinic and agreed to participate. They were diagnosed with PPA on the basis of having a predominant and progressive deterioration in language in the absence of major

Table 1
PPA variants and demographic information

Patient ID	Age (years)	Gender	PPA variants	Locus of impairment
1	62	Male	sv	1
2	56	Female	sv	1
3	68	Male	sv	1
4	84	Female	nfv	2
5	62	Female	lv	3
6	70	Male	nfv	4
7	58	Male	lv	3
8	67	Female	lv	3
9	74	Female	nfv	1
10	66	Female	lv	3
11	60	Female	sv	1
12	84	Female	nfv	3
13	70	Male	lv	3
14	62	Male	sv	1
15	74	Female	sv	1
16	67	Female	lv	3
17	71	Male	lv	3
18	70	Male	sv	1
19	72	Female	lv	3
20	71	Female	lv	1
21	70	Female	unclassifiable	1
22	73	Female	lv	1
23	69	Female	unclassifiable	1
24	51	Male	lv	1
25	79	Female	unclassifiable	3
26	62	Female	nfv	3
27	57	Male	sv	1
28	55	Female	nfv	4
29	63	Female	lv	4
30	73	Male	sv	1

PPA variants: sv = semantic; nfv = nonfluent/agrammatic; lv = logopenic.
Locus of impairment: 1 = semantics & orthography; 2 = Phonology to Orthography Conversion (POC); 3 = partially impaired POC, partially impaired access to orthographic word forms; 4 = impairment at the level of the Graphemic Buffer.

change in personality, behavior or cognition other than praxis for at least two years [6]. Participants were classified, when possible, as one of the variants of PPA according to recent guidelines [7]. However, several participants were only anomic and dysgraphic, and did not meet criteria for any of these variants. PPA variants and demographics are included in Table 1. All participants completed a battery of language and spelling tests together and had a high resolution T1 weighted image (T1-WI) brain scan, within 1 month post testing. Six participants were followed up one year later where they repeated the scan and testing.

2.2. Language testing

A battery of tests was used to classify participants' overall language impairments and aid classification into the global PPA variant groupings, as described in Gorno-Tempini et al. [7]. These included 1) *speech production*: analysis of the Cinderella story, elicited with a series of pictures; naming of nouns and verbs; repetition of sentences; a sentence formulation test using scrambled words or anagrams of sentences; 2) *reading*: oral reading; reading aloud of regular and irregular words; 3) *language comprehension*: a short form of the Pyramids and Palm Trees Test [19], and a spoken word to picture matching test. For detailed analyses of spelling the Johns Hopkins Dysgraphia Battery was administered to all participants (see [8] for details of the stimuli). Within each subtest of this battery stimuli control for a multitude of variables including word frequency, length and grammatical class. For example, in the word length subtest, 4, 5, 6, 7, and 8-letter words are matched for frequency, length in syllables, and grammatical word class.

Spelling error classifications: Errors were classified as phonologically plausible errors (PPEs) if each letter produced by the participant was a valid instance of the phoneme (speech sound) in the corresponding stimulus at that position. For example, for the stimulus "cactus" phonologically plausible errors included kaktis, kactos, caktess, cacktuss, etc. Phonologically implausible nonword errors were nonwords in which at least one letter did not correspond to the phonology of the stimulus (e.g. "cactus" → kaptess). Semantic errors were semantically related to the word (e.g. "cactus" → plant or desert). Phonologically similar word errors (e.g. bear → pear) shared at least 50% of phonemes, and excluded morphologically related errors (e.g. read → "reading"). Morphological errors included derivational errors (e.g. baking → baker) and inflectional errors (e.g., baking → baked, the latter of which did not change the grammatical word class).

Determining the locus of impairment within the spelling system: Our *a priori* framework for identifying the level of impairment within the spelling system included the types of errors in each spelling task that were expected and the pattern of errors across tasks. Nevertheless, the precise criteria are somewhat difficult to define because the errors also depend in part on the severity as well as the locus of impairment. Even when criteria can be defined, often a patient may not meet every single criterion and yet will overall have the impression of having a pattern of performance that can be nicely explained by assuming a deficit to a particular component of the spelling process. So, we refer readers to criteria for each deficit outlined in Beeson and Hillis [8], but these will be best illustrated in each case below.

We identified lexical effects or word length effects in spelling using Fisher's exact tests, comparing correct versus incorrect responses on lists contrasting the relevant contrast, matched for the other variables that might affect performance. The patient's first response was scored; there were no time limits for responding.

2.3. Imaging analysis

MPRAGE T1-WIs (TR/TE = 8.4/3.9 ms) were acquired using a 3T whole body MRI scanner (Philips Medical Systems, Best, The Netherlands), with axial orientation and a image matrix of 256×256 mm. Half of the participants were scanned with a field of view (FOV) of 230×230 mm and 120 slices of 1 mm thickness; and half had FOV of 212×212 mm and 140 slices of 1.1 mm thickness. To measure the volume of each anatomical region we performed an atlas-based analysis (ABA). In brief, the ABA consists on transforming a brain image (the atlas) and the anatomical parcellation defined in this atlas to each participant's brain. As a result, a specific parcellation is created for each individual and, therefore, each participant's brain can be fully and automatically parceled in multiple regions of interest (ROIs). In this study, the ABA analysis was made possible due the high accuracy of the mapping algorithm, the large deformation diffeomorphic metric mapping – LDDMM [13]. As we showed in previous studies [9–11], the accuracy of this automated parcellation rivals the manual delineation of structures, considered as gold standard.

A schematic diagram of the imaging post-process, performed using DiffeoMap (Li, X.; Jiang, H.; and Mori, S.; Johns Hopkins University, www.MriStudio.org or mri.kennedykrieger.org), is shown in Fig. 1. The images were first normalized to the ICBM-DTI-81 coordinates [12] using a 12-parameter affine transformation and further transformed non-linearly to a single-subject template using LDDMM. The dual-contrast LDDMM [13] was based on T1-WIs and cerebrospinal fluid (CSF) maps. The JHU-MNI "Eve" was chosen as the Atlas. This is a single-subject template in the ICBM-DTI-81 space, extensively parceled and labeled to 159 regions. Details of this parcellation are described in our previous article [14]. Because of the reciprocal nature of the LDDMM, the transformation results can be used to warp the parcellation map to the original MRI data, thus automatically parceling each brain into the 159 sub-regions. After sub segmenting the cortex and the associated white matter in peripheral ROIs using

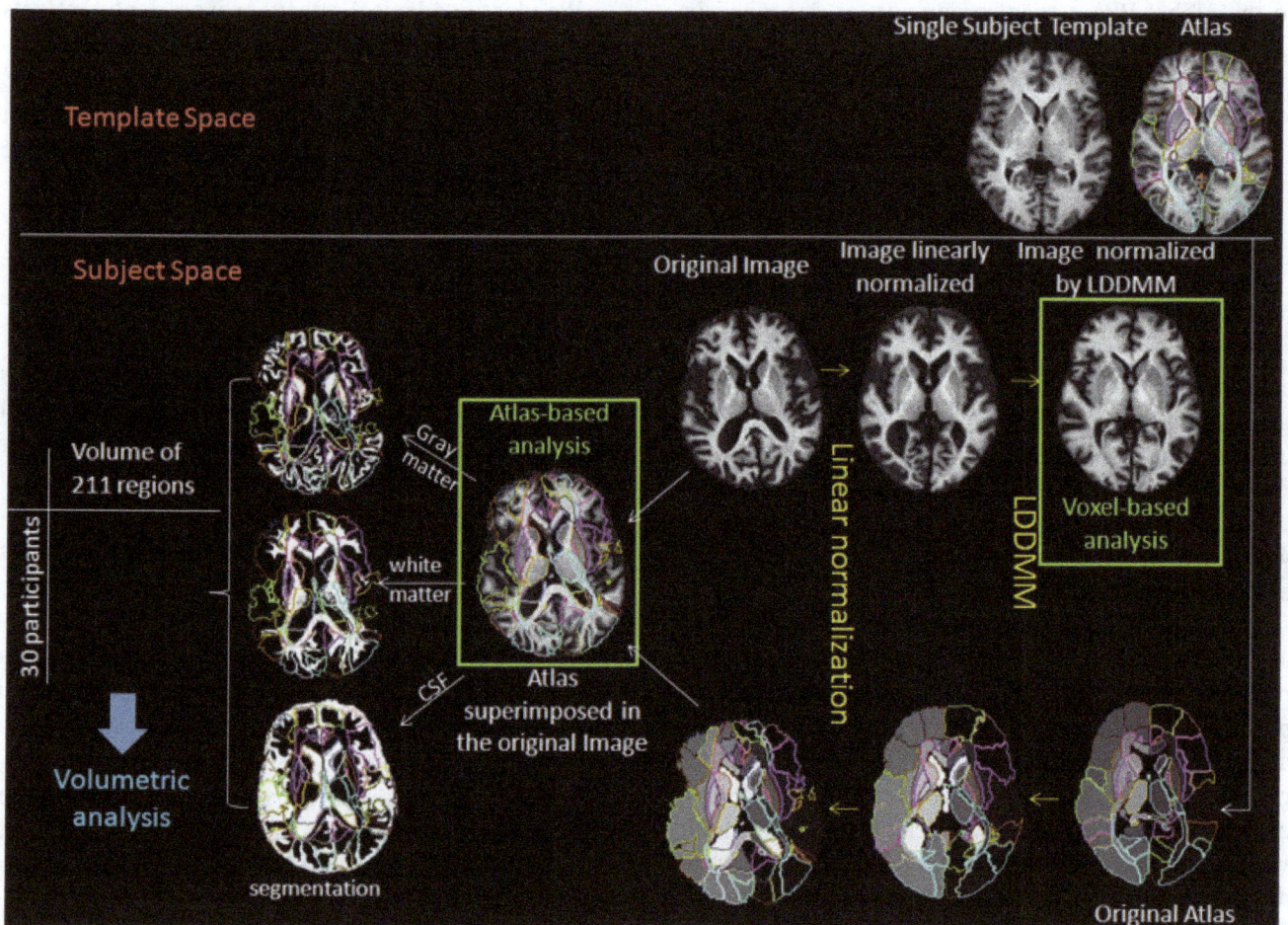

Fig. 1. Image post-processing. Using linear transformations and large deformation diffeomorphic metric mapping (LDDMM), we mapped each participant's brain to the atlas space. After this procedure, all brain images were transformed to a shape similar to that of the atlas, where is possible to perform voxel-based analysis. Using the reciprocal attribute of LDDMM, the parcellation map was transformed to each original MRI. This allows automated segmentation of the original images into 159 subregions. For cortical areas where there is a large amount of anatomical variability, the cortex and the white matter were further divided in each participant using SPM8 segmentation. This resulted in a matrix of participants by volume of 211 regions that was used for the volumetric analysis.

tissue maps obtained from SPM8, we finally obtained 3 dimensional 211 ROIs for each participant.

The post-processing of the six participants for whom longitudinal imaging data were collected followed the same procedure except in these cases we did not use "Eve" as the target but each participant's first T1-WI. Here we were interested in mapping volumetric within-subject changes over time and relating this to their corresponding changes in spelling. As a quantitative metric of local volume changes, we used the Jacobian determinant (i.e., the local expansion factor) of the LDDMM deformation fields. The Jacobian maps indicate local tissue expansion (Jacobian > 1) or shrinkage (Jacobian < 1) relative to the template [15,16] that allows identification of localized volume increases/reductions at the voxel level.

The native differences in the ROIs volumes were evaluated using ANOVA. Age, gender and image pro-tocol were co-variates of no interest. In a second set of analyses, the ROIs volumes were normalized by the total brain volume to exclude any confounding effects of total intracranial volume. The level of statistical significance was set at p-value < 0.01 throughout unless otherwise reported.

3. Results

First we report three distinct patterns of spelling impairments among the PPA participants that can be explained by proposing disruption at the level of one or two cognitive representations or processes within the complex spelling system. Then we report the group's structural imaging results for participants who made predominantly phonologically plausible errors (i.e. rely on phonology to orthography conversion) versus those who made predominantly implausible errors (impaired phonology to orthography conversion as well as partially impaired access to orthographic word forms).

3.1. Pattern 1: Impairment at the level of orthography and semantics

When either access to semantics or access to orthographic word forms (or both) is impaired, we would expect reliance on sublexical phonology-to-orthography conversion mechanisms. Of course, there might be an interaction between lexical and sublexical mechanisms, such that participants use a combination of information to access lexical representations when they have partial impairment of one or the other mechanism [17, 18]; we address that issue in more detail in the subsequent sections. Here we describe three PPA participants who seemed to rely almost entirely on sublexical mechanisms to spell. It is important to highlight that orthography to phonology conversion (OPC) was spared, because participants were able to spell pseudowords.

Case 1 is a 62 year old man with 20 years of education who was first evaluated about four years after the onset of anomia. He had noticed deterioration in word retrieval and spelling but was still working in a highly verbal job. At that time, he showed preservation of word and sentence comprehension, sentence repetition, and conceptual semantics. He lived independently and remained successfully employed in a high level of occupation.

His performance on the Johns Hopkins Dysgraphia Battery could be explained by selective impairment at the level of accessing orthographic word forms, with reliance on sublexical phonology-to-orthography conversion mechanisms to spell. Nearly all (92.3%) of his errors were phonologically plausible (e.g. sparrow $\rightarrow$ sparo; courage $\rightarrow$ currage; palace $\rightarrow$ pallis; bought $\rightarrow$ bot; about $\rightarrow$ abowt; become-> becum; career $\rightarrow$ currear). Furthermore, he spelled pseudowords more accurately than words (91.2% vs. 63.1; $p < 0.005$); regular words more accurately than irregular words (93.3 vs. 63.8%; $p < 0.005$). At that time, there was no difference in spelling accuracy for concrete vs. abstract words (52.4 vs. 57.1%) or any effect of word length (e.g. 4-letter vs. 8-letter words: 64.3 vs. 42.9%).

One year later, Case 1 showed deterioration in his word and sentence comprehension. He scored only 3/17 correct on a word/picture verification test, on which virtually all non-neurologically impaired adults make no errors. He correctly accepted most targets as the name of the object, but also incorrectly accepted nearly all semantically related words (e.g. "knife" for fork) as the name of the object. On a 15 item version of the Pyramid and Palm Trees Test [19], a picture association test, he scored on 12/15 (normal performance is ceiling). He continued to live independently, but made errors in daily life (e.g., offered his credit card when asked for his insurance card). His speech remained fluent, grammatical, and well articulated. He was able to carry on a social conversation, but produced few specific nouns. He made frequent semantic paraphasic errors and circumlocutions when speaking. He named verbs (40%) more accurately than nouns (13%). At this time point he met the criteria for semantic variant PPA (svPPA) and his spelling had deteriorated substantially as well. He still spelled pseudowords more accurately than words (79.4% vs. 57.1%; $p = 0.03$); and there was no effect of concreteness, grammatical word class, or frequency. All responses showed some attempt to apply phonology to orthography conversion mechanisms. Figure 2 shows deterioration of his accuracy on subtests of the Dysgraphia Battery over the course of one year. Related to his dramatic deterioration in semantics, the imaging data showed significant areas of brain atrophy between the two testing sessions, primarily in the left frontal and temporal regions.

Case 2 is a 56 year old right handed woman with a master's degree who was in graduate school when she developed progressive difficulty with word retrieval and understanding what she was reading. She remained independent in daily activities for several years, but needed to discontinue her studies. She was eventually diagnosed with svPPA on the basis of her impaired word comprehension with spared speech articulation and speech fluency. She was scanned and tested twice on the dysgraphia battery, one year apart, although not all lists were given the second time due to her significant deterioration over that time. Her speech was fluent and grammatical. She remained very pleasant and cooperative, although it was difficult for her to understand words and the directions for new tasks. Her husband needed to take over the cooking, driving, and housework, because she also developed difficulties understanding the meanings of objects.

On both testing occasions, the majority of her spelling errors were phonologically plausible. PPE's constituted 82.6% of errors at time 1 and 80.0% of her errors at time 2. Errors included: ocean $\rightarrow$ ousean, strange $\rightarrow$ strainge, column $\rightarrow$ callem, sought $\rightarrow$ saut, thief $\rightarrow$ theaf, jerk $\rightarrow$ jurck. Orthographic probability did not significantly affect accuracy, although she was more accurate for high probability than low probably

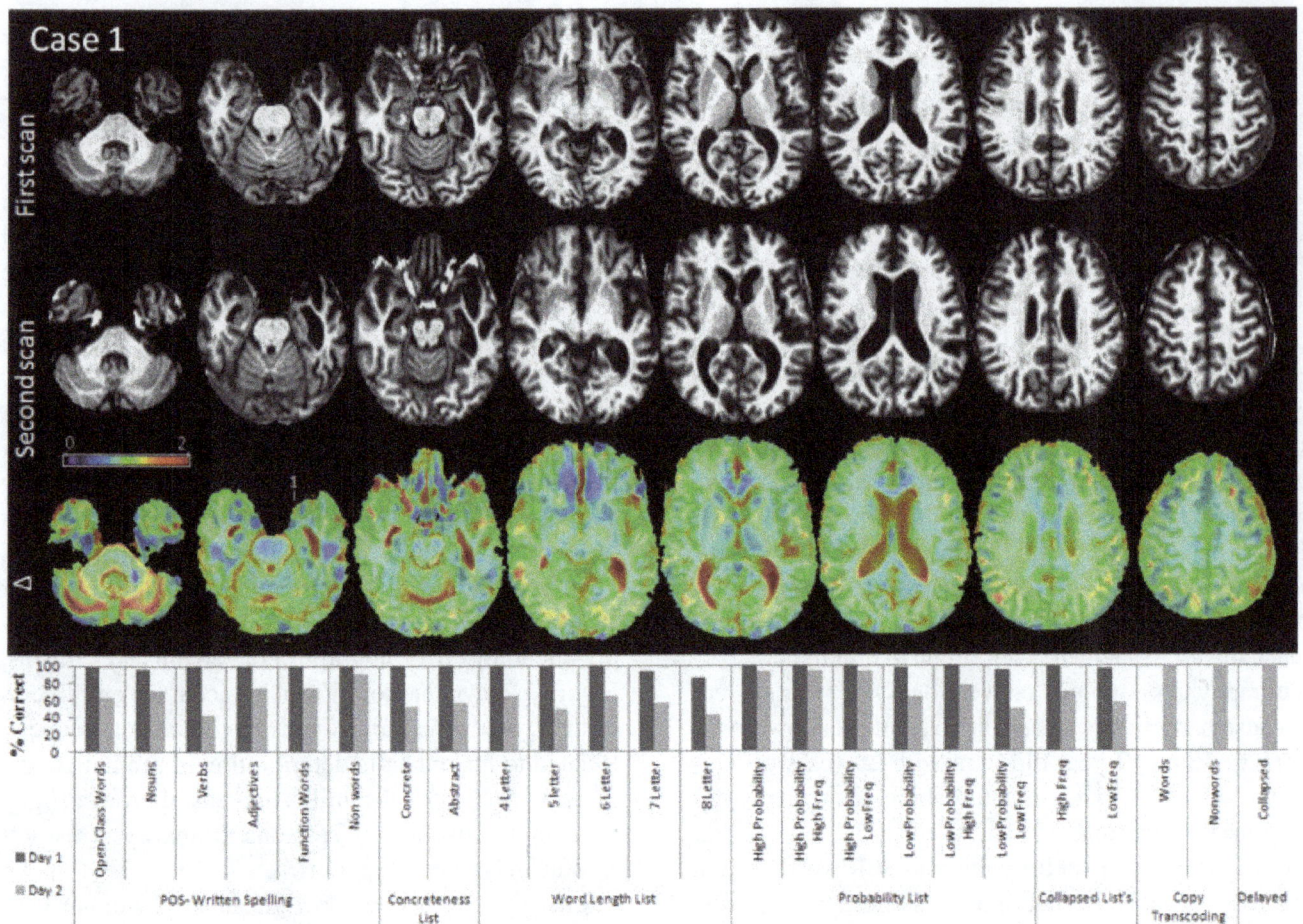

Fig. 2. Longitudinal volumetric analysis of Case 1. Note the enlargement of lateral ventricles, particularly at left, between the first and the second scans, spaced by 1 year. Δ is the color-coded for the Jacobians determinants from LDDMM and shows how each voxel expanded (red, > 1) or shrieked (blue, < 1) overtime. Note the "expansion" of the ventricles, in agreement with the visual impression, and also the atrophy (blue patches) in frontal and temporal areas. The bottom row shows the results of spelling on various subtests of the Dysgraphia Battery Test, 1 year apart.

words: 83.3% vs. 71.2% at time point 1; this list was not administered at time 2. The only variables to significantly affect accuracy were lexicality and concreteness. She spelled pseudowords significantly more accurately than words (97.1% vs. 76.2%, $p = 0.007$ at time 1; 73.6% vs. 42.9%, $p = 0.004$ at time 2) and abstract words more accurately than concrete words (81.0 vs. 71.4% at time 1; 76.2% vs. 33.3%, $p = 0.01$) at time 2. Figure 3 shows deterioration of her accuracy on subtests of the Dysgraphia Battery and the progression of brain atrophy temporal, parietal (particularly left) and subregions of basal ganglia over the course of 1 year.

Case 3 is a 68-year-old man with a college education who was tested 8 years after onset of aphasia, when he met criteria for svPPA. He had fluent, grammatical, but "empty" speech with little content and only a shallow awareness of his difficulty communicating. He had impaired word and sentence comprehension. He lived with his wife, but was independent in daily ac-

tivities, including driving. His performance fell somewhere between the first and second pattern shown by Case 1. Only 38% of his errors were phonologically plausible errors (e.g., center → senter; ready → readie), but many others were "close" (e.g., complete → compleade; fluid → floude; future → fercher; frequent → freacken). He spelled pseudowords more accurately than words (38.2% vs. 9.5% correct; $p < 0.001$). However, there were no significant effects of any tested parameters for words, because his performance was essentially at floor. For example, there was no difference between regular and irregular words because both were very poorly spelled (10% correct for each). Abstract words were spelled slightly more accurately than concrete words (14% vs. 0 correct), but there was no effect of word length (0% correct for both 4- and 8-letter words). His profile suggested an attempt to rely on phonology to orthography conversion mechanisms to spell.

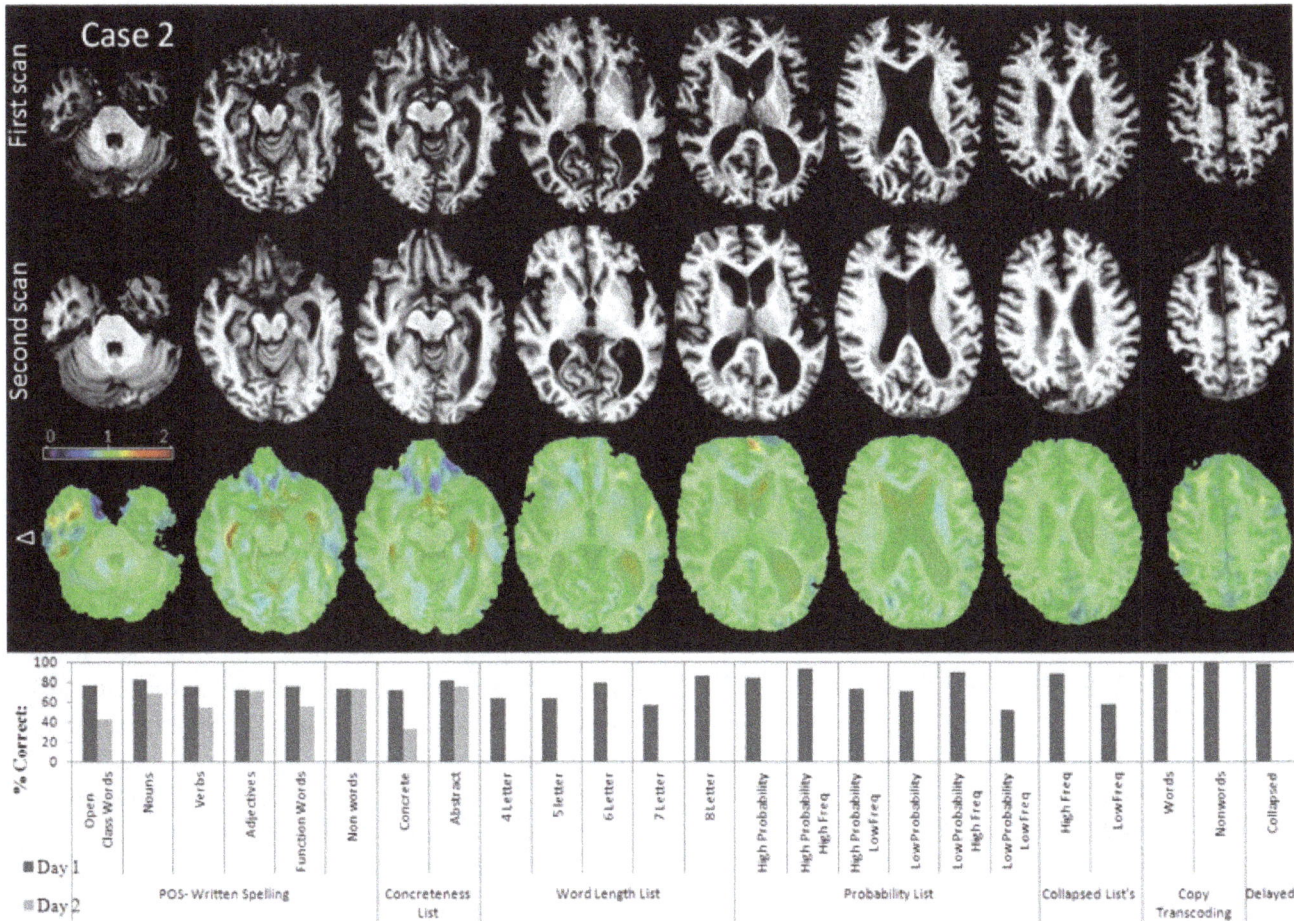

Fig. 3. Longitudinal volumetric analysis of Case 2. Again, first and second scans are spaced by 1 year and Δ shows how each voxel changed overtime (red (> 1) = expansion; blue (< 1) = shrinkage). Note the enlargement of CSF spaces (ventricles and sulci) and the atrophy of temporal, parietal (particularly left) and subregions of basal ganglia. The bottom row shows the results of spelling on various subtests of the Dysgraphia Battery Test, 1 year apart.

In summary, these 3 PPA cases' spelling profiles are similar and consistent with those of chronic stroke participants previously reported in the literature. For example, patient JJ, reported by Hillis and Caramazza [17], had a category-specific semantic impairment, affecting naming and comprehension of all categories except animals (and to a lesser degree, also sparing fruits and vegetables). He had no special premorbid expertise, familiarity, or fondness for animals according to his wife; he had no pets and had not visited a zoo in his adult life. Nevertheless, he was remarkably accurate in naming and word/picture matching for all types of animals (77–100%) compared to inanimate objects (8–33% correct), but he spelled to dictation non-animal names correctly (for regular names) or plausibly (e.g. 'carrot' → cairit, 'kangaroo' → cangarue). He made the same sorts of errors in written naming (e.g. ostrich → ostrage), although he also made semantic errors (e.g. bean → pea) or mixed semantic + PPE (e.g. carrot → cyoucumber) in written naming for non-animals.

Virtually all of his errors in spelling to dictation (and reading) were PPEs. He occasionally spelled or read-aloud irregular words that he only partially understood. This was interpreted as evidence that access to lexical representations for output can be achieved through a summation of partial information from the semantic system and partial information from phonology-to-orthography and orthography-to-phonology conversion mechanisms. JJ's stroke affected a large part of the left anterior and inferior, middle, and superior temporal cortex, and basal ganglia, see [17].

3.2. Pattern 2: Severe impairment at the level of phonology to orthography conversion (and partially impaired access to orthographic word forms for output)

Case 4 is an 84 year old woman 9 years post onset of nonfluent/agrammatic variant PPA (nfvPPA), who had a master's degree in a health care related field. She lived independently in a retirement community. She had effortful, poorly articulated, telegraphic speech, and named objects more accurately than actions. Sentence production was agrammatic. She had asyntactic comprehension, but followed conversation well. On the Dysgraphia Battery, she showed nearly the opposite pattern to the previously described participants. She spelled words more accurately than pseudowords (51.2 vs. 0%; $p < 0.05$). Only 1.6% of her errors could be considered PPEs. Her most common error type (43.2%) was semantic (e.g. beauty → pretty; happy → laughter; tiny → little; jury → plea; college → graduation; bought → store; moose → deer; debt → money). Her other errors consisted of phonologically implausible words (10.3%), phonologically similar words (21.1%; e.g. belief → between; should → short; offense → often; palace → place), or "don't know" (23.8%). There was a non-significant trend toward concrete words to be spelled more accurately than abstract words (76.2 vs. 47.6%), again the opposite pattern to that seen in the participants described above who had svPPA. There was no effect of word length (e.g. 4-letter vs. 8-letter: 50.0 vs. 57.1%). The only variable to significantly affect spelling accuracy was grammatical word class: she spelled nouns significantly more accurately than verbs at both time point 1 (67.9% vs. 35.7% correct; $p = 0.02$) and again 1 year later (25.0% vs. 3.6% correct; $p = 0.02$).

This identical pattern has been reported in an acute stroke patient RCM [5]. RCM had very poor phonology to orthography conversion (POC) and made semantic errors in spelling to dictation and written, despite intact word comprehension and oral naming of the same items. She also showed an effect of concreteness, spelled nouns better than verbs, and showed no effects of other variables. RCM had a lesion in the left posterior inferior frontal cortex (Broca's area). This pattern of performance, with both impaired access to POC mechanism and written word forms (especially verbs) for output was also described in an additional group of stroke patients with acute ischemia in Broca's area [20]. In these patients, impaired spelling of words and pseudowords was associated with infarct and/or hypoperfusion in voxels within Brodmann's areas 44/45 (Broca's area), the area of cortical atrophy classically associated with nfvPPA, see [7]. In a separate large acute stroke study [3], damage to the left supramarginal gyrus, Brodmann's area 40, was also associated with this spelling profile.

3.3. Pattern 3: Partially impaired access to orthographic word forms and partially impaired phonology to orthography conversion mechanisms

In some cases, there is nearly equal impairment of lexical and sublexical mechanisms. Participants make some phonologically plausible errors (PPEs) and at least as many implausible errors. They make phonologically related word errors also, probably because partial information from OPC mechanisms can be used to access both target words and phonologically related words in the lexicon. Because they have intact semantics, their intact semantic features also activate both the target word and semantically related words in the lexicon, so that semantically related words may be activated. Words that are both semantically and phonologically related to the target are common errors, resulting from an interaction from partial information from (impaired) POC mechanisms and an intact lexical-semantic system, activating representations whose access is impaired.

To illustrate, *Case 5* is a 62 year old woman 6 years since onset of logopenic variant PPA (lvPPA), characterized by fluent, grammatical speech, with intact word comprehension but poor sentence repetition. She lived with her husband, but was independent in daily activities. She was very pleasant and interactive, and initially had good recall of events. She made frequent circumlocution and phonemic paraphasic errors and hesitations when speaking.

On the dysgraphia battery, she spelled words and pseudowords with approximately equal accuracy (65.5 vs. 61.8% accuracy). There was no significant difference between high and low regularity words (80.0 vs. 83.8% correct). There was no significant effect of word length; she correctly spelled 85.7% of 4-letter vs. 92.9% of 8-letter words.

Only 15.2% of her errors were phonologically plausible errors (e.g. rooster → rouster; pigeon → picheon). The majority of her errors were phonologically similar word errors (e.g. bright → bride, brick; chain → chant) or phonologically/semantically similar words including morphological errors (e.g. jury → juror, absence → absent; speak → speech; begin → begun). These types of errors have been proposed to occur as a result of an interaction between partial information from the semantic system and partial information from the impaired orthography-to-phonology conversion mechanisms, while accessing lexical representations semantically or phonologically related to the target. There-

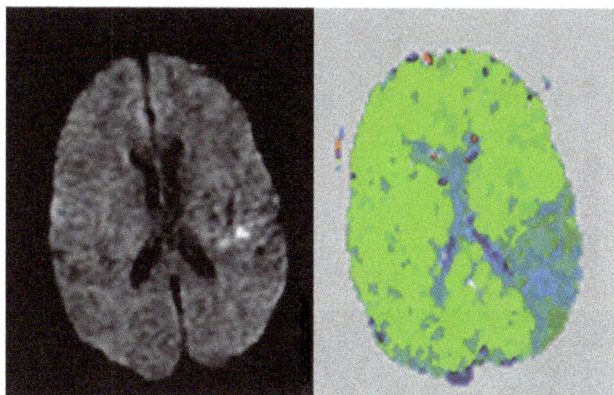

Fig. 4. Diffusion-weighted image (left) and Perfusion-weighted image (right) showing an area of hypoperfusion in the posterior temporal and inferior parietal cortex in an acute stroke patient who showed a pattern of performance in spelling similar to Case 5, attributable to partially impaired access to orthographic word forms and partially impaired access to orthography-to-phonology conversion mechanisms.

fore, some lexical representations that are both semantically and phonologically related to the target will be activated nearly as much as the target itself is activated. When the target lexical orthographic representation is unavailable due to damage at that level, the semantically and phonologically related representation might be activated for output instead [5].

Stroke participants sometimes show similar patterns of performance. For example, the patient whose scans are shown in Fig. 4 had fluent, grammatical but anomic speech, with disproportionately impaired reading and spelling, but intact auditory comprehension. Sentence repetition was impaired. This individual produced phonologically similar word errors in spelling (e.g. axe → axel) at the acute stage of stroke, as well as some phonologically implausible nonwords (e.g. church → chorch). Interestingly, this patient's area of ischemia, in the left inferior parietal lobule and superior temporal cortex is the same brain region where participants with lvPPA show the most focal atrophy. The previously described stroke patient RCM, whose frontal lesion spared the left temporo-parietal cortices also showed a similar pattern of performance in spelling after she improved in POC mechanisms after rehabilitation. This is consistent with the hypothesis that partially spared POC mechanisms can interact with partially spared lexical mechanisms for accessing word forms for output.

3.4. Impairment at the level of the graphemic buffer

In other cases equal impairment in spelling of words and pseudowords could be due to functional disruption at the level the graphemic buffer, a short-term memory system for holding a series of graphemes on-line while the word is spelled aloud or written. In such a case, we would expect all spelling tasks to be equally affected except direct copying of words or pseudowords [21]. Delayed copy transcoding entails showing the patient a word or pseudoword briefly, and then asking them to write the word from memory in the opposite case (upper vs. lower case). Even if they do not know how to spell the word, or do not have a lexical representation as in the case of pseudowords, they should normally be able to retain the sequence of graphemes long enough to spell the word. Participants with impairment at this level have trouble retaining the sequence of graphemes long enough to spell the word or pseudoword, even if they do accurately access the correct spelling (the lexical representation), both in oral and written spelling tasks. They make more errors per letter on longer words than shorter words, because longer words put more stress on the buffer. Because the buffer affects output after the lexical representation is accessed or the spelling is assembled, there are no significant effects of lexical parameters such as word frequency, concreteness, regularity, or grammatical word class (if the impairment is the only deficit in the spelling system), other than word length in graphemes. Errors are phonologically implausible nonword errors, consisting of insertions, deletions or transpositions of letters [21,22].

Case 6 presented with such a profile. He is a 70-year-old man with college education first tested when he was 3 years post onset of nfvPPA. He was tested a second time a year later, by which time he was almost mute. There was no significant effect of lexicality (words vs. pseudowords (34.5% vs. 32.4%); orthographic probability (high vs. low: 93.3 vs. 81.3%), concreteness (concrete vs. abstract: 76.2 vs. 47.6%). More than 73% of his errors were phonologically implausible errors (PINs) the first time he was tested, and 79% of his errors were also PINs a year later on his second testing. These errors included deletions (e.g. priest → priet; caught → cauht), substitutions (e.g. decent → deciet), transpositions (e.g. nature → natuer), and mixed errors (e.g. fierce → furrage; above → aveu). He made similar errors on pseudowords (e.g. donsept → dorseat; croid → crier).

Stroke participants who show this identical pattern of errors have been described in the literature [21–24]. These participants have tended to have focal lesions involving the posterior parietal cortex [25] or visual association cortex [26]. However, in a recent study of 331 participants with acute left hemisphere ischemic stroke evaluated with various spelling tests and magnet-

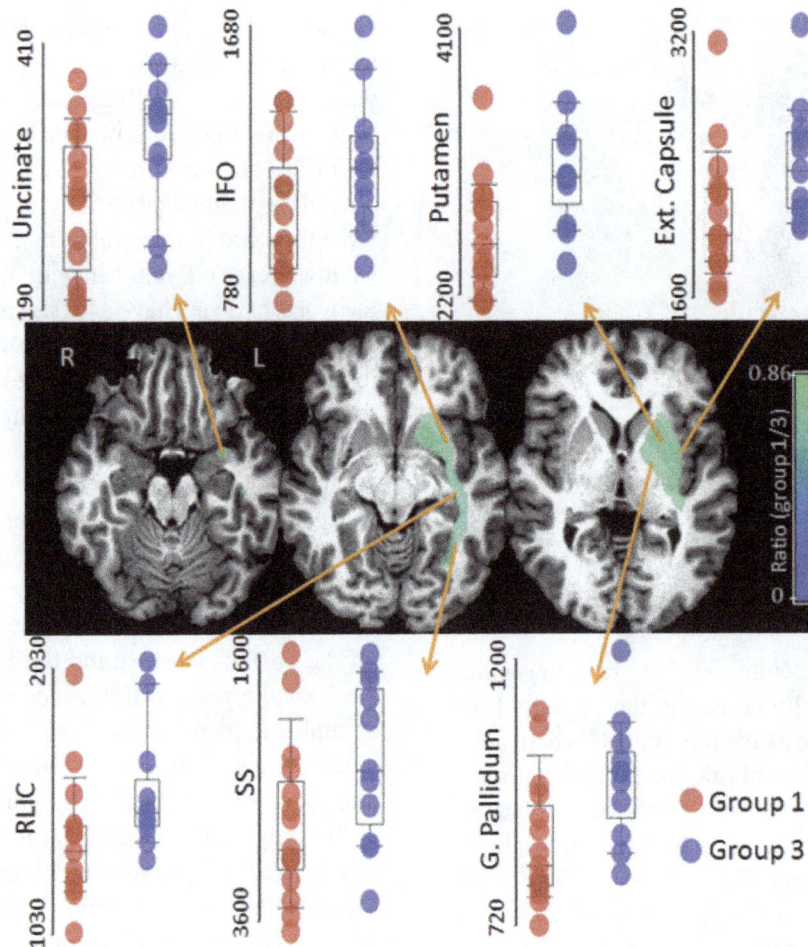

Fig. 5. Comparison between participants who made phonologically plausible errors (PPEs, group 1) and those who made a mixture of PPEs and implausible errors (group 3). Colors overlaid to T1-WI represent the ratio (group 1/3) of the volumes of the areas that showed statistical significant differences between groups ($p < 0.01$). Participants who made PPEs had greater atrophy of uncinate, inferior frontal occiptal fasciculus (IFO), saggital stratum (SS, that includes geniculostriate pathway and inferior longitudinal fasciculus), globus pallidum (G Pallidum), putamen, retrolenticular portion of internal capsule (RLIC) and external capsule, all in the left hemisphere.

ic resonance diffusion and perfusion-weighted imaging a voxel-wise statistical map showed that ischemia in posterior and inferior frontal and parietal cortices, subcortical white matter underlying left prefrontal cortex, lateral occipital gyrus, and caudate was associated with spelling impairments at the level of the graphemic buffer [27]. Functional imaging studies also provide evidence for an extensive network of occipital, parietal, and inferior frontal regions supporting a "visual-spatial sketch pad" as might be needed for any sort of buffer system for holding information that has inherently spatial extent [28–32]. Data from stroke participants who make errors that increase as a function of the number of letters from the center of the word toward the contralesional side, irrespective of the task (spelling, reading, backward spelling, mirror-reversed reading) provide evidence that information at the level of the graphemic buffer does have spatial extent [33].

3.5. Group imaging data

Participants were divided into 4 groups. Group 1 (15 participants) included those who made predominantly PPEs, due to severe impairment at the level of semantics and/or the orthographic word form, and relied on phonology-to-orthography conversion mechanisms for spelling. Cases 1–3 described in the previous sections fell into this group. Group 2 (of which there was only 1 participant, Case 4 outlined above) made mostly semantic errors, and showed the pattern sometimes referred to as "deep dysgraphia". Group 3 (11 participants) made a mixture of PPEs and implausible errors, with frequent phonologically similar word errors, due to partially impaired access to orthographic word forms and partially impaired phonology to orthography conversion mechanisms, exemplified by Case 5 above. Finally, Group 4 (3 participants) showed impairment at the level of the graphemic buffer, exemplified by Case 6 above.

Figure 5 shows comparison for the two largest groups, 1 and 3. There were statistically significant volumetric differences in 7 brain regions, all in the left hemisphere. These included uncinate, inferior fronto-occipital fasciculus, and sagittal stratum (including geniculostriate pathway and inferior longitudinal fasciculus). All 7 regions were significantly more atrophied in group 1 vs. group 3. The results remained significant when regional volumes were normalized by the total brain volume.

4. Discussion

The above cases illustrate that the patterns of dysgraphia previously described after focal vascular lesions (stroke) can also be identified in neurodegenerative cases of PPA. Interestingly, there does not seem to be a one-to-one correspondence between the variant of PPA and the form of dysgraphia, but there are some correspondences between the location of brain atrophy associated with a particular variant of PPA and the affected component of the spelling system, that are consistent with the post-stroke dysgraphia literature.

For example, the combination of severely impaired POC mechanisms and impaired access to orthographic word forms (especially for verbs), with semantic errors in spelling despite good word comprehension was observed only in a nfvPPA patient, who had focal atrophy in posterior left inferior frontal cortex (BA 44/45). This same pattern of dysgraphia has been reported in detailed case studies of stroke participants with focal strokes in BA 44/45 [5,20]. Milder impairments in POC were observed in combination with impaired access to access to orthographic word forms in lvPPA participants, who have atrophy in left inferior parietal cortex. These participants made mostly phonological similar word errors. Similar patterns of dysgraphia have been observed in stroke participants with ischemia in left inferior parietal cortex.

Interestingly, the only PPA participants with impairment at the level of the graphemic buffer had nfvPPA. nfvPPA classically affects the posterior inferior frontal cortex, and this region was identified as critical for the graphemic buffer in a recent study of 331 participants with acute left hemisphere ischemic stroke evaluated with various spelling tests and magnetic resonance diffusion-weighted imaging and perfusion-weighted imaging [27]. That study revealed ischemic damage to many regions including posterior and inferior frontal and parietal cortex, subcortical white matter underlying prefrontal cortex, lateral occipital gyrus, and caudate were associated with acquired spelling impairments at the level of the graphemic buffer. All these regions have been associated with working memory functions (bilaterally), in functional neuroimaging studies.

Most notably, we found that left hemisphere brain regions where atrophy correlated with impairments in access to orthographic word forms and semantics (with reliance on phonology-to-orthography to produce phonologically plausible spellings of words) included the uncinate, inferior fronto-occipital fasciculus, sagittal stratum (including geniculostriate pathway and inferior longitudinal fasciculus), and other deep grey and white matter structures. These tracts have connections with the anterior and inferior temporal lobe and peri-rhinal cortex – areas of cortex known to be affected in svPPA [7]. Furthermore, these same white matter tracts have been found to be disproportionately atrophied in svPPA compared to other variants of PPA. Indeed, most of the participants with this pattern of dysgraphia (9/15) were classified as having svPPA. Others were not classifiable, on the basis that they did not meet criteria for any of the variants, but had only dysgraphia and anomia. One hypothesis is that this pattern of performance may turn out to be an early sign of svPPA. Surface dyslexia is one of the supporting features of svPPA [7]; "surface dysgraphia" may also turn out to be an important early diagnostic symptom.

Most current concepts of the neural networks underlying language include critical nodes for object semantics within the temporal cortex (often including a semantic hub in the anterior temporal lobe – the temporal pole, anterior portion of the superior and middle temporal gyrus and fusiform gyrus anterior to Brodmann's area 37) [34,38–45], and often a more distributed posterior frontal, middle temporal and inferior parietal network underlying action semantics [46]. In previous studies we proposed that access to orthographic word forms for output often depends on an interaction between (or summation of) partial information from semantics and partial information from POC mechanisms [17,18]. Connections between these semantic nodes in temporal cortex and areas critical for access to orthographic word forms (including posterior frontal cortex) and POC mechanisms (such as posterior frontal cortex, angular gyrus, and perhaps supramarginal gyrus) could be essential for such interactions. Disruption of these white matter tracts would plausibly result in reliance on a single component (e.g. POC mechanisms), depending on which component is preserved. In svPPA, POC mechanisms might be preserved because (as previous evidence indicates) POC mechanisms depend on posterior frontal cortex and inferior parietal cortex – regions that are relatively preserved in svPPA.

Considering the computational demands of spelling to dictation participants who make phonologically plausible errors on this task may do so because 1) the distributed components of the orthographic word form are *not accessible* together, or 2) the word form is not being activated appropriately from the impaired semantic representation (or from the spoken input), or 3) the orthographic word form (the "representation") is degraded in some way. Although it would be empirically difficult to distinguish these causes of PPEs, one can imagine that disruption of white matter tracts, leading to impaired connections between critical nodes of a network, could lead to any of these 3 causes of such errors.

Although there was not a one-to-one correspondence between the dysgraphia type and the PPA variant, at a group level the majority of participants with Pattern 1 (reliance on POC mechanisms) had svPPA, and the majority of participants with Pattern 3 (impaired POC mechanisms as well as partially impaired access to orthographic word forms) had lvPPA. The majority of participants with impairment at the level of the graphemic buffer (Type 4) had nfvPPA. The only patient with abolished POC mechanisms and production of predominantly semantic errors in writing (Type 2) also had nfvPPA. These results indicate that the dysgraphia subtype might provide a diagnostic clue early in the course of PPA. For example, Case 1 did not initially meet criteria for svPPA as he had intact word and object comprehension, but had predominantly PPEs in spelling. Later he developed severe word and object comprehension deficits with clear svPPA. Likewise, Case 2 initially did not meet criteria for svPPA, because of intact word and object comprehension. At that time, she did show the Type 1 pattern of performance, with predominantly PPE's. Later, when she maintained this pattern of performance in spelling, albeit with lower spelling accuracy, she was diagnosed with svPPA.

Identification of the cognitive and neural substrates that are impaired in cases of dysgraphia in PPA can not only provide a better understanding of the neural substrates of spelling, but may also provide clues to more effective treatment approaches. Although PPA is a progressive condition, intervention can be helpful in at least temporarily improving production of trained sets of words in both speech [47] and writing [48], which in turn may improve the individual's quality of life, sense of accomplishment and perhaps contribute to their maintenance of language functions over time. Other reasonable goals of treatment might be to reduce the rate of language decline and to provide effective alternative communication strategies.

Acknowledgments

The research reported in this paper was supported by NIH (NIDCD), through RO1 DC 05375 and RO1 DC 03681 (AEH); UL1 RR 025005 from NCRR/NIH and NIH Roadmap for Medical Research (AVF), and UK MRC Clinical Scientist Fellowship G0701888 (JC). We gratefully acknowledge this support and the involvement of the participants.

References

[1] M.L. Henry, P.M. Beeson, A.J. Stark and S.Z. Rapcsak, The role of left perisylvian cortical regions in spelling, *Brain Lang* **100**(1) (Jan 2007), 44–52.

[2] P.M. Beeson, S.Z. Rapcsak, E. Plante, J. Chargualaf, A. Chung, S.C. Johnson et al., The neural substrates of writing: A functional magnetic resonance imaging study, *Aphasiology* **17** (2003), 647–665.

[3] L.E. Philipose, R.F. Gottesman, M. Newhart, J.T. Kleinman, E.H. Herskovits, M.A. Pawlak et al., Neural regions essential for reading and spelling of words and pseudowords, *Ann Neurol* **62**(5) (Nov 2007), 481–492.

[4] A.E. Hillis, S. Chang, E. Breese and J. Heidler, The crucial role of posterior frontal regions in modality specific components of the spelling process, *Neurocase* **10**(2) (Apr 2004), 175–187.

[5] A.E. Hillis, B.C. Rapp and A. Caramazza, When a rose is a rose in speech but a tulip in writing, *Cortex* **35**(3) (Jun 1999), 337–356.

[6] M.M. Mesulam, Slowly progressive aphasia without generalized dementia, *Ann Neurol* **11**(6) (Jun 1982), 592–598.

[7] M.L. Gorno-Tempini, A.E. Hillis, S. Weintraub, A. Kertesz, M. Mendez, S.F. Cappa et al., Classification of primary progressive aphasia and its variants, *Neurology* **76**(11) (15 Mar 2011), 1006–1014.

[8] P. Beeson and A.E. Hillis, Comprehension and production of written words, in: *Language Intervention Strategies in Aphasia and Related Neurogenic Communication Disorders*, (4th ed.), R. Chapey, ed., Baltimore: Williams and Wilkens, 2001, pp. 572–604.

[9] A.V. Faria, A. Hoon, E. Stashinko, X. Li, H. Jiang, A. Mashayekh et al., Quantitative analysis of brain pathology based on MRI and brain atlases–applications for cerebral palsy, *Neuroimage* **54**(3) (1 Feb 2011), 1854–1861.

[10] A.V. Faria, J. Zhang, K. Oishi, X. Li, H. Jiang, K. Akhter et al., Atlas-based analysis of neurodevelopment from infancy to adulthood using diffusion tensor imaging and applications for automated abnormality detection, *Neuroimage* **52**(2) (23 Apr 2010), 415–428.

[11] K. Oishi, A. Faria, H. Jiang, X. Li, K. Akhter, J. Zhang et al., Atlas-based whole brain white matter analysis using large deformation diffeomorphic metric mapping: application to normal elderly and Alzheimer's disease participantstlas, *Neuroimage* **46**(2) (Jun 2009), 486–499.

[12] S. Mori, K. Oishi, H. Jiang, L. Jiang, X. Li, K. Akhter et al., Stereotaxic white matter atlas based on diffusion tensor imaging in an ICBM template, *Neuroimage* **40**(2) (1 Apr 2008), 570–582.

[13] C. Ceritoglu, K. Oishi, X. Li, M.C. Chou, L. Younes, M. Albert et al., Multi-contrast large deformation diffeomorphic metric mapping for diffusion tensor imaging, *Neuroimage* **47**(2) (15 Aug 2009), 618–627.

[14] K. Oishi, K. Zilles, K. Amunts, A. Faria, H. Jiang, X. Li et al., Human brain white matter atlas: identification and assignment of common anatomical structures in superficial white matter, *Neuroimage* **43**(3) (15 Nov 2008), 447–457.

[15] W.R. Riddle, R. Li, J.M. Fitzpatrick, S.C. DonLevy, B.M. Dawant and R.R. Price, Characterizing changes in MR images with color-coded, *Jacobians Magn Reson Imaging* **22**(6) (Jul 2004), 769–777.

[16] M.K. Chung, K.J. Worsley, T. Paus, C. Cherif, D.L. Collins, J.N. Giedd et al., A unified statistical approach to deformation-based morphometry, *Neuroimage* **14**(3) (Sep 2001), 595–606.

[17] A.E. Hillis and A. Caramazza, Mechanisms for accessing lexical representations for output: evidence from a category-specific semantic deficit, *Brain Lang* **40**(1) (Jan 1991), 106–144.

[18] A.E. Hillis and A. Caramazza, Converging evidence for the interaction of semantic and phonological information in accessing lexical information for spoken output, *Cogn Nuropsychol* **12** (1995), 187–227.

[19] D. Howard and K. Patterson, Inventors. Pearson, assignee, The Pyramid and palm trees test, 1992.

[20] A.E. Hillis, J.T. Kleinman, M. Newhart, J. Heidler-Gary, R. Gottesman, P.B. Barker et al., Restoring cerebral blood flow reveals neural regions critical for naming, *J Neurosci* **26**(31) (2 Aug 2006), 8069–8073.

[21] A. Caramazza, G. Miceli, G. Villa and C. Romani, The role of the Graphemic Buffer in spelling: evidence from a case of acquired dysgraphia, *Cognition* **26**(1) (Jun 1987), 59–85.

[22] A. Caramazza and G. Miceli, Orthographic structure, the graphemic buffer and the spelling process, in: *Brain and Reading: MacMillan/Wenner-Gren*, C. von Euler, I. Lundberg and G. Lennerstrand, eds, 1989.

[23] L. Posteraro, P. Zinelli and A. Mazzucchi, Selective impairment of the graphemic buffer in acquired dysgraphia: a case study, *Brain Lang* **35**(2) (Nov 1988), 274–286.

[24] A.E. Hillis and A. Caramazza, The graphemic buffer and attentional mechanisms, *Brain Lang* **36**(2) (Feb 1989), 208–235.

[25] S.Z. Rapcsak and P.M. Beeson, Neuroanatomical correlates of spelling and writing, in: *Handbook of Adult Language Disorders: Integrating Cognitive Neuropsychology*, A.E. Hillis, ed., Neurology, and Rehabilitation Philadelphia: Psychology Press, 2002, pp. 71–99.

[26] A.E. Hillis, A. Kane, E. Tuffiash, N. Beauchamp, P.B. Barker, M.A. Jacobs et al., Neural substrates of the cognitive processes underlying spelling: Evidence from MR diffusion and perfusion imaging, *Aphasiology* **16** (2002), 425–438.

[27] L. Cloutman, L. Gingis, M. Newhart, C. Davis, J. Heidler-Gary, J. Crinion et al., A neural network critical for spelling, *Ann Neurol* **66**(2) (Aug 2009), 249–253.

[28] J.S. Bedwell, M.D. Horner, K. Yamanaka, X. Li, H. Myrick, Z. Nahas et al., Functional neuroanatomy of subcomponent cognitive processes involved in verbal working memory, *Int J Neurosci* **115**(7) (Jul 2005), 1017–1032.

[29] S. Crottaz-Herbette, R.T. Anagnoson and V. Menon, Modality effects in verbal working memory: differential prefrontal and parietal responses to auditory and visual stimuli, *Neuroimage* **21**(1) (Jan 2004), 340–351.

[30] J. Jonides, E.H. Schumacher, E.E. Smith, R.A. Koeppe, E. Awh, P.A. Reuter-Lorenz et al., The role of parietal cortex in verbal working memory, *J Neurosci* **18**(13) (1 Jul 1998), 5026–5034.

[31] C. Wendelken, S.A. Bunge and C.S. Carter, Maintaining structured information: an investigation into functions of parietal and lateral prefrontal cortices, *Neuropsychologia* **46**(2) (31 Jan 2008), 665–678.

[32] Y. Xu and M.M. Chun, Dissociable neural mechanisms supporting visual short-term memory for objects, *Nature* **440**(7080) (2 Mar 2006), 91–95.

[33] A. Caramazza and A.E. Hillis, Lexical organization of nouns and verbs in the brain, *Nature* **349**(6312) (28 Feb 1991), 788–790.

[34] Y. Bi, T. Wei, C. Wu, Z. Han, T. Jiang and A. Caramazza, The role of the left anterior temporal lobe in language processing revisited: Evidence from an individual with ATL resection, *Cortex* **47**(5) (May 2011), 575–587.

[35] R.J. Binney, K.V. Embleton, E. Jefferies, G.J. Parker and M.A. Ralph, The ventral and inferolateral aspects of the anterior temporal lobe are crucial in semantic memory: evidence from a novel direct comparison of distortion-corrected fMRI, rTMS, and semantic dementia, *Cereb Cortex* **20**(11) (Nov 2010), 2728–2738.

[36] M.A. Lambon Ralph, L. Cipolotti, F. Manes and K. Patterson, Taking both sides: do unilateral anterior temporal lobe lesions disrupt semantic memory? *Brain* **133**(11) (Nov 2010), 3243–3255.

[37] K. Patterson, P.J. Nestor and T.T. Rogers, Where do you know what you know? The representation of semantic knowledge in the human brain, *Nat Rev Neurosci* **8**(12) (Dec 2007), 976–987.

[38] G. Pobric, E. Jefferies and M.A. Ralph, Amodal semantic representations depend on both anterior temporal lobes: evidence from repetitive transcranial magnetic stimulation, *Neuropsychologia* **48**(5) (Apr 2010), 1336–1342.

[39] T.T. Rogers, J. Hocking, U. Noppeney, A. Mechelli, M.L. Gorno-Tempini, K. Patterson et al., Anterior temporal cortex and semantic memory: reconciling findings from neuropsychology and functional imaging, *Cogn Affect Behav Neurosci* **6**(3) (Sep 2006), 201–213.

[40] M.F. Schwartz, D.Y. Kimberg, G.M. Walker, O. Faseyitan, A. Brecher, G.S. Dell et al., Anterior temporal involvement in semantic word retrieval: voxel-based lesion-symptom mapping evidence from aphasia, *Brain* **132**(Pt 12) (Dec 2009), 3411–3427.

[41] W.K. Simmons and A. Martin, The anterior temporal lobes and the functional architecture of semantic memory, *J Int Neuropsychol Soc* **15**(5) (Sep 2009), 645–649.

[42] D. Tranel, Impaired naming of unique landmarks is associated with left temporal polar damage, *Neuropsychology* **20**(1) (Jan 2006), 1–10.

[43] D. Tranel, H. Damasio and A.R. Damasio, A neural basis for the retrieval of conceptual knowledge, *Neuropsychologia* **35**(10) (Oct 1997), 1319–1327.

[44] K. Tsapkini, C.E. Frangakis and A.E. Hillis, The function of the left anterior temporal pole: evidence from acute stroke and infarct volume, *Brain* **134**(10) (17 Jun 2011), 3094–3105.

[45] G.M. Walker, M.F. Schwartz, D.Y. Kimberg, O. Faseyitan, A. Brecher, G.S. Dell et al., Support for anterior temporal involvement in semantic error production in aphasia: new evidence from VLSM, *Brain Lang* **117**(3) (Jun 2011), 110–122.

[46] D. Kemmerer, D. Rudrauf, K. Manzel and D. Tranel, Behavioral patterns and lesion sites associated with impaired processing of lexical and conceptual knowledge of actions, *Cortex* (18 Nov 2010).

[47] M. Newhart, C. Davis, V. Kannan, J. Heidler-Gary, L. Cloutman and A.E. Hillis, Therapy for naming deficits in two variants of primary progressive aphasia, *Aphasiology* **23** (2009), 823–834.

[48] B. Rapp and B. Glucroft, The benefits and protective effects of behavioural treatment for dysgraphia in a case of primary progressive aphasia, *Aphasiology* **23**(2) (2009), 236–235.

12

Demonstrating the qualitative differences between semantic aphasia and semantic dementia: A novel exploration of nonverbal semantic processing

Krist A. Noonan[a], Elizabeth Jefferies[b], Sheeba Eshan[a], Peter Garrard[c] and
Matthew A. Lambon Ralph[a,*]
[a]School of Psychological Sciences, University of Manchester, Manchester, UK
[b]Department of Psychology, University of York, York, UK
[c]Stroke and Dementia Research Centre, St George's University of London, London, UK

Abstract. Semantic dementia (SD) implicates the anterior temporal lobes (ATL) as a critical substrate for semantic memory. Multi-modal semantic impairment can also be a feature of post-stroke aphasia (referred to here as "semantic aphasia" or SA) where patients show impaired regulatory control accompanied by lesions to the frontal and/or temporo-parietal cortices, and thus the two patient groups demonstrate qualitatively different patterns of semantic impairment [1]. Previous comparisons of these two patient groups have tended to focus on verbal receptive tasks. Accordingly, this study investigated nonverbal receptive abilities via a comparison of reality decision judgements in SD and SA. Pictures of objects were presented alongside non-real distracters whose features were altered to make them more/less plausible for the semantic category. The results highlighted a number of critical differences between the two groups. Compared to SD patients, SA patients: (1) were relatively unimpaired on the two alternative forced choice (2AFC) decisions despite showing a comparable degree of semantic impairment on other assessments; (2) showed minimal effects of the plausibility manipulation; (3) were strongly influenced by variations in the regulatory requirements of tasks; and (4) exhibited a reversed effect of familiarity – i.e., better performance on less commonly encountered items. These results support a distinction between semantic impairments which arise from impaired regulatory processes (e.g., SA) versus those where degraded semantic knowledge is the causal factor (e.g., SD). SA patients performed relatively well because the task structure reduced the requirement for internally generated control. In contrast, SD patients performed poorly because their degraded knowledge did not allow the fine-grained distinctions required to complete the task.

Keywords: Semantic representation, semantic control, aphasia, semantic dementia, feature reality task

1. Introduction

Semantic cognition is fundamental to our everyday lives because it allows us to activate and utilise conceptual knowledge in a flexible, time- and context-

appropriate fashion. This requires comprehension of objects in terms of their core similarities and differences and not just their superficial characteristics [2, 3]. In addition, semantic cognition (rather than semantic memory alone) requires executive regulation to focus on which specific aspects of our rich semantic database are appropriate for the task in hand [4, 5]. Semantic dementia (SD), a condition associated with bilateral anterior temporal lobe (ATL) degeneration, is the purest example of degraded semantic knowledge [6]. SD patients exhibit a frequency graded loss of semantic knowledge across all testing modalities

*Address for correspondence: Prof. M.A. Lambon Ralph, Neuroscience and Aphasia Research Unit (NARU), Zochonis Building, School of Psychological Sciences, University of Manchester, Oxford Road, Manchester, M13 9PL, UK.
E-mail: matt.lambon-ralph@manchester.ac.uk.

(e.g., pictures, words, sounds, smells) and gradually lose the fine-grained knowledge required to distinguish between similar concepts [7–9]. This supports the idea that the ATL bilaterally is a critical substrate for semantic representations and SD represents a 'dimming' of semantic acuity [10]. Multimodal semantic impairments can also emerge in the context of stroke aphasia (referred to here as semantic aphasia or SA) where damage is restricted to the left hemisphere, in areas outside the ATL [1]. Recent investigations show that these patients do not have degraded knowledge, but that their semantic performance is modulated by the requirement for regulatory control [5,11–13]. These earlier studies utilised verbally-based tasks in order to manipulate key control-related factors or used more inherently complex open-ended assessments of object use. Given that both patient groups exhibit nonverbal as well as verbal comprehension impairment, a dedicated comparison of the nature of nonverbal receptive skills in SD and SA is required. Accordingly, this paper directly compares both patient groups on a multimodal feature reality task to examine the hypothesis that, in line with the results from verbal assessment, the two patient groups present with qualitatively different patterns of nonverbal semantic performance.

Since the earliest observations of SD it has been recognised that conceptual loss is graded in nature [14]. Aside from the benefits derived by frequently encountered items, concepts with the highest proportion of shared features (i.e., the most *typical* concepts from a semantic category) tend to survive the longest and exert a strong influence on residual semantic processing. In picture naming, this is evident in patients' errors, where the names of frequent and typical category members are often erroneously produced and inappropriately overextended (e.g., *cat* for a picture of a *squirrel*). SD patients also produce many superordinate errors, where they identify pictures as belonging to a particular category but are unable to produce the specific name (e.g., *squirrel* → "*animal*"). Recent computational models of the ATL provide a principled explanation for these findings. Rogers et al. [15] conceptualised the bilateral ATL as a semantic hub that extracts amodal structure from multimodal experience (see also [3,16]). Importantly, in this model, concepts with many shared features contribute the most towards change in connection weights and lead to the entrenchment of broad category boundaries which are highly resistant to damage [17]. Distinctive features (e.g., a *squirrel's* bushy tail; an *elephant's* trunk) that allow discrimination between similar category members are the most vulnerable to damage because they lack the redundancy provided by consistent collateral activation. Many of the key typicality findings in the SD literature have been simulated by this model including patterns of longitudinal naming performance [i.e., the way that responses become more general over time: 8]) and the tendency to omit specific features in delayed picture copying [e.g., drawing a camel without its hump; 15].

In line with this framework, Garrard and Carroll [18] demonstrated that SD patients were poor at making alternative forced-choice reality decision judgements when the distracter was characterised by a feature that was not possessed by the pictured item, but was applicable to the item's semantic neighbours. More specifically, SD patients had difficulty choosing the real object when the non-real distracter items had a colour, sound or environmental context consistent with other real semantic items (e.g., colour condition: greater difficulty choosing a *red strawberry* when accompanied with a *green strawberry*, than when paired with a *blue strawberry*). Critically, impairment on this task correlated strongly with background tests of semantic knowledge and patients were highly consistent across conditions, supporting the idea that the progressive 'dimming' of amodal semantic representations was the causal factor in each of these tasks.

The nature of the semantic impairment in SA is quite different. Although patients with SA can show an equivalent degree of impairment across verbal and non-verbal versions of semantic tasks, degraded representations do not appear to be the causal factor. In contrast to SD patients, individuals with SA (1) show variable performance across tests requiring different types of semantic judgements [e.g., naming vs. associative decisions; 1]; (2) are sensitive to refractory/access variables [i.e., speed of presentation, item repetition and semantic blocking; 12]; (3) exhibit minimal or no effects of frequency/familiarity [12]; (4) demonstrate strong effects of cues in picture naming, object use and synonym judgement [1,5,11,13]; and (5) have lesions in prefrontal (PFC) and/or the pMTG-to-angular gyrus region (temporo-parietal junction (TPJ), sparing the ATL [1,19]. These results indicate that, following lesions to the PFC or TPJ, patients develop increased sensitivity to competition within the semantic system: although their semantic representations are not severely degraded (and in fact may not be impaired at all), access to this knowledge is deregulated following impaired semantic control. This pattern has been replicated by repetitive transcranial magnetic stimulation studies in control participants [20]. Functional neuroimag-

Table 1
Demographic information for SA patients

Patient	Age	Sex	Education (leaving age)	Neuroimaging summary	PFC	TPJ	Aetiology of CVA	Aphasia type
JD	81	M	16	Infarction of putamen and internal capsule. Compression of L lateral ventricle.	†	†	Haemorrhage	Mixed transcortical
NY	65	M	15	L frontal-temporal-parietal	√	√		Conduction
PG	62	M	18	L frontal and capsular (CT)	√	†	Subarachnoid haemorrhage	TSA
HN	78	M	14	L occipital-temporal	×	√	Ischemia	Anomic/TSA
SC	78	M	16	L occipital-temporal (& R frontal-parietal)	×	√	Haemorrhage	Anomic/TSA
BB	57	F	16	L frontal & capsular (CT)	√	√	Subarachnoid haemorrhage	Mixed transcortical
ME	39	F	16	L occipital-temporal	×	√	Subarachnoid haemorrhage	TSA
KA	76	M	14	L frontal-temporal-parietal	√	√	Thomboembolic/partial haemorrhage	Global
LS	73	M	15	L temporal-parietal-frontal	√	√		TSA

Patients are arranged in order of composite semantic score (see Table 2). Aphasia classifications were derived from the Boston Diagnostic Aphasia Examination [BDAE; 48]. JD withdrew from the study before the BDAE could be administered therefore classification was based on background assessments of fluency, repetition and comprehension. TSA = Transcortical sensory aphasia. Neuroimaging summaries are based on visual inspection of CT/MRI scans, except in the cases of PG and JD where only written reports of clinical scans were available. PFC = lesion involves left prefrontal cortex; TPJ = lesion involves left temporoparietal junction; †= neuroradiological information is not sufficient to make a definitive statement regarding the extent of cortical damage.

ing studies of healthy participants are also consistent with this view. For example, the process of orientating attention to particular semantic categories, processing the non-literal meaning of metaphors and retrieving the less dominant meanings of ambiguous words gives rise to activation in both TPJ and inferior PFC regions [21–23]. Anatomically, these two cortical areas (i.e., PFC and TPJ) are strongly connected by the arcuate and superior longitudinal fasciculi, and may form a distributed but functionally coherent system [24,25].

Although the nature of the semantic impairment in SD and SA is very different, reflecting degraded semantic representations and impaired semantic control respectively, both types of impairment affect nonverbal as well as verbal comprehension. Garrard and Carroll [18] used a series of novel, nonverbal reality decision judgements to probe the nature of nonverbal semantic processing in semantic dementia and in this study we compared these results to those obtained for a group of SA patients. In doing so, this study is the first to investigate the impact of *feature* typicality in SA. As noted above, SD patients lack knowledge of the specific features of objects and will base their decisions on more general information. For this reason, SD patients are highly susceptible to 'plausible' distracter items which have a strong overlap with the target and other semantic neighbours [18]. SA patients should be less vulnerable to 'plausible' distracters because they retain intact semantic representations that include the unique features

of items. In addition, SA patients will benefit from the use of a 2AFC format because this form of assessment reduces the requirement for internally-generated control and minimises competition between potential response choices. These patients may therefore be relatively unimpaired when making reality judgements, even when they are matched to SD patients for other semantic test results.

2. Participants

A total of nine SA patients took part in the study. Their ages ranged from 39 to 81, with a mean of 67 years. On average the patients completed eleven years of education. All of the patients had chronic impairments resulting from a CVA at least one year prior to testing. Patients were selected to show multimodal semantic deficits affecting the comprehension of words and pictures (see Table 2). The group included patients with fluent and less fluent profiles (Table 1 provides background aphasialogical and demographic information). Neuroradiological investigations (where available) confirmed that the SA patients had left hemisphere lesions in the PFC and/or the TPJ regions. Figure 1 presents MRI scans for SC, NY, HN, ME and LS as well as CT scans for BB and KA. MRI was not performed in PG or JD due to contraindications, although

Table 2
Background neuropsychology for the Semantic Aphasic patients

	Max	Normal cut off	JD	NY	PG	HN	SC	BB	ME	KA	LS
Semantic tests											
Composite semantic score			0.97	0.91	0.84	0.65	0.55	−0.20	−1.07	−1.20	−1.45
WPM	64	62	64	60*	58*	50	59*	54*	50*	26*	37*
Picture Naming	64	59	49	55*	46*	50	28*	10*	5*	0*	5*
CCTp	64	51	38	36*	44*	44	46*	38*	13*	46*	16*
Background Neuropsychology											
VOSP Screening	20	15	20	19	20	19	20	20	19	20	18
VOSP Position Discrimination	20	18	20	20	20	19	17*	18	15*	14	16*
VOSP Number Location	10	7	10	10	9	9	0*	8	2*	6	8
Corsi span forward			4	4	5	4	3	5	3	5	3
Corsi span backward			3	4	2	4	3	0	2	2	2
Digit span forward	−	5	5	3*	6	6	6	5	6	0*	4*
Digit span backward	−	2	2	2	2	2	2	0*	3	NT	1*
Brixton Spatial Anticipation Test (correct)	55	28	28	34	26*	27*	25*	23*	11*	6*	14*
TEA: elevator counting (no distraction)	7	6	7	3*	3*	7	7	4*	7	TA	3*
TEA: elevator counting (distraction)	10	3	6	2*	0*	9	1*	0*	9	NT	2*
Hayling sentences: A (errors)	15	−	1	3	3	1	5	3	1	TA	8
Hayling sentences: B (errors)	15	−	6	8	1	12	6	6	3	TA	6
Raven's coloured matrices (correct)	−	−	30	28	27	20	28	32	16	17	24
WCST (no. categories)	6	1	1	2	0*	NT	6	1	0*	1	0*

Patients are arranged in order of their composite semantic scores derived from the three background tests of semantic processing (i.e., WPM, picture naming, CCTp). WPM = word to picture matching; CCTp = picture version of the Camel and Cactus Test [7]; VOSP = Visual Object and Space Perception battery [26]; TEA = Test of Everyday Attention [32]; WCST = Wisconsin Card Sorting Test [30,31]. *denotes impaired performance. NT = not tested. TA = testing abandoned.

written reports of previous CT scans were available for both cases.

The SA group was compared with 12 SD cases recruited from specialist memory clinics in London and Cambridge. Ages ranged from 56 to 73, with a mean of 64 years. On average, patients completed 13 years of education. These patients were first described by Garrard and Carroll [18]. Their data are re-reported here in order to license a direct comparison to those obtained for the SA patients. All SD cases fulfilled all of the published criteria for SD [6]. Patients presented with word-finding difficulties in the context of fluent speech and were impaired on tests of single word comprehension and semantic knowledge. In contrast, phonology, syntax, nonverbal reasoning and visuo-spatial processing were relatively well preserved. They all showed relatively circumscribed atrophy of the anterior temporal lobes.

Twelve control participants were selected from a volunteer database to match as closely as possible the age and educational level of the patient groups. This group ranged in age from 41 to 78, with a mean of 67 years. Controls completed, on average, 12 years of full-time education.

3. Background neuropsychological assessment

3.1. General neuropsychological tests

Visual-spatial processing in both groups was assessed using the Visual Object and Space Processing battery [VOSP: 26]. Working memory in the SA group was examined using forward and backward digit span [27] and the Corsi block-tapping task [28]. A range of additional tests were used to assess executive/attentional functions in the SA group: (1) the Ravens Coloured Progressive Matrices test of nonverbal reasoning [29], (2) the Wisconsin Card Sorting test [30,31], (3) Elevator Counting with and without distraction from the Test of Everyday Attention [32], (4) the Brixton Spatial Rule Attainment task [33] and

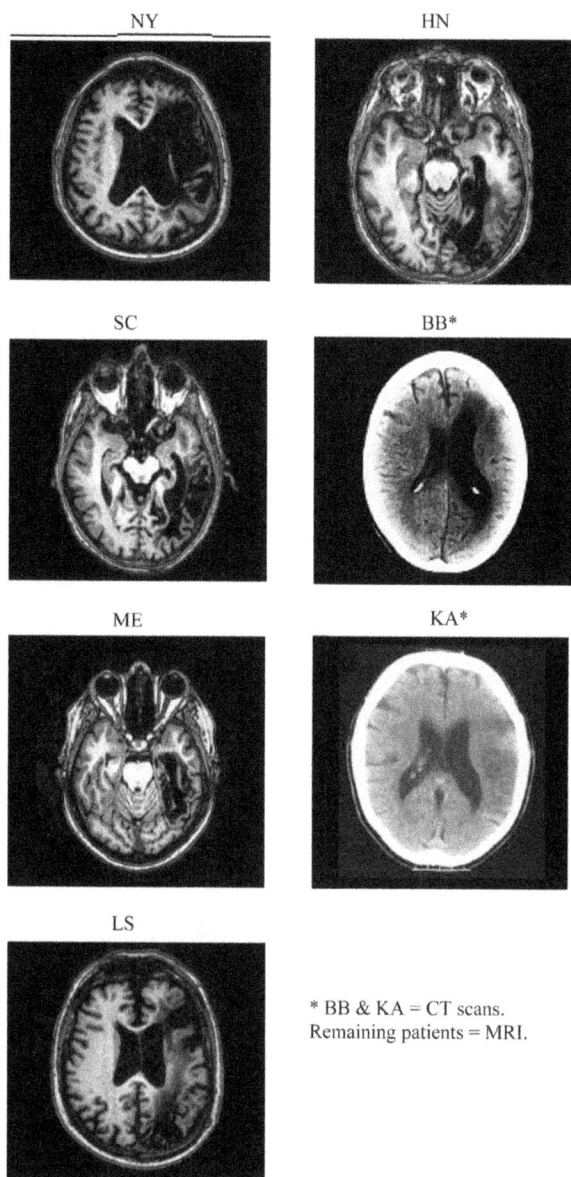

Fig. 1. Neuroimaging for the SA patients.

* BB & KA = CT scans.
Remaining patients = MRI.

(5) the Hayling Sentence Completion test [33] which contrasts the production of appropriate sentence endings (e.g., "It is hard to admit when one is... *wrong*") with nonsensical endings that require the prepotent word to be suppressed (e.g., "Most sharks attack very close to... *cups*").

3.2. Results

Tables 2 and 3 presents the background data for SA and SD patients, respectively. Visual-spatial processing was relatively preserved in the SA group: only three patients failed one or more subcomponents of the VOSP. Evidence of mild visual-spatial problems was also evident in three SD patients. Some SA patients showed additional problems on the memory span tasks (i.e., corsi block-tapping and digit span). However, all SA patients showed evidence of impaired executive/attentional processing.

3.3. Background semantic memory assessments

The presence of multimodal semantic impairment was assessed using a battery of semantic tests which tapped different input and output modalities for the same 64 items [7]. There were four test components:

1. Spoken word-picture matching (WPM): The patients were required to match a verbally presented word to a target picture presented alongside nine semantically related foils. The pictures were black and white line drawings taken from the Snodgrass and Vanderwart [34] corpus.
2. Picture naming: The patients named these drawings presented individually.
3. Camel and Cactus Test [CCT'; Bozeat et al. 7]: This test of semantic associations is similar to the Pyramid and Palm Trees test [35]. Patients were asked to decide which of four pictures was most associated to a probe picture: e.g., "camel" with "cactus", "rose", "tree" or "sunflower"?

A composite score reflecting each patient's overall semantic abilities was derived from these three semantic tests using factor analysis. This score was computed separately for each patient group, with larger numbers representing better semantic performance. All tables are ordered by this score.

3.4. Background semantic test results

Tables 2 and 3 show that every patient, regardless of group, was impaired on all background semantic tasks. SA and SD patients showed no quantitative difference in their level of impairment across picture naming, WPM and CCTp (all t values < 1; see Fig. 2). As expected given their amodal semantic breakdown, SD patients showed strong correlations across all three semantic tasks ($r > 0.84$, $p < 0.001$). In line with underlying poor executive-semantic control [1], the SA patients were far less consistent, showing a correlation between the two tasks which required identity matching (e.g., WPM and naming: $r = 0.72$, $p < 0.03$) but not between CCTp and WPM or CCTp and naming ($r > 0.45$, $p > 0.2$). SA patients also showed correlations between their semantic test performance and measures

Table 3
Background neuropsychology for the Semantic Dementia patients

	Max	Normal cut off	JM	NG	BG	AN	VH	RW	DW	TW	WM	IB	FO	AT
Semantic tests														
Composite semantic score			1.06	1.02	0.97	0.82	0.49	0.28	0.05	−0.80	−0.95	−1.41	−1.51	−
WPM	64	62	61*	59*	61*	62	59*	56*	49*	38*	18*	19*	11*	NT
Picture Naming	64	59	48*	60*	41*	41*	38*	39*	33*	8*	10*	5*	1*	0*
CCTp	64	51	54	46*	55	49*	41*	35*	35*	27*	33*	19*	23*	NT
Background Neuropsychology														
VOSP Screening	20	15	19	19	20	20	20	18	18	NT	20	NT	NT	19
VOSP Position Discrimination	20	18	20	10*	19	20	20	20	19	NT	20	NT	NT	NT
VOSP Number Location	10	7	10	10	6*	10	10	6*	10	NT	10	NT	NT	NT
GNT	30	−	3*	NT	6*	1	11*	0	0	0	0	0	0	0
MMSE	30	26	28	NT	27	27	27	24	25	23	21	23	NT	15

Patients are arranged in order of their composite semantic scores derived from the three background tests of semantic processing (i.e., WPM, picture naming, CCTp). PM = word to picture matching; CCTp = picture version of the Camel and Cactus Test [7]; VOSP = Visual Object and Space Perception battery [26]; GNT = Graded Naming Test [49]; MMSE = Mini-mental State Exam [50]* denotes impaired performance. NT = not tested. TA = testing abandoned.

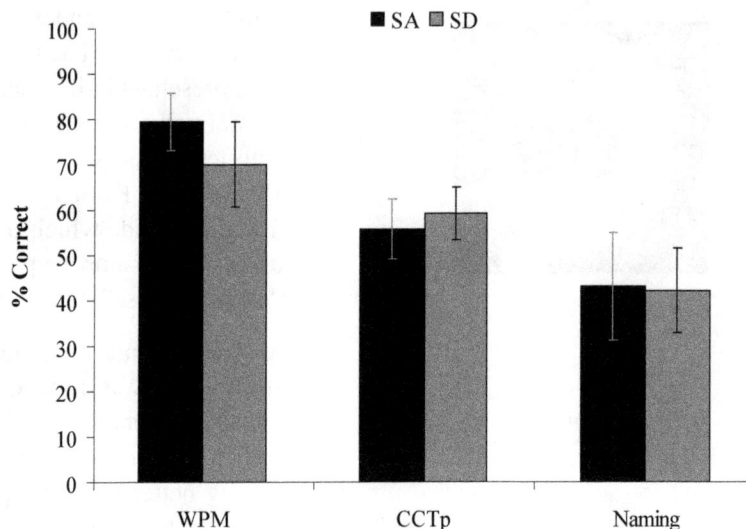

Fig. 2. Background semantic scores.

of executive/attentional control. Scores on the Brixton spatial anticipation test (number correct) and Raven's Coloured Matrices correlated with the composite semantic scores for this group (one-tailed: $r = 0.92, p < 0.001$; $r = 0.59$, $p < 0.05$, respectively), while the correlation between semantic severity and backwards Corsi approached significance ($r = 0.51$, $p = 0.08$ one-tailed).

4. Experimental task – Feature Reality Task

4.1. Method

Participants were presented with pairs of pictures and asked to indicate the 'more real-looking' of the two.

The two pictures in each presentation differed along a single feature dimension (i.e., colour, environmental context, sound or motion). The real pictures were presented alongside either plausible or implausible distracter images. Plausible distracters were constructed by manipulating one of the target object's features such that it was typical of other exemplars from the targets semantic category. In contrast, implausible distracters possessed features which not were typical of the targets' neighbours. Thirty-three concrete concepts were used in this experiment, selected from a range of living and non-living categories. Each item appeared in at least two of the four experimental conditions (see Table 4). Specific details about each of the four conditions are provided below.

4.2. Condition 1: Colour

Twenty-nine concepts were presented as coloured line drawings. Each appropriately coloured line drawing was presented twice – once with a duplicate coloured in a typical way for that semantic category (e.g., *grey elephant* presented with a *brown elephant*) and once with an atypically coloured distracter (e.g., *pink elephant*).

4.3. Condition 2: Environmental Context

Twenty-nine pictures were superimposed on an environmental context. The real items were presented in their most common context (e.g., *horse* in a *field*). Distracter items were presented on either a plausible context (e.g. *horse* in a *desert*) or implausible context (e.g., *horse* in a *shopping centre*).

4.4. Condition 3: Sound

Twenty-six black and white line drawings were accompanied by sounds. Plausible distracter images were taken from the same domain as the target – and produced similar types of sound (e.g., the target *dog* presented alongside a picture of a *cat*). Pictures from the opposing semantic domain – which were associated with very different sounds – were used as implausible distracters (e.g., the target *dog* presented alongside a picture of an *alarm clock*).

4.5. Condition 4: Motion

Twenty concepts were presented as of pairs of animations, each showing the same item involved in two distinct kinds of motion. For example, a *cow* was depicted as chewing and swinging its tail from side to side in the target animation but as rearing up on its hind legs in the manner of a *horse*, in the distracter image. The plausibility manipulation was not incorporated into the motion test.

5. Results

5.1. Overall accuracy

Figure 3 shows the performance of the patients and controls on the four conditions of the feature reality task. A 3 (group) by 4 (condition) ANOVA revealed a main effect of group (F (2,30) = 23.25, $p < 0.001$); post hoc comparisons showed the control group performed better than both patient groups, while SA patients performed better than SD patients (Bonferroni $p < 0.05$). There was no effect of condition.

Table 4
Familiarity ratings for items in the FRT

Item	Mean Familiarity	Colour	Context	Sound	Motion
Apple	4.9				
Banana	4.48				
Bee	2.43				
Cat	3.62				
Clock	4.86				
Cow	2.29				
Crab	1.38				
Dog	3.52				
Duck	2.48				
Egg	4.47				
Elephant	1.43				
Fire Engine	2.86				
Frog	2.14				
Guitar	2.23				
Hammer	2.9				
Helicopter	2.57				
Horse	2.86				
Kangaroo	1.38				
Mouse	1.9				
Orange	4				
Penguin	1.38				
Piano	3.33				
Pig	1.86				
Pigeon	3.76				
Saw	2.33				
Scissors	4.48				
Snowman	2.1				
Suitcase	3.76				
Tap					
Tiger	1.33				
Tortoise	1.38				
Trumpet	1.67				
Windmill	1.71				

5.2. Plausibility effects

The effect of distracter plausibility was investigated using a 3 (group) by 2 (distracter plausibility) ANOVA. Plausible distracters resulted in less accurate performance overall (F (1,30) = 58.35, $p < 0.001$). This effect was most evident in the SD group, resulting in a group by plausibility interaction (F (2,30) = 8.89, $p = 0.001$; see Fig. 4). Bonferroni comparisons confirmed that the plausibility effect was strongest in the SD group (t (11) = 5.6, $p < 0.001$) but also present to a lesser extent in the SA (t (8) = 4.1, $p < 0.01$) and control (t (11) = 3.8, $p < 0.01$) groups.

Given the excellent performance of the SA patients, we also examined the effects of the plausibility manipulation on RT using a 2 (SA vs. control group) by 2 (distracter plausibility) ANOVA. Incorrect responses and outliers (outside 2 SDs) were not included in the analysis. Although RT did not differ significantly between groups (F (1,19) < 1), there was a group by plausibility interaction (F (1,19) = 8.1, $p = 0.01$, see Fig. 5). RT was not affected by distracter plausibility

■ Colour ■ Context ▨ Sound □ Motion

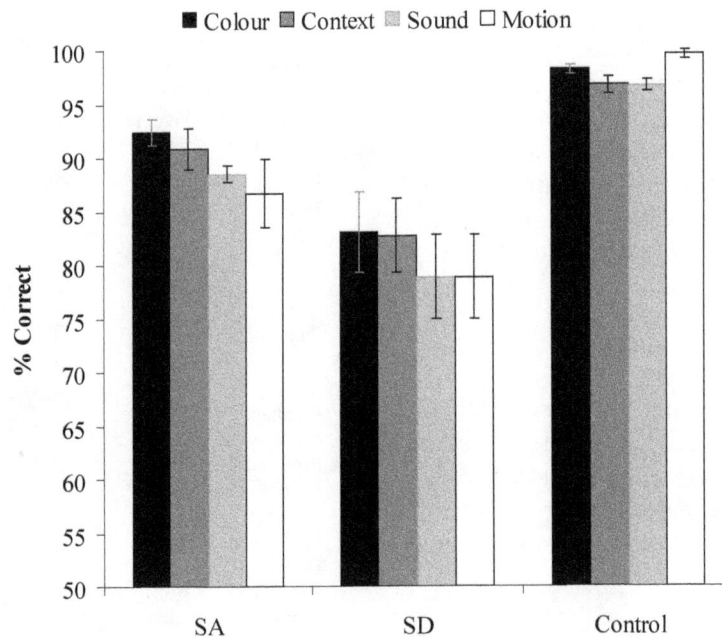

Fig. 3. Overall accuracy on the FRT.

■ Plausible ▨ Implausible

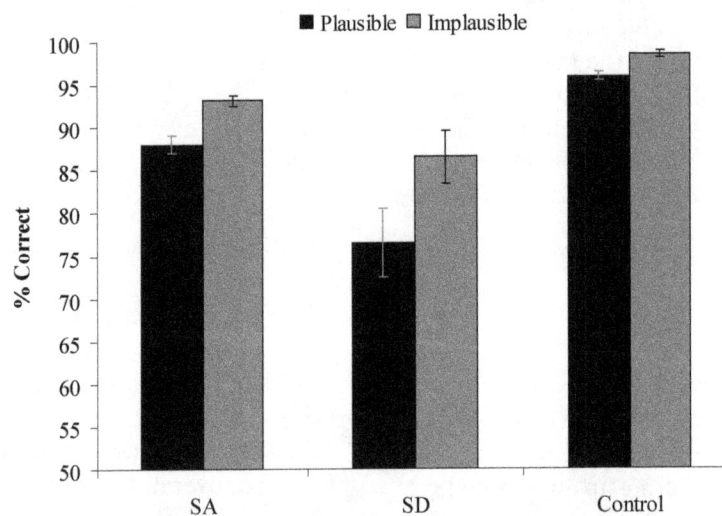

Fig. 4. Distracter plausibility and FRT accuracy.

in the SA group ($t < 1$), but a strong effect was present in the control group ($t(11) = 4.1$, $p < 0.005$ Bonferroni corrected). Individually, none of the SA patients showed a significant difference between plausible and implausible trials ($t < 1$). In contrast, 7/12 controls were significant slower on plausible trials ($t = 3–1.6$, $p < 0.05$ one-tailed).

5.3. Correlations between FRT components and background tasks

The SA group showed minimal correlations between the various sub-tasks within the FRT, in fact only one

of six possible correlations was significant (i.e., motion and context: $r = 0.69$, $p < 0.05$). Furthermore, none of the FRT sub-tasks correlated with any of the three background tests of semantic knowledge (naming: $r < 0.24$, $p > 0.5$; WPM: $r < 0.34$, $p > 0.2$; CCTp: $r < 0.41$, $p > 0.1$) or the composite semantic severity score ($r < 0.16$, $p > 0.6$). A similar pattern of non-significant correlations were observed when overall performance on each FRT sub-task was compared with scores on the background executive measures ($r < 0.4$, $p > 0.1$). In contrast, the SD group showed strong correlations between 3/4 of the FRT sub-tasks – i.e.,

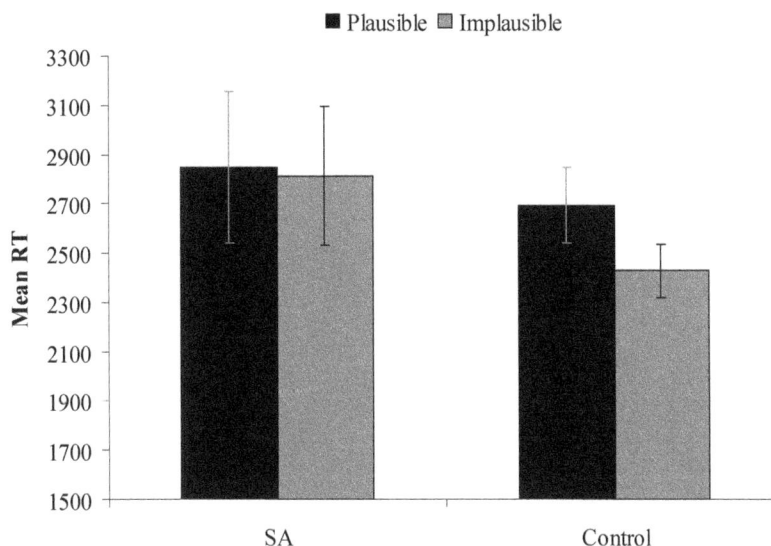

Fig. 5. FRT reaction times.

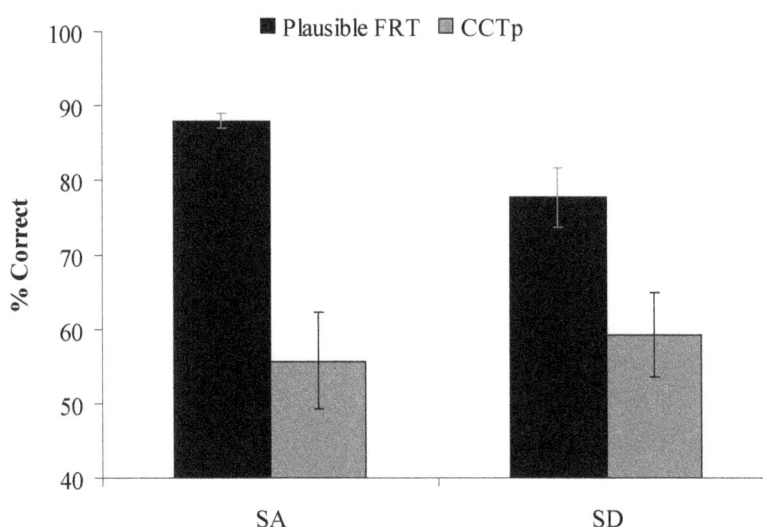

Fig. 6. Differential effects of regulatory demand on accuracy in SA and SD.

colour, context and sound all correlated with each other: $r > 0.73$, $p < 0.001$). These three conditions were also strongly correlated with composite semantic severity scores ($r > 0.69$, $p < 0.05$) and performance on each of the background semantic tasks ($r > 0.69$, $p < 0.05$). In contrast, the motion sub-task did not correlated with any of the other FRT sub-tasks or performance on the background semantic measures ($r = -0.29$–0.13, $p > 0.3$).

5.4. The relationship between regulatory constraints and task performance

To investigate whether the differential plausibility effects in SA and SD arose from the semantic control demands of the tasks, patient performance on plausible trials was directly compared with the two background receptive tasks (i.e., WPM and CCTp). The CCTp places higher demands on semantic elaboration and inhibitory control because it is necessary to work out which aspect of an object's meaning is relevant on any given trial. For example, we know many things about *camels* and *cacti* so selecting the correct response requires the ability to focus on the relevant desert relationship. In contrast, WPM involves more straightforward identify matching and therefore might place fewer demands on semantic control. The 2AFC format of the FRT task might also reduce demands on semantic control leading to better performance in the SA than the SD group. Therefore, a group by task interaction

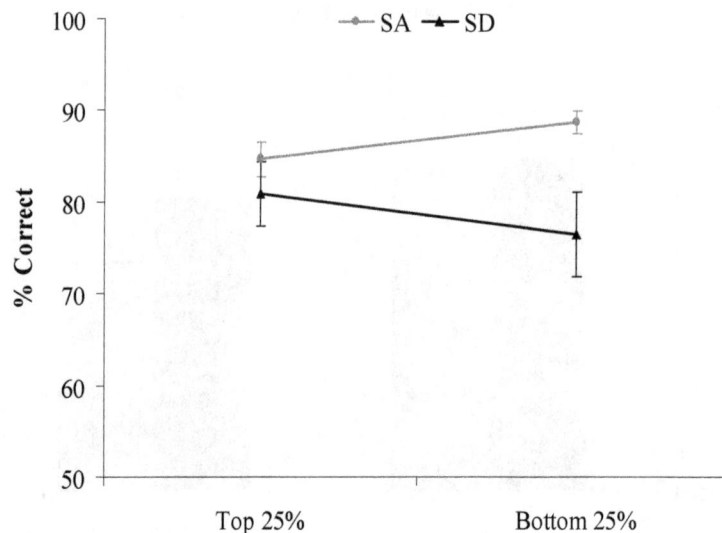

Fig. 7. Differential familiarity effects in SA and SD.

might be expected when the highly constrained FRT is compared with CCTp but not WPM. Both groups did better on the FRT task than the background measures (F (1,18) = 54, $p < 0.001$). However, as predicted, a group by task interaction emerged when plausible FRT trials were compared with the CCTp (F (1,18) = 4, $p = 0.06$). No interaction was present for the WPM comparison (F (1,18) < 1). The results suggest that group differences in FRT performance are underpinned by the minimal regulatory requirements of this task, combined with relative preservation of the specific features of concepts in the SA vs. SD group.

5.5. Familiarity effects

Previous work indicated that SA patients are less influenced by familiarity/frequency than SD patients [36]. This issue was examined using a series of logistic regression analyses which aimed to predict individual item accuracy. A combined group analysis including, familiarity, patient group and a group by familiarity interaction term significantly predicted behaviour (χ^2 (3) = 82.9, $p < 0.01$). Overall performance was influenced by both familiarity (Wald = 6.2, $p < 0.05$) and patient group (Wald = 35.96, $p < 0.001$), and a significant interaction emerged between these variables (Wald = 10.78, $p < 0.001$). Analysis on each group separately revealed that SA patients were influenced by familiarity (Wald = 5.16, $p < 0.05$), but counter intuitively, they were less likely to make an accurate judgement as item familiarity increased (Exp(B) 0.84, C.I.$_{95}$, 0.74–0.97). In contrast, SD patients showed the opposite pattern; the odds of making a correct judgement

increased with item familiarity (Exp(B) 1.13, C.I.$_{95}$, 1.07–1.24, Wald = 6.22, $p = 0.05$). In each of the above models, the predictive power and directionality of the familiarity effect was unaffected by the inclusion of distracter plausibility and patient identity as independent predictors (i.e., Wald values for familiarity remained within a similar range: 9.42–3.26, $p < 0.05$). A separate ANOVA analysis comparing performance on the most and least familiar items (i.e., top and bottom 25% of items) also yielded a group by familiarity interaction (F (1,19) = 5.2, $p < 0.03$, see Fig. 7). SA patients were less accurate on the high frequency items (t (8) = 1.9, $p = 0.04$ one tailed), while the opposite pattern approached significance in the SD patients (t (11) = 1.7, $p = 0.06$ one tailed).

6. Discussion

This study investigated the nonverbal semantic performance of two groups of patients with multimodal semantic impairment, semantic aphasia (SA) and semantic dementia (SD), on a reality decision judgement task. The patients were required to select the correct colour, context, sound or motion for objects in a two alternative forced choice (2AFC) test. In addition, three of these tasks manipulated the plausibility of distracter items. Plausible distracters were typical of the object's semantic category (e.g., a *red tomato* vs. a *green tomato*, which is the typical colour for plants). Therefore, this manipulation examined the ability to base judgements on the specific features of objects while avoiding incorrect shared features. By directly comparing the SA and SD groups on these tasks, this study of nonverbal semantic processing casts light on the nature of semantic deficits that follow left frontal and/or temporoparietal infarcts in SA and anterior temporal lobe atrophy in SD. It has been suggested that the semantic impairment in these groups has a different underlying cause: deregulated semantic control in SA and degraded conceptual representations in SD [1]. As a consequence, SA patients might be less affected by the plausibility manipulation than the SD group; their intact semantic representations and the relatively constrained 2AFC test format should allow relatively accurate performance. SD patients, in contrast, are highly sensitive to the plausibility manipulation due to their loss of specific fine-grained knowledge [14,15]. The results of this study upheld these predictions and highlighted significant differences between the semantic profiles of SA and SD. The main points are summarised below:

1. SA patients performed better than SD on reality decision judgements even though both groups performed similarly on background tests of semantic knowledge.
2. The SA patients were relatively insensitive to the plausibility manipulation in both accuracy and RT, in sharp contrast to the SD patients.
3. The type of semantic processing required in a task strongly influenced SA patients' performance, whereas SD patients were consistent across all measures.
4. SD patients showed a beneficial affect of familiarity. In contrast, SA patients were *less* likely to produce a correct response as item familiarity increased.

This differential performance can be explained by considering the aetiology of each group's semantic impairment coupled with the regulatory constraints imposed by the semantic tasks.

6.1. Reality decision judgements in SD

SD patients present with a highly specific and progressive impairment of semantic memory which follows atrophy and hypometobolism focussed on the bilateral ATL [6,37]. They fail a broad range of verbal and nonverbal semantic measures regardless of the nature of the stimuli [i.e., words, pictures, sounds, and smells; 7, 9]. SD patients show a profile of semantic performance which is consistent with degraded representations being the causal underlying deficit – they show strong item consistency across different seman-

tic tasks and minimal effects of cueing [7,13]. One key additional feature of their profile helps to explain the current findings; In SD the loss of fine-grained semantic knowledge (e.g., the knowledge that *strawberries* are *red*) is more vulnerable than more general superordinate information (e.g., *strawberries* are *plants*). Patients show greater difficulties on tasks that require access to specific semantic knowledge, such as sorting pictures into specific vs. general categories [15]. Moreover, when drawing items from memory, SD patients not only omit idiosyncratic features (e.g., drawing a rhino without its horn) but also make intrusion errors, including features which are typical of other category members [e.g., drawing a duck with four legs; 38]. With the progressive loss of specific features (e.g., the *rhino's* horn), the semantic system is left representing category structure in terms of the most frequently encountered similarities shared across category members [15,17]. This is why the SD group are highly sensitive to the plausibility manipulation when making reality judgements in this study. When the target (e.g., *red strawberry*) is presented alongside a plausible distracter (e.g., *green strawberry*), SD patients are likely to select the stimulus which has the largest overlap with the remaining similarity structure coded in the partially degraded semantic network. Implausible distracters (e.g., *blue strawberry*) share less similarity with category members – because their features are generally not typical for other semantic neighbours – therefore, they can be more easily rejected. Consequently, our results support the hypothesis that the bilateral ATL is a critical substrate for semantic representations [3,39,40] and degeneration of this bilateral network leads to the large effects of plausible distracters seen on the FRT task. In SA, however, the ATL is spared and patients do not show a profile consistent with degraded semantic knowledge. So what can account for the multimodal comprehension impairment in this group?

6.2. Reality decision judgements in SA

SA patients present with a number of characteristics which suggest their impaired performance stems from an inability to regulate conceptual knowledge as opposed to degraded semantic representations per se. SA patients are highly sensitive to the executive demands of semantic tasks – indeed, on a range of measures, their performance has been shown to reflect the ease with which target items can be selected whilst competing information is ignored [1,4,5,11] Similarly, item consistency – the ability to access the same concept on different occasions – is low when the nature of the task changes (e.g., naming vs. associative decisions). Finally, semantic impairment in SA correlates with domain-general executive/control problems – as measured by standardised tests of reasoning and cognitive flexibility [i.e., Ravens Coloured Matrices and the Wisconsin Card Sorting Test; 1]. In this study, the SA patients performed comparatively well on the experimental task because it placed minimal demands on self-generated regulation of semantic activation. The 2AFC format provided strong constraints on the target response and helped to minimise competition from accompanying choices. The insensitivity of the SA patients to the plausibility of distracters suggests that the specific features of items were not severely degraded, in contrast to SD. Previous investigations of cueing effects support this interpretation by showing that SA patients are much better at retrieving semantic information when their response space is constrained, even when the task requires access to specific semantic knowledge [5,13]. Our findings are, therefore, consistent with the interpretation that SA patients' comprehension problems arise from difficulties regulating and shaping activation. The extent to which this impairment will affect overall performance is mediated by the nature of the task and the amount of constraint it places on intrinsic semantic control.

The deficient semantic control hypothesis is consistent with the nature of the lesions in the SA group which affect left PFC and TPJ regions [1,19]. These areas show coupled activation on a range of executive and attentional tasks in functional neuroimaging studies [41,42]. Similarly, they are both activated when semantic tasks place a high demand on regulatory control – studies looking at the resolution of conflict when dealing with ambiguous material frequently show activation in these two areas [22,23,43], while additional studies have suggested an important role of inferior frontal and/or temporoparietal areas in the selection/retrieval and allocation of attention to semantic representations [21,44,45].

6.3. Differential effects of familiarity in SA & SD

We found that SA patients were less likely to make correct judgements as item familiarity increased, while SD patients showed better performance with increasing item familiarity. A number of previous investigations have shown that SA patients are insensitive to familiarity/frequency. In their original case-series comparison, Jefferies & Lambon Ralph [1] found the SA group showed no familiarity effects on any of the semantic tests, a finding replicated in subsequent work on refractory effects [12]. Conversely, strong effects of familiarity/frequency are consistent characteristics of SD [1, 46]. The benefits of familiarity/frequency in SD can be explained with reference to the underlying principles of PDP models. Items which are encountered frequently present the model with greater opportunity to learn and distinguish between similar exemplars [17,47]. In contrast, familiarity/frequency may have a negative effect in SA by increasing regulatory demand. Recent studies have shown that highly familiar/frequent items are generally encountered in a larger variety of environmental contexts, therefore regulatory control is required to focus selectively on the relevant aspects of knowledge that are appropriate for a given task [36].

7. Conclusions

The nature of the semantic impairment in SA and SD interacted with the regulatory demands of the FRT to produce qualitatively different semantic performance in the two groups of patients. The SA patients, supported by their intact semantic knowledge and a task structure which reduced competition at an individual trial level, performed well overall and showed minimal effects of the feature plausibility manipulation. However, their underlying regulatory impairment emerged in their reversed sensitivity to familiarity. SD patients in contrast, exhibited a profile which was best explained in terms of degraded semantic knowledge; they were highly sensitive to the feature plausibility manipulation and performed better on high familiarity items. This provides further support for the proposal that semantic cognition is underpinned by two principle components: semantic representations and regulatory control processes which regulate and shape activation within the semantic system.

Acknowledgments

We are indebted to the patients and their carers for their generous assistance with this study. We would like to thank Rachel Byrne, Linda Collier and Claire Slinger for referring some of the patients to us. The work was supported by a programme grant from the MRC (G0501632) and an MRC studentship to KAN.

References

[1] E. Jefferies and M.A. Lambon Ralph, Semantic impairment in stroke aphasia versus semantic dementia: A case-series comparison, *Brain* **129** (2006), 2132–2147.

[2] M.A. Lambon Ralph and K. Patterson, Generalization and Differentiation in Semantic Memory: Insights from Semantic Dementia, *Ann NY Acad Sci* **1124** (2008), 61–76.

[3] M.A. Lambon Ralph et al., Coherent concepts are computed in the anterior temporal lobes, *Proceedings of the National Academy of Sciences* **107** (2010), 2717–2722.

[4] F. Corbett et al., Different impairments of semantic cognition in semantic dementia and semantic aphasia: evidence from the non-verbal domain, *Brain* **132** (2009), 2593–2608.

[5] K. Noonan et al., Elucidating the nature of deregulated semantic cognition in semantic aphasia: Evidence for the roles of prefrontal and temporoparietal cortices, *Journal of Cognitive Neuroscience* **22** (2010), 1597–1613.

[6] J.R. Hodges et al., Progressive fluent aphasia with temporal lobe atrorphy, *Brain* **115** (1992), 1783–1806.

[7] S. Bozeat et al., Non-verbal semantic impairment in semantic dementia, *Neuropsychologia* **38** (2000), 1207–1215.

[8] J.R. Hodges, K.S. Graham and K. Patterson, Charting the progression in semantic dementia: Implications for the organisation of semantic memory, *Memory* **3** (1995), 463–495.

[9] S. Luzzi et al., Distinct patterns of olfactory impairments in Alzheimer's disease, semantic dementia, frontotemporal dementia and corticobasal degeneration, *Neuropsychologia* **45** (2007), 1823–1831.

[10] M.A. Lambon Ralph, C. Lowe and T. Rogers, Neural basis of category-specific semantic deficits for living things: evidence from semantic dementia, HSVE and a neural network model, *Brain* **130** (2007), 1127–1137.

[11] F. Corbett, E. Jefferies and M.A. Lambon Ralph, Deregulated semantic cognition follows prefrontal and temporo-parietal Damage: Evidence from the impact of task constraint on non-verbal object use, *Journal of Cognitive Neuroscience* **0** (in press), 1–11.

[12] E. Jefferies et al., Refractory effects in stroke aphasia: A consequence of poor semantic control, *Neuropsychologia* **45** (2007), 1065–1079.

[13] E. Jefferies, K. Patterson and M.A. Lambon Ralph, Deficits of knowledge versus executive control in semantic cognition: Insights from cued naming, *Neuropsychologia* **46** (2008), 649–658.

[14] E.K. Warrington, The selective impairment of semantic memory, *Quarterly Journal of Experimental Psychology* **27** (1975), 635–657.

[15] T.T. Rogers et al., The structure and deterioration of semantic memory: A neuropsychological and computational investigation, *Psychological Review* **111** (2004), 205–235.

[16] G. Pobric, E. Jefferies and M.A. Lambon Ralph, Category-specific versus category-general semantic impairment induced by transcranial magnetic stimulation, *Current Biology* **20** (2010), 964–968.

[17] T.T. Rogers and J.L. McClelland, *Semantic Cognition*, (1st ed.), London: Bradford Book, 2004.

[18] P. Garrard and E. Carroll, Lost in semantic space: a multimodal, non-verbal assessment of feature knowledge in semantic dementia, *Brain* **129** (2006), 1152–1163.

[19] M.L. Berthier, Unexpected brain-language relationships in aphasia: Evidence from transcortical sensory aphasia associated with frontal lobe lesions, *Aphasiology* **15** (2001), 99–130.

[20] C. Whitney et al., The Neural Organization of Semantic Control: TMS Evidence for a Distributed Network in Left Inferior Frontal and Posterior Middle Temporal Gyrus, *Cerebral Cortex* (2010).

[21] T.C. Cristescu, J.T. Devlin and A.C. Nobre, Orientating attention to semantic categories, *NeuroImage* **33** (2006), 1178–1187.

[22] S.S. Lee and M. Dapretto, Metaphorical vs. literal word meanings: fMRI evidence against a selective role of the right hemisphere, *NeuroImage* **29** (2006), 536–544.

[23] M.-Z. Zempleni et al., Semantic ambiguity processing in sentence context: Evidence from event-related fMRI, *NeuroImage* **34** (2007), 1270–1279.

[24] P. Gloor, The temporal lobe and limbic system, New York: Oxford University Press, 1997.

[25] G.J.M. Parker et al., Lateralization of ventral and dorsal auditory-language pathways in the human brain, *NeuroImage* **24** (2005), 656–666.

[26] E.K. Warrington and M. James, The Visual Object and Space Perception Battery. Bury St Edmunds: Thames Valley Test Company, 1991.

[27] D. Wechsler, Wechsler Memory Scale – Revised (WMS-R), New York: Psychological Corporation, 1987.

[28] M.D. Lezak, D.B. Howieson and D.W. Loring, Neuropsychological Assessment, Oxford: Oxford University Press, 2004.

[29] J.C. Raven, *Coloured Progressive Matrices Sets A, AB, B.*, London: H. K. Lewis, 1962.

[30] B. Milner, Effects of different brain lesions on card sorting: the role of the frontal lobes, *Archives of Neurology* **9** (1964), 100–110.

[31] D.T. Stuss et al., Wisconsin card sorting test performance in patients with focal frontal and posterior brain damage: effects of lesion location and test structure on separable cognitive processes, *Neuropsychologia* **34** (2000), 388–402.

[32] I.H. Robertson et al., *The Test of Everyday Attention*, London: Thames Valley Test Company, 1994.

[33] P.W. Burgess and T. Shallice, *The Hayling and Brixton Tests*. Bury St Edmunds: Thames Valley Test Company, 1997.

[34] J.G. Snodgrass and M. Vanderwart, A standardized set of 260 pictures: Norms for name agreement, image agreement, familiarity and visual complexity, *Journal of Experimental Psychology: Human Learning and Memory* (1980), 174–215.

[35] D. Howard and K. Patterson, Pyramid and palm trees: a test of semantic access from pictures and words, Bury Saint Edmunds: Thames Valley Test Company, 1992.

[36] P. Hoffman, T. Rogers and M.A. Lambon Ralph, SA-squared: Semantic ambiguity accounts for the missing word frequency effect in semantic aphasia, in press.

[37] P.J. Nestor, T.D. Fryer and J.R. Hodges, Declarative memory impairments in Alzheimer's disease and semantic dementia, *NeuroImage* **30** (2006), 1010–1020.

[38] S. Bozeat et al., A duck with four legs: Investigating the structure of conceptual knowledge using picture drawing in semantic dementia, *Cognitive Neuropsychology* **20** (2003), 27–47.

[39] R.J. Binney et al., The inferolateral aspects of the anterior temporal lobe are crucial in semantic memory: Evidence from a novel direct comparison of distortion-corrected fMRI, rTMS and semantic dementia, *Cerebral Cortex*, in press.

[40] K. Patterson, P.J. Nestor and T. Rogers, Where do you know what you know? The representation of semantic knowledge in the human brain, *Nature Reviews Neuroscience* **8** (2007), 976–987.

[41] F. Collette et al., Exploration of the neural substrate of executive functioning by functional imaging, *Neuroscience* **139** (2006), 209–221.

[42]   H. Garavan et al., A Parametric Manipulation of Central Executive Functioning, *Cereb Cortex* **10** (2000), 585–592.

[43]   J.M. Rodd, M.H. Davis and I.S. Johnsrude, The Neural Mechanisms of Speech Comprehension: fMRI studies of Semantic Ambiguity, *Cereb Cortex* **15** (2005), 1261–1269.

[44]   S.L. Thompson-Schill et al., Role of left inferior prefrontal cortex in retrieval of semantic knowledge: A reevaluation, *Proceedings of the National Academy of Science* **94** (1997), 14792–14797.

[45]   A.D. Wagner et al., Recovering meaning; Left prefrontal cortex guides controlled semantic retrieval, *Neuron* **31** (2001), 329–338.

[46]   E. Jefferies et al., Comprehension of concrete and abstract words in semantic dementia, *Neuropsychology* **23** (2009), 492–499.

[47]   J.L. McClelland and T.T. Rogers, The Parallel Distributed Processing Approach to Semantic Cognition, *Nature Reviews Neuroscience* **4** (2003), 310–322.

[48]   E. Kaplan, H. Goodglass and S. Weintraub, *Boston Naming Test*, Philadelphia: Lea and Febiger, 1983.

[49]   E.K. Warrington, The Graded Naming Test: A Restandardisation, *Neuropsychological Rehabilitation* **7** (1997), 143–146.

[50]   M.F. Folstein, S.E. Folstein and P.R. McHugh, "Mini-mental state": A practical method for grading the cognitive state of patients for the clinician, *Journal of Psychiatric Research* **12** (1975), 189–198.

13

Verbal and nonverbal memory in primary progressive aphasia: The Three Words-Three Shapes Test

Sandra Weintraub[a,b,*], Emily Rogalski[a], Emily Shaw[a], Sabrina Sawlani[a], Alfred Rademaker[c], Christina Wieneke[a] and M.-Marsel Mesulam[a,d]

[a]*Cognitive Neurology and Alzheimer's Disease Center, Northwestern University Feinberg School of Medicine, Chicago, IL, USA*

[b]*Department of Psychiatry and Behavioral Sciences, Northwestern University Feinberg School of Medicine, Chicago, IL, USA*

[c]*Department of Preventive Medicine, Northwestern University Feinberg School of Medicine, Chicago, IL, USA*

[d]*Ken and Ruth Davee Department of Neurology , Northwestern University Feinberg School of Medicine, Chicago, IL, USA*

Abstract. *Objectives:* To investigate cognitive components and mechanisms of learning and memory in primary progressive aphasia (PPA) using a simple clinical measure, the Three Words Three Shapes Test (3W3S).

Background: PPA patients can complain of memory loss and may perform poorly in standard tests of memory. The extent to which these signs and symptoms reflect dysfunction of the left hemisphere language versus limbic memory network remains unknown.

Methods: 3W3S data from 26 patients with a clinical diagnosis of PPA were compared with previously published data from patients with typical dementia of the Alzheimer type (DAT) and cognitively healthy elders.

Results: PPA patients showed two bottlenecks in new learning. First, they were impaired in the effortless (but not effortful) on-line encoding of verbal (but not non-verbal) items. Second, they were impaired in the retrieval (but not retention) of verbal (but not non-verbal) items. In contrast, DAT patients had impairments also in effortful on-line encoding and retention of verbal and nonverbal items.

Conclusions: PPA selectively interferes with spontaneous on-line encoding and subsequent retrieval of verbal information. This combination may underlie poor memory test performance and is likely to reflect the dysfunction of the left hemisphere language rather than medial temporal memory network.

1. Introduction

The diagnosis of PPA is based on the *presence* of aphasia in the earliest stages of illness but also on the *absence* of impairment in other cognitive domains, including episodic memory, reasoning, and visuospatial functions [1–5]. However, the clinician is frequently faced with patients and families who report "memory loss" even though there is usually little indication that daily living activities are being undermined by impaired episodic memory. Is the reported 'memory' impairment a secondary manifestation of the aphasia or is there an amnestic component in PPA? This is a challenging question to address through neuropsychological assessment because many of the relevant tasks require verbal instructions, contain verbal stimuli and/or require a verbal response. For example, one of the

*Corresponding author: Sandra Weintraub, PhD, Northwestern Cognitive Neurology and Alzheimer's Center, 320 E. Superior, Searle 11-467, Chicago, IL 60611, USA.

E-mail: sweintraub@northwestern.edu.

most common tests of dementia severity, the Mini Mental State Examination (MMSE) [6] relies heavily on language processing. Thus, although the MMSE has served to characterize severity in a variety of clinical dementia syndromes where language is not the primary deficit, it may overestimate the extent of functional impairment in PPA. This dissociation between test scores and daily function was demonstrated in a study comparing patients with PPA, patients with dementia of the Alzheimer type (DAT) and patients with behavioral variant frontotemporal dementia on the Activities of Daily Living Questionnaire (ADLQ) [7], an informant completed assessment of activities of daily living. Despite similar MMSE scores in the three groups, the PPA group scored consistently better on subscales of the ADLQ than the other two groups. The relative preservation of episodic memory and executive function in the PPA patients likely accounted for their ability to function at a higher level, despite the language impairment [8]. Thus, the principled assessment of memory and learning in PPA has important implications for the rigorous confirmation of the diagnosis and also for the comprehensive assessment of functional capacity.

The ability to recall an experience requires the perceptual encoding and on-line holding of the constituent information, its subsequent transformation into distributed off-line neural representations that sustain long-term retention, and the ability for the binding and coherent reactivation of these representations during voluntary recall. The mediotemporal limbic system plays its pivotal role in episodic memory by binding and then coherently activating distributed information pertaining to recent multimodal events [9]. This system is not a primary target of pathology in PPA. However, some of the distributed information belonging to recent experience, such as modality-specific word-forms and object representations, are encoded in perisylvian and inferotemporal areas that do become the targets of initial atrophy in PPA. It is therefore reasonable to assume that PPA may be associated with material- and modality-specific impairments of new learning despite the overall preservation of episodic memory for recent experiences. A selective loss of verbal memory is frequently mentioned in the literature on PPA but is rarely documented with parallel verbal and non-verbal tasks. The current study was undertaken to investigate if memory and learning for visually presented words and shapes are affected differently in PPA and, if so, whether this dissociation encompasses all or only some of the component processing stages.

We had designed a six-item memory test, the Three Words Three Shapes Test (3W3S), to specifically ass-

es verbal and non-verbal memory as well as the constituent stages of perceptuomotor encoding, on-line holding, retention, recall, retrieval and recognition [10]. A systematic scoring method was subsequently devised so that the 3W3S test could be used to discriminate between age-related memory loss and amnesia associated with DAT [11]. The 3W3S Test was designed to fulfill the need for a simple test that could be used in moderate stages of illness so that patients would not show the floor effects that are common when using most standard memory measures [12]. In addition, there were several unique attributes built into the test. First, most memory tests confound material (verbal vs nonverbal) with modality (auditory vs visual). For example, verbal memory is most often tested in the auditory modality with oral word lists or stories, while non verbal memory is tested in the visual modality by reproduction of geometric designs or picture recognition. In order to keep the modality consistent, words and shapes were both presented as visual stimuli in the 3W3S Test. Secondly, we required that all stimuli be copied prior to assessing memory to ensure that there were no primary writing or drawing deficits that could affect subsequent recall performance. A third innovation was to have an incidental encoding condition. Thus, participants were not forewarned to remember the stimuli as they copied them and recall was tested immediately after copying. This condition assesses the amount of information that can be encoded without effort, a type of memory that has greater ecological validity than memory based on rote learning. Following incidental recall of the six items, a number of effortful encoding (i.e., rote learning) trials were presented to bring the participant to a criterion level before testing delayed recall. Delayed recall was then tested and compared to the recognition of the items in order to assess the specific contribution of retrieval versus retention failure to overall explicit memory.

2. Methods

2.1. Study design

The study design was a retrospective analysis of test performance on the Three Words Three Shapes test in the context of a clinical evaluation for PPA. Data from the PPA participants were compared with previously published data from individuals with DAT and cognitively healthy elders.

Table 1
Cognitive operations indexed by 3W3S scores

Copy	Perceptuomotor aspects of the task
Incidental encoding	Capacity for effortless, spontaneous encoding of information and its on-line holding for immediate reproduction
Effortful encoding	Capacity for effortful, deliberate encoding of information and its on-line holding for immediate reproduction
Delayed recall	Amount of information that has been transferred to and retrieved from off-line storage
Recognition	Amount of information that has been transferred to off-line storage and retained in a form that can sustain recognition
Difference between effortful encoding and delayed recall	Represents the amount of information that fails to be transferred from on-line to off-line storage in a form that can be retained and reproduced
Difference between recognition and delayed recall	Represents the memory impairment that can be attributed to a deficit of retrieval rather than retention

2.2. Subjects

The sample consisted of 26 patients participating in a research project on PPA at the Northwestern University Cognitive Neurology and Alzheimer's Disease Center (DNADC). Informed consent was obtained on a research protocol approved by the Institutional Review Board at Northwestern University to participate in a three-day study, which included neuropsychological testing, experimental tests of language processing and structural neuroimaging. They had agreed to review of their clinical records with HIPAA assurances for information pertinent to their condition and participation in research. Comparison data from the previously published study had been obtained on 21 patients with a diagnosis of DAT and 14 cognitively normal controls.

All PPA patients had been given a root diagnosis of PPA [1,3,4] based on clinical evaluation in a memory disorders clinic. In addition, all patients had been subtyped on the basis of clinical impression on examination. Some had also been subtyped on the basis of an algorithm developed for this purpose based on measures of fluency, single word comprehension, naming and grammatical competence [13] and in all cases this subtyping was in agreement with the clinical assessment. One group was designated as agrammatic (PPA-G, N = 10) based on prominent deficits in grammatical processing and preserved single word comprehension and naming; a second group was designated as logopenic (PPA-L, N = 7) based on preserved grammatical processing and single word comprehension and reduced speech fluency and naming; a third group was labeled semantic (PPA-S, N=7) on the basis of impaired single word comprehension and naming and preserved grammar. Two patients could not be classified because the severity of their symptoms resulted in deficits in multiple components of language processing.

2.3. Materials and procedures

3W3S had been administered to participants as part of their evaluation in a behavioral neurology clinic. As previously described [11], the stimuli consist of three simple geometric designs and three words, one under each of the designs, horizontally distributed on a letter-sized page, in portrait orientation. (Test and scoring forms can be downloaded from our website www.brain.northwestern.edu).

Table 1 lists the conditions of the 3W3S test and the corresponding operations each measures. Patients are first asked to copy the three designs and the words directly beneath the stimuli. Participants are not forewarned to remember the stimuli but immediately after copying them, the page is removed and they are given a blank sheet and asked to reproduce what they just copied (Incidental Encoding trial). If the patient remembers at least five of the six stimuli, Delayed Recall is tested as described below. If on the Incidental Encoding trial the subject recalls fewer than five stimuli, the original stimulus sheet is presented for a 30-second study with the explicit instruction to try to remember the six stimuli in order to reproduce them from memory (Effortful Encoding trial). If after the first such trial the subject recalls five of the six stimuli, Delayed Recall is tested (below). If fewer than five stimuli are reproduced correctly, these trials are repeated up to a total of five or until five of the six stimulus items are reproduced correctly. Figure 1 shows a sample from a patient (number 17, Table 2).

Delayed recall was tested once, following either Incidental Encoding if criterion had been reached at that point, or following the last Effortful Encoding trial. Because of the constraints of the clinical examination, delay intervals ranged from 10 to 40 minutes, with a mean of 19.92 ± 5.91 minutes (median and mode = 20). Multiple choice recognition was tested following

Table 2
Demographics and clinical test scores of PPA sample

Subject ID	Gender	Subtype	Education years	Age at visit	Symptom duration (Years)	WAB AQ 100	WAB Rep 100	BNT score 60	PPVT 36	NAT 10	CDR sum boxes	Global CDR score
1	Male	NS/L	15	70	2	92	90	59	35	9	0	0
2	Male	NS/G	15	64	8.5	–	–	–	–	–	–	–
3	Male	NS/L	18	63	2	97.1	89	58	36	10	0.5	0
4	Female	Severe	12	63	4	41.2	32	9	NA		2.5	0.5
5	Female	NS/L	18	62	3	88.7	95	22	ND	ND	1.5	0.5
6	Male	NS/G	12	58	2	–	–	–	–	–	–	–
7	Female	NS/L	16	74	2	–	–	49	–	–	–	–
8	Female	Semantic	12	54	3.5	82.4	97	8	–	–	1	0.5
9	Male	Semantic	20	64	5	88.2	92	14	31	9	1	0.5
10	Female	NS/L	16	78	4.5	69.5	54	10	32	9	0	0
11	Male	NS/G	17	54	4	50	72	4	32	1	2.5	0.5
12	Female	NS/G	16	64	5	38.6	19	3	25	–	–	–
13	Female	NS/L	14	78	3.5	62.6	50	39	29	–	1.5	0.5
14	Male	NS/G	16	70	3.5	78.1	74	43	33	4	1	0.5
15	Female	NS/G	14	81	2	93.7	90	56	–	–	1.5	0.5
16	Male	NS/G	13	76	4	71.6	78	50	ND	ND	1.5	0.5
17	Female	Semantic	16	52	2.5	–	–	–	–	–	–	–
18	Male	Semantic	20	64	2	87.4	97	6	31	10	1	0.5
19	Female	NS/G	19	62	3	76.2	60	24	35	6	1	0
20	Male	NS/G	14	57	4	77.7	92	44	28	4	1.5	0.5
21	Female	NS/L	18	64	1.5	83.2	95	59	33	8	0	0
22	Male	Semantic	15	60	4	–	–	–	–	–	–	–
23	Female	Semantic	18	56	2	75.5	84	3	14	10	3	0.5
24	Female	Semantic	16	56	4	–	–	16	–	–	4	1
25	Female	NS/G	18	57	4	76.7	70	41	34	5	3.5	0.5
26	Male	Severe	14	58	4	60.3	45	20	–	–	2	0.5
		MEAN	15.84	63.81	3.44	74.54	73.75	28.95	30.57	7.08	1.53	0.40
		St Dev	*2.34*	*8.16*	*1.47*	*16.68*	*23.24*	*20.85*	*5.63*	*3.00*	*1.12*	*0.26*
		N				*20.00*	*20.00*	*22.00*	*14.00*	*12.00*	*20.00*	*20.00*

WAB = Western Aphasia Battery-Revised; AQ = Aphasia Quotient; Rep = Repetition; BNT = Boston Naming Test; PPVT-Peabody Picture Vocabulary Test; NAT = Northwestern Anagram Test; CDR = Clinical Dementia Rating; NS = Non semantic PPA subtype; G = agrammatic subtype; L = logopenic subtype; St Dev: standard deviation; N = number of observations on which means and standard deviations are based for each clinical measure.

the delay trial, unless the patient spontaneously and accurately recalled the stimuli. Nineteen of the patients were administered the Recognition condition; the rest had reproduced that stimuli correctly on delayed recall. They were asked to select the three words and three designs that they recalled from the test from among a set of 10 words and 10 designs.

Each condition was scored using previously developed criteria [11]. Each word had a total possible score of 5, 15 points for all the words; each design had a total score of 5, 15 for all the designs. Inter-rater reliability was established for the scoring criteria. Two raters were trained to use the scoring criteria. Each coded all 26 test protocols. A comparison of all scoring points for each condition indicated 100% agreement for the words. For the shapes the Kappa coefficient was 0.84, considered a level of almost perfect agreement. In instances where there was disagreement, however, the scores were discussed and consensus achieved.

2.4. Analyses

Analyses were designed to compare the PPA, DAT and control groups with respect to the components of verbal and nonverbal episodic memory assessed with 3W3S. Of particular interest was the comparison between effortful encoding and delayed recall, which would reflect the extent to which retrieval was affected, and the comparison between delayed recall and recognition which would provide information about the retention of information over time (Table 1). These distinctions were tested with ANOVA comparing performance of the PPA group with prior data derived from patients with DAT and cognitively healthy controls previously reported [11]. In the original 3W3S study, participants were tested at three delay intervals, five-, 15-, and 30-minutes following either the incidental encoding or the last Effortful Encoding trial. Results had shown that there was a significant reduction in the

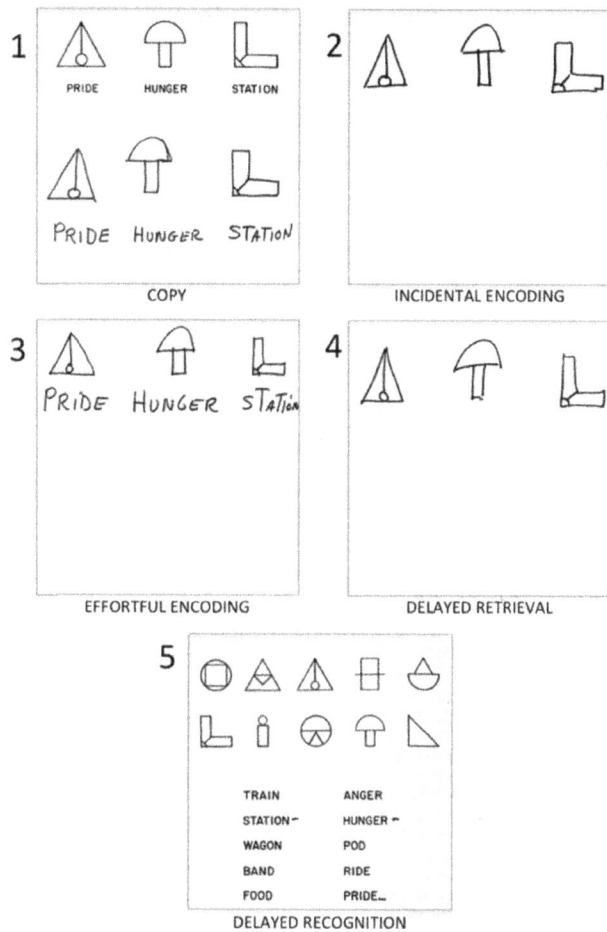

Fig. 1. Sample of performance from a patient with primary progressive aphasia (number 17, Table 2). 1) Copy. The patient was able to accurately copy all of the six stimuli. 2) Incidental encoding trial. The patient correctly reproduced all the shapes but none of the words. 3) Effortful encoding. With only one additional exposure and the instruction to remember all the stimuli, the patient could reproduce all the shapes and the words. 4) Delayed retrieval. After 10 minutes, the patient recalled all the shapes and none of the words. 5) Delayed recognition. The recognition form contains 10 shapes and 10 words, including the original 6 stimuli. Immediately after the delayed recall condition, in which she obtained a perfect score for shapes but could not recall any of the words, she recognized the three words.

amount of information retrieved after the initial delay of five minutes with no further loss over remaining delay intervals [11]. For purposes of comparison with data from the present study, the 15-minute delayed recall condition was used from the original cohort since it was closest in duration to our 20-minute average for the PPA participants.

Two additional ANOVA's were conducted within the PPA group to compare verbal and nonverbal memory: one on the entire group of PPA patients and a second comparing the three PPA subtypes. Two patients were too impaired to be subtyped (see below) and were excluded from this analysis.

3. Results

3.1. Demographics and clinical tests

Table 2 shows individual PPA participants' demographics and clinical test scores. Because of the retrospective nature of the study, not all individuals in the PPA group were administered the same battery of clinical tests at the same time as they were tested with 3W3S. Table 2 indicates the numbers of subjects on which each mean score is based.

Of the twenty-six patients included in this study 12 were male and 14 female. The average age was 63.81 ± 8.16 years and average education level was 15.85 ± 2.34 years. There was a large age range from 52 to 81 years. In the PPA group, symptom duration varied from 1.5 to 8.5 years with a mean of 3.44 ± 1.47 years. Seven of the PPA participants were subtyped as semantic, 17 as non semantic (10 agrammatic and 7 logopenic) and two could not be subtyped (Table 2, subjects 4 and 26) due to the severe nature of their condition resulting in more generalized language deficits. The previously published DAT and control samples were somewhat older (DAT mean $= 66.38 \pm 3.10$ years; control mean $= 70.86 \pm 2.20$ years) and less well educated (DAT mean education $= 12.90 \pm 0.51$ years; control mean education $= 13.79 \pm 0.68$ years). Dementia severity, as measured by the Blessed Dementia Scale [14] was within the mild-moderate range (mean $= 10.03 \pm 1.07$, of a possible 37; higher score = greater impairment) similar to the aphasia severity range for the PPA sample.

The average WAB AQ, a measure of aphasia severity was 74.54 ± 16.68, indicating a moderate level overall, but considerable variability. Scores ranged from 41.2 (severely impaired) to 97.2 (very mildly impaired). Although the average score on the Boston Naming Test was very low (28.95 ± 20.85) the range was from 3 to 59. Scores on the Peabody Picture Vocabulary Test (36 items) ranged from 14 to 36, mean $= 30.57 \pm 5.63$. Only 14 participants had been administered the 10-item form of the Northwestern Anagram Test (NAT-10) a measure of grammatical processing and the average score was 7.08 ± 3.00.

Dementia severity was measured by the mean Global Score on the Clinical Dementia Rating (CDR) scale [15] and was 0.40 ± 0.26 (very mildly impaired). The CDR Sum of Boxes score [16], which provides an expanded scoring range for the CDR, also indicated a very minimal level of dementia severity (mean $= 1.53 \pm 1.12$). In early stages, patients with PPA typically do not have the memory and orientation deficits that figure prominently in dementia of the Alzheimer type and that are the focus of the CDR. The CDR is also based on the level of impairment of judgment and problem solving, functioning in home and hobbies, and ability in community affairs. Patients with PPA, aside from their aphasia, do not have early impairments in these areas. Thus, despite the range of aphasia severity, all the patients in the sample were able to perform the 3W3S.

3.2. Three words three shapes performance

3.2.1. Comparison among study groups

Table 3 shows mean scores and standard deviations of 3W3S performance by condition for the PPA, DAT and healthy control groups. As previously reported, elderly controls perform near ceiling on all components of this test, explained by our effort to design an instrument with a reduced level of difficulty for patients with dementia. The results are presented as they address each of the episodic memory components measured. Significance levels were interpreted with Bonferroni corrections for multiple pairwise comparisons ($p = 0.016$).

3.2.2. Perceptuomotor components

There were no significant differences between PPA, DAT and healthy controls on the Copy condition, indicating that perceptuomotor components of the task were sufficient to direct attention to and support adequate rendering of the stimuli. Thus, low scores in subsequent conditions could not be explained by more primary perceptuomotor dysfunction.

3.2.3. Incidental encoding

This condition represents the capacity for online spontaneous and effortless encoding for immediate recall. Under this condition, the PPA group's performance was worse than controls for words ($p < 0.001$) but similar to DAT patients ($p = 0.37$) (mean PPA = 4.63 ± 4.78; mean NC = 12.14 ± 3.23; mean DAT = 5.95 ± 6.59). In contrast, their Incidental Encoding score for shapes was not significantly different from that of controls ($p = 0.062$) and superior to that of DAT patients ($p < 0.0001$) (mean PPA = 8.88 ± 4.77; mean NC = 11.79 ± 3.56; mean DAT = 4.33 ± 2.37.

3.2.4. Effortful encoding

With the explicit instruction to commit the stimuli to memory, that is to engage in effortful encoding,

PPA patients required more trials than NC (mean = 1.96 ± 1.00 vs 0.43 ± 0.51; $p = 0.0002$) but fewer trials than DAT patients (mean = 3.10 ± 1.58, $p = 0.0015$) to reach criterion. At the last acquisition trial the three groups did not differ in their scores for words. However effortful encoding of shapes was similar in PPA and control groups and both groups had significantly higher scores for shapes than the DAT group (both $p < 0.0001$). These results indicate that after a few additional trials, PPA patients are able to immediately retrieve words and shapes at a level similar to controls while patients with DAT have more difficulty with immediate retrieval of shapes than words.

3.2.5. Delayed retrieval

Following the delay interval, PPA patients had lower scores than controls for word recall (mean PPA = 7.79 ± 5.84 vs mean controls = 13.43 ± 2.62, $p = 0.0004$) but similar scores to controls for shape recall (mean PPA = 12.29 ± 3.34; mean controls = 14.29 ± 1.38, $p = 0.18$). However, PPA patients had higher scores for both words and shapes than DAT patients (mean DAT Words = 2.05 ± 3.43; Shapes = 5.05 ± 6.16; both $p < 0.0001$). These results imply that there is a material specific effect for word retrieval after a delay in PPA when compared with cognitively healthy controls but superior performance to patients with amnestic DAT regardless of material.

3.2.6. Delayed recognition

On multiple choice recognition, a measure of retentive memory, PPA patients obtained near ceiling scores for both words and shapes, better than DAT patients ($p < 0.0001, 0.0014$, respectively), and similar to controls ($p = 0.65, 0.96$, respectively).

3.2.7. Within-group analysis of all PPA patients

ANOVA was conducted to identify material specific (words and shapes) and task components (i.e., copy, recall) deficits within the PPA group. PPA patients' scores for shapes was higher than for words on the incidental and delayed recall conditions ($p = 0.0004, 0.0015$, respectively, Table 3). Words and shapes scores were similar on all the other conditions, namely, copy, effortful encoding, and delayed recognition. These results indicate that when retrieval is aided by effortful encoding or by the absence of a delay, retentive memory is as good for words as it is for shapes.

Three within group comparisons were of particular interest for identifying the bottleneck for performance in the PPA patients. First, comparing the last effort-

Table 3
3W3S scores for PPA, DAT, NC

Subject group	Copy		Incidental recall		Last acquisition		Delayed recall**		Recognition		Effortful encoding trials (#)
	W	S	W	S	W	S	W	S	W	S	
PPA (N = 26)											
Mean	14.96	14.83	4.63	8.88	12.57	13.24	7.79	12.29	14.25	14.93	1.96
SD	0.20	0.48	4.78	4.77	4.08	2.45	5.84	3.34	1.29	0.32	1.00
DAT (N = 21)											
Mean	15.00	14.81	5.95	4.33	13.00	7.95	2.05	5.05	5.28	11.11	3.10
SD	0.00	0.33	6.59	2.37	3.95	4.60	3.43	6.16	6.30	6.08	1.58
NC (N = 14)											
Mean	15.00	14.93	12.14	11.79	14.50	14.36	13.43	14.29	13.57	15.00	0.43
SD	0.00	0.27	3.23	3.56	1.40	1.39	2.62	1.38	3.63	0.00	0.51

PPA = Primary Progressive Aphasia; DAT = Dementia of the Alzheimer type; NC = Normal Control.
*Data for DAT (aka probable AD) and NC groups taken from Weintraub et al., 2000.
**Delay For PPA = 20.42 minutes (SD = 6.41); Delay for NC and PrAD = 15 minutes.

Table 4
3W3S: Difference scores (shapes minus words) for non semantic and semantic PPA subtypes

	Non semantic	Non semantic	Difference	Semantic	Semantic	Difference	Non semantic vs semantic
	Words mean (sem)	Shapes mean		Words mean (sem)	Shapes mean (sem)		p-value
Copy	14.94 (0.05)	14.76 (0.12)	−0.1765	15.00 (0.08)	15.00 (0.18)	**0.000**	0.39
Incidental	6.12 (1.07)	10.18 (1.14)	**4.0588***	1.43 (1.67)	8.57 (1.78)	**7.1429****	0.27
Acquisition	12.58 (0.71)	13.29 (0.58)	0.7059	14.86 (1.11)	13.57 (0.90)	−1.2857	0.31
Delay	10.71 (1.06)	12.59 (0.68)	1.8824	2.71 (1.65)	13.57 (1.06)	**10.8571*****	**0.0011**
Recognition	14.63 (0.30)	14.91 (0.08)	0.2816	14.57 (0.44)	15.00 (0.12)	**0.4286**	0.76

Sem = standard error of the mean. *$p = 0.012$; **$p = 0.005$; ***$p = 0.0001$.

ful encoding trial (last acquisition) with delayed recall provides information about retrieval failure while a comparison between effortful encoding and recognition provides information about retention failure. There was a statistically significant difference between effortful encoding and delayed recall scores for words ($p = 0.0003$) but not for shapes ($p < 0.038$, Bonferroni correction for multiple pairwise comparisons $= p < 0.005$). There was no significant difference between effortful encoding and delayed recognition scores for words but there was a significant difference for shapes ($p = 0.003$) with recognition superior (Table 3). This implies that retention for words and shapes is preserved despite problems with word retrieval.

The third comparison of interest was between copy and incidental encoding scores to determine what is retained online without conscious effort. In this instance, patients with PPA had lower scores on incidental encoding than on copy for both words and shapes, suggesting that, without the explicit instruction to remember the information, they are not as efficient in retaining both types of material. However, in the analyses reported earlier, comparing PPA and DAT participants, the PPA group outperformed the DAT group for this type of encoding of shapes.

3.2.8. Comparison of PPA subtypes

Similar analyses to the one described above for the entire PPA group were conducted separately on the semantic and the non semantic PPA subgroups and both groups were compared. Table 4 shows 3W3S mean scores for both subtypes. Of interest is the fact that when words and shapes were compared across all conditions for the non semantic PPA group, the only comparison that approached significance ($p = 0.012$, Bonferroni correction for multiple comparisons $= p < 0.01$) was a lower score for words than shapes in the incidental encoding condition. For all other test component comparisons, words and shapes scores did not differ significantly. In contrast, comparisons within the semantic group showed significant differences between words and shapes on both incidental encoding and delayed recall conditions ($p = 0.005$, $p = 0.0001$, respectively).

Semantic and non semantic groups were compared in an analysis that contrasted the *difference scores* between words and shapes scores in each condition. Positive numbers reflect worse word than shape performance while negative numbers reflect the reverse and zero implies no difference. In this comparison, the only statistically significant difference was in the delayed recall condition, where the difference between words and shapes was far greater in the semantic than in the non semantic group (mean semantic difference between words and shapes=10.86; mean non semantic difference = 1.88, $p = 0.0011$).

4. Discussion

The present study investigated episodic memory in patients with primary progressive aphasia (PPA) using the 3W3S Test, a simple test of verbal and non verbal retentive memory that can be used during routine outpatient clinic assessments. Performance was compared to previously published data from patients with amnestic dementia of the Alzheimer type and cognitively healthy controls [11]. The goal of the present study was to determine if explicit memory in PPA patients is influenced by the type of information to be remembered (verbal vs nonverbal) and if there are retrieval and/or retention deficits. To this end, the ability to reproduce words and shapes was tested under conditions of copying, incidental encoding, effortful encoding, delayed recall and recognition, with all stimuli in the visual modality.

The PPA patients had no perceptuomotor impediment to the performance of the task as shown by perfect copying scores. Incidental recall, indicative of the effortless (spontaneous) on-line encoding and subsequent reproduction of the items, was low for both types of items but more so for the words. This impairment was largely overcome during effortful on-line encoding as shown by the much higher scores at the end of the acquisition stage when compared to the incidental recall scores. Once the information entered on-line storage in a form that could sustain item reproduction, it was successfully transferred to off-line storage, as shown by the stability of performance when acquisition and recognition scores are compared. However, the PPA patients also showed a material-specific impairment in the retrieval of verbal items as shown by the declining performance when the recognition scores were compared to the delayed recall scores. In contrast, the DAT patients did not show consistent material-specific impairments and displayed abnormalities also at the stages of effortful on-line encoding (for non-verbal items) and retention (for verbal items).

Incidental recall, not commonly assessed in the clinical examination, tests the capacity for spontaneous on-line encoding and very short-term storage for purposes of immediate recall. The incidental recall condition used in this report can be considered to test a type of working memory but differs from standard working memory test methods in that the latter typically include the explicit instruction for recall. On this condition, patients with PPA could reproduce the shapes at a level close to controls and superior to the DAT patients. However, incidental word encoding was poorer than that of the controls and similar to that of DAT patients. This implies that verbal working memory, especially under conditions of automatic processing, is specifically impaired in PPA. In DAT, this type of short-term storage is impaired for both words and shapes.

This failure of verbal working memory was overcome by the Effortful Encoding trials where deliberate encoding resulted in successful on-line holding and immediate recall of both words and shapes. The DAT group required more trials than the PPA and control groups to reach criterion in the Effortful Encoding stage while the PPA group required more trials than the control group. All three groups were equally successful in the immediate reproduction of words and shapes through effortful encoding. However, the larger number of exposures required by the DAT patients to reach criterion and the lesser difference between scores of delayed recall and recognition in that group are consistent with a greater defect in the acquisition and retention of new information than in the PPA group.

A comparison of 3W3S performance between semantic and non semantic subtypes showed that the former group was more impaired for word recall than the latter but only in the delayed recall condition, perhaps consistent with the spread of atrophy to medial temporal areas in that group [17]. We conducted a previous study in which PPA patients viewed words and pictures in an incidental recognition memory task and gave abnormally high false positive response rates compared with cognitively normal individuals, primarily to semantically related words [18]. The number of target stimuli and distracters in that study was much greater than the 6 stimuli on the 3W3S task and this additional load may have contributed to the emergence of false-positive responses, a phenomenon that was not observed in the current study.

Although a number of studies have examined episodic memory in patients with various forms of progressive aphasia ([19–21]; also see [22] for a review and meta-analysis) none have made a direct comparison between the same number of verbal and non verbal stimuli within a single modality, namely, visual. Many studies have used standard tests that demand sophisticated language skills for comprehension of instructions. A number of case studies have documented the preservation of autobiographical memory but typically have required spoken responses. The Three Words Three Shapes Test therefore fills a gap for the need for a brief, convenient measure of memory that can be used even in moderate to severe stages of PPA.

One potential weakness of this study has to do with the nature of the stimuli. Created initially on the spot as a bedside test, the stimuli were not carefully controlled for imageability of words, verbalization of shapes, multiplicity of meanings for each word (e.g., "pride" and "station" have more than one meaning) and potential associations between the words and shapes. It was possible, then, that, for example, the pair including the word "Hunger" and a line drawing that looks like a mushroom could be recalled more easily than the others. We examined the data to determine if this had occurred and found only one example of incidental recall and one different example of delayed recall where the [Mushroom]-Hunger pair was the only one remembered. In all other instances where this pair was recalled, other pairs were also recalled. Thus, the word recall deficit in PPA overpowered any advantage offered by the implicit association between words and shapes.

There are a number of therapeutic implications from the results of the current study. First, on-line encoding, a necessary precursor for off-line storage and retention, was enhanced when the PPA patients were specifically asked to effortfully learn the information. This suggests that providing explicit encouragement to pay attention and multiple exposures (i.e., repetition of the information) for the purpose of remembering might enhance subsequent recall, even of verbal information. Another therapeutic strategy is to provide cues to aid retrieval. The PPA patients had no difficulties with recognition, suggesting that explicit cues can promote retrieval of information that might otherwise appear lost. For example, a "Communication Notebook", a collection of pictures, phrases, calendars, and other materials in a small format that a patient can use to activate information that is not quickly retrievable (http://www.brain.northwestern.edu/ppa/treatment.html) may provide benefical cues for retrieval.

The demonstration that a patient does not have a multimodal loss of new learning, and that the apparent memory loss is confined to an impairment of verbal retrieval, is critical for confirming the accuracy of the PPA diagnosis. The 3W3S test permits the objective demonstration of this pattern and contributes to our understanding of the intersection of memory and language.

Acknowledgments

This study was supported by grants R01DC008552 from the National Institute on Deafness and other Communication Disorders, 5KL2RR025740 from the National Center for Research Resources, and by grant AG13854 (Alzheimer's Disease Core Center) from the National Institute on Aging. Disclosures of Funding from NIH and others.

References

[1] M.L. Gorno-Tempini, A.E. Hillis, S. Weintraub et al., Classification of primary progressive aphasia and its variants, *Neurology* **76**(11) (15 Mar 2011), 1006–1014.

[2] M. Mesulam, Slowly progressive aphasia without generalized dementia, *Ann Neurol* **11**(6) (1982), 592–598.

[3] M. Mesulam, Primary progressive aphasia, *Ann Neurol* **49**(4) (2001), 425–432.

[4] M. Mesulam, Primary progressive aphasia–a language-based dementia, *N Engl J Med* **349**(16) (16 Oct 2003), 1535–1542.

[5] M. Mesulam, Primary progressive aphasia: a 25-year retrospective, *Alzheimer Dis Assoc Disord* **21**(4) (Oct-Dec 2007), S8–S11.

[6] M.F. Folstein, S.E. Folstein and P.R. McHugh, "Mini-mental state", A practical method for grading the cognitive state of patients for the clinician, *J Psychiatr Res* **12**(3) (1975), 189–198.

[7] N. Johnson, A. Barion, A. Rademaker, G. Rehkemper and S. Weintraub, The Activities of Daily Living Questionnaire: a validation study in patients with dementia, *Alzheimer Dis Assoc Disord* **18**(4) (Oct–Dec 2004), 223–230.

[8] A.H. Wicklund, N. Johnson, A. Rademaker, B.B. Weitner and S. Weintraub, Profiles of decline in activities of daily living in non-Alzheimer dementia, *Alzheimer Dis Assoc Disord* **21**(1) (Jan–Mar 2007), 8–13.

[9] M.M. Mesulam, From sensation to cognition, *Brain* **121**(Pt 6) (1998), 1013–1052.

[10] S. Weintraub and M.-M. Mesulam, Mental state assessment of young and elderly adults in behavioral neurology, in: *Principles of Behavioral Neurology*, M.-M. Mesulam, ed., Philadelphia, PA: FA Davis, 1985, pp. 71–123.

[11] S. Weintraub, G.M. Peavy, M. O'Connor et al., Three words three shapes: A clinical test of memory, *J Clin Exp Neuropsychol* **22**(2) (Apr 2000), 267–278.

[12] J.J. Locascio, J.H. Growdon and S. Corkin, Cognitive test performance in detecting, staging, and tracking Alzheimer's disease, *Arch Neurol* **52**(11) (Nov 1995), 1087–1099.

[13] M. Mesulam, C. Wieneke, E. Rogalski, D. Cobia, C.K. Thompson and S. Weintraub, Quantitative template for subtyping primary progressive aphasia, *Archives of Neurology* **66**(12) (Dec 2009), 1545–1551.

[14] G. Blessed, B.E. Tomlinson and M. Roth, The association between quantitative measures of dementia and of senile change in the cerebral grey matter of elderly subjects, *Br J Psychiatry* **114** (1968), 797–811.

[15] J.C. Morris, The Clinical Dementia Rating (CDR): Current version and scoring rules, *Neurology* **43** (1993), 2412–2414.

[16] S.E. O'Bryant, S.C. Waring, C.M. Cullum et al., Staging dementia using Clinical Dementia Rating Scale Sum of Boxes

scores: a Texas Alzheimer's research consortium study, *Arch Neurol* **65**(8) (Aug 2008), 1091–1095.

[17] E. Rogalski, D. Cobia, T.M. Harrison, C. Wieneke, S. Weintraub and M.M. Mesulam, Progression of language decline and cortical atrophy in subtypes of primary progressive aphasia, *Neurology* **76**(21) (24 May 2011), 1804–1810.

[18] E. Rogalski, D. Blum, A. Rademaker and S. Weintraub, False recognition of incidentally learned pictures and words in primary progressive aphasia, *Neuropsychologia* **45**(2) (28 Jan 2007), 368–377.

[19] K.S. Graham, J.S. Simons, K.H. Pratt, K. Patterson and J.R. Hodges, Insights from semantic dementia on the relationship between episodic and semantic memory, *Neuropsychologia* **38**(3) (2000), 313–324.

[20] M. Grossman, J. Mickanin and K. Onishi, Progressive nonfluent aphasia: language, cognitive and PET measures contrasted with probable Alzheimer's disease, *Journal of Cognitive Neuroscience* **8** (1996), 135–154.

[21] J.R. Hodges and K.S. Graham, Episodic memory: insights from semantic dementia, *Philos Trans R Soc Lond B Biol Sci* **356**(1413) (29 Sep 2001), 1423–1434.

[22] K.K. Zakzanis, The neuropsychological signature of primary progressive aphasia, *Brain Lang* **70**(1) (15 Oct 1999), 70–85.

14

Treatment for apraxia of speech in nonfluent variant primary progressive aphasia

M.L. Henry[a,*], M.V. Meese[b], S. Truong[c], M.C. Babiak[a], B.L. Miller[a] and M.L. Gorno-Tempini[a]

[a]Memory and Aging Center, Department of Neurology, University of California, San Francisco, CA, USA
[b]Alta Bates Medical Center, El Cerrito, CA, USA
[c]San Francisco State University, San Francisco, CA, USA

Abstract. There is a growing body of literature examining the utility of behavioral treatment in primary progressive aphasia (PPA). There are, however, no studies exploring treatment approaches to improve speech production in individuals with apraxia of speech (AOS) associated with the nonfluent variant of PPA. The purpose of this study was to examine a novel approach to treatment of AOS in nonfluent PPA. We implemented a treatment method using structured oral reading as a tool for improving production of multisyllabic words in an individual with mild AOS and nonfluent variant PPA. Our participant showed a reduction in speech errors during reading of novel text that was maintained at one year post-treatment. Generalization of improved speech production was observed on repetition of words and sentences and the participant showed stability of speech production over time in connected speech. Results suggest that oral reading treatment may offer an efficient and effective means of addressing multisyllabic word production in AOS associated with nonfluent PPA, with lasting and generalized treatment effects.

Keywords: Apraxia of speech, treatment, speech therapy, nonfluent PPA, primary progressive aphasia

1. Introduction

Primary progressive aphasia (PPA) is a degenerative neurological condition in which speech and language functions are disrupted, while other cognitive abilities remain relatively spared. The disorder results from atrophy in regions of the brain that sub-serve language. Three clinical variants of PPA are now widely accepted. These include a semantic variant, with verbal and nonverbal semantic deficits, a logopenic variant, with anomia and phonological working memory problems, and a nonfluent/agrammatic variant, with agrammatism and/or apraxia of speech [1,2].

PPA has been linked to several types of neuropathology, including tau or ubiquitin/TDP-43 positive frontotemporal lobar degeneration and Alzheimer's Disease [3,4]. While the prevalence of PPA is not known,

frontotemporal dementia, which may manifest in PPA, is now recognized as a common cause of dementia affecting individuals under the age of 65 [5,6].

Relative to individuals with aphasia resulting from stroke, individuals with PPA are under-referred for speech-language pathology services [7]. Further, they are less likely to be offered behavioral treatment, in part due to lack of understanding of the disorder by referring and treating clinicians, and also due to negative assumptions regarding the feasibility and utility of behavioral treatment in patients with neurodegenerative disease. Treatment research focused on individuals with PPA has addressed restitutive treatments designed to rehabilitate impaired speech-language processes, augmentative/alternative approaches to treatment, and interventions designed to address activity and participation limitations (for reviews, see [8,9]).

Word-finding deficits (for a review, see [8]) as well as sentence production [10] and written language impairments [11] have been the object of restitutive treatments. At present, there is modest evidence supporting the utility of speech-language treatment in PPA. Re-

*Corresponding author: Maya L. Henry, Memory and Aging Center, Department of Neurology, University of California, San Francisco, CA, USA. E-mail: mhenry@memory.ucsf.edu.

search reports have shown gains on language measures, which were largely restricted to treated language domains and certain treatment approaches appear to slow the progression of language deficits for specifically-trained behaviors [12]. Much remains to be learned, however, with regard to the treatment paradigms that may be beneficial for the clinical variants and stages of PPA. In addition, the long-term benefits of treatment in this population have yet to be elucidated.

The majority of research on speech-language treatment in PPA has involved individuals with semantic variant. The logopenic and nonfluent variants have received less attention. Treatment studies addressing nonfluent variant PPA have focused on linguistic deficits associated with the disorder, including verb and sentence production [13], phonological processing [14], and lexical retrieval [15]. The motor speech deficits, or more specifically, apraxia of speech (AOS), observed in nonfluent variant have not, to our knowledge, been examined with systematic treatment research. This is unfortunate, given that a gradual decline in motor planning ability for speech, or AOS, can be the most prominent and debilitating feature of nonfluent variant PPA [16].

A 2006 review of the AOS treatment literature by Wambaugh and colleagues [17] revealed that the vast majority of published AOS treatment cases were stroke patients and most of those were classified as severely apraxic. There are relatively few treatment studies examining the utility of treatment in mildly apraxic patients, perhaps because these individuals are largely intelligible and have fairly functional spoken communication. In contrast to many stroke patients with AOS, motor speech deficits in nonfluent variant are often quite mild during initial stages of the disease, and sometimes are the only deficit for a number of years. Thus, treatment approaches designed for individuals with AOS due to stroke, who are often profoundly apraxic, may not be appropriate for AOS in the context of nonfluent variant PPA. However, in PPA, AOS can be expected to worsen over time and early intervention, when the disorder is mild, may be beneficial in slowing the progression of deficits and/or providing strategies for communication in the face of a worsening impairment of motor programming for speech.

In this study, we attempted to remediate speech production for multisyllabic words via structured oral reading of text. It is a well-documented feature of AOS that production breaks down with words of increasing length and articulatory complexity [18]. Multisyllabic word production was our patient's primary difficulty and therefore, this was the level at which treat-

ment efforts were directed. Oral text reading has been used therapeutically in individuals with aphasia with or without apraxia of speech, with benefits observed in written and spoken language [19,20]. Written word forms have also been incorporated as a supplement to other treatment approaches in acquired AOS, and have been described as a means of "intersystemic facilitation" wherein a relatively intact system or modality is used to facilitate improvement in an impaired system or modality [16]. In the case of oral reading to promote speech production, relatively preserved visual processing of orthography and conversion between orthography and phonology prior to motor implementation may serve to facilitate motor planning and execution for speech. In effect, orthography may serve to cue speech sound production by serving as a visual guide to the correct sequence of phonemes and syllables.

To our knowledge, there are no treatment studies examining oral reading as a primary means of rehabilitating speech production in AOS. In mild AOS, where production of multisyllabic words may be the most pronounced difficulty, oral reading can provide a context within which to elicit production of these words, which may not occur frequently in spontaneous speech. Oral reading also allows for rehearsal of multisyllabic word production in the context of connected speech rather than in isolation. Here we describe a single-subject treatment study wherein we implemented a novel treatment approach for a case of mild AOS in the nonfluent variant of PPA. Goals of the study were a) to determine whether structured oral reading practice can improve production of multisyllabic words read aloud, b) to examine generalization to untrained speech behaviors and contexts, and c) to assess long-term effects of training on oral reading and speech production.

2. Methods

2.1. Participant

The participant, GA (fictitious initials), was a 73 year-old right-handed woman. She spoke English as her second (after German) but primary language. GA studied English in school and began using it as her primary language 52 years prior to this study. She obtained 20 years of education and worked for an insurance brokerage before retiring at age 55. GA had no history of developmental disorders of speech and language. At the start of treatment, she had a five-year history of progressive impairment of speech production.

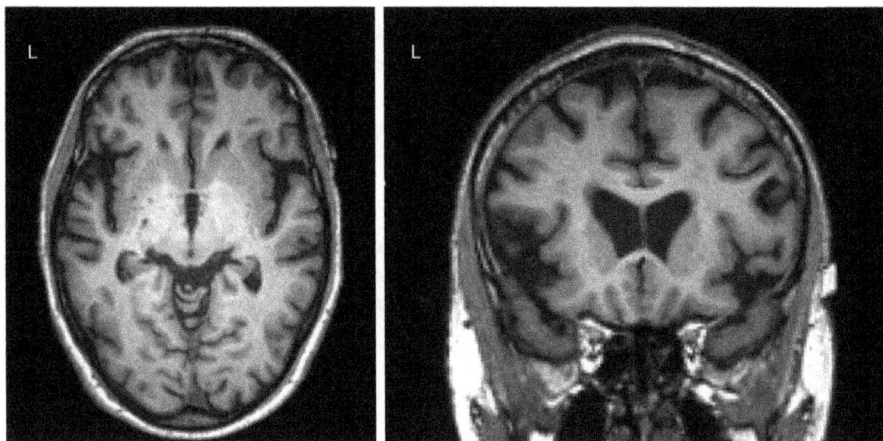

Fig. 1. Structural MRI scan obtained three months prior to initiation of treatment.

She participated in yearly research evaluations at the Memory and Aging Center (MAC) at UCSF for three years prior to her enrollment in the treatment study reported here. A consensus diagnosis of nonfluent variant primary progressive aphasia was reached by a team of clinicians (neurologist, neuropsychologist, and speech-language pathologist) at her initial visit according to published clinical criteria [1,21]. A structural MRI scan was obtained three months prior to initiation of treatment (Fig. 1). The scan revealed frontal/insular as well as temporoparietal atrophy in the left hemisphere. At the time treatment was initiated, the patient's major complaint concerned difficulty with production of multisyllabic words and an overall slowness and effortfulness of speech production, which she observed to be worsening gradually over time.

2.1.1. Pre-treatment speech and language evaluation

Pre-treatment speech and language assessment showed relatively fluent, grammatical spoken language (Table 1). The Motor Speech Evaluation [22] revealed that speech production was slow in rate with vowel and consonant distortions; sound insertions, deletions, and transpositions; pauses between words and syllables; increasing errors with increasing word length; and reduced prosodic variation. This pattern is consistent with an impairment of motor planning for speech production, or AOS [16,17,23]. Dysarthria was not noted. Syntax comprehension and production were examined using in-house assessments (for details, see [24]). On the production task, which involves generation of sentences in response to pictured scenes, as well as the comprehension task, which requires matching an auditorily-presented sentence to one of two pictures, GA performed at ceiling. Semantic processing, as measured by the picture version of the Pyramids and Palm

Trees Test [25] and the Boston Naming Test [26], was spared. Reading and spelling of single words and nonwords on the Arizona Battery of Reading and Spelling (ABRS) [27] was normal.

Repetition was tested at the word and sentence level in order to assess motor speech at increasing levels of difficulty. Word repetition was examined with a list of one- and three-syllable words used previously to test speech production ability in stroke patients [28]. Words were presented auditorily and repeated five times in succession by GA. Repeated word production was spared for monosyllables, but was impaired for trisyllabic words. On a sentence repetition task adapted from Bayles [29], repetition of short sentences was near ceiling, whereas repetition of longer sentences was impaired.

Oral reading of text was examined using passages 10–14 (most difficult passages) of the Gray Oral Reading Test (GORT-4). Pre-treatment assessment of oral reading confirmed difficulty with production of multisyllabic words in sentence context. In fact, 95% of speech errors occurred on multisyllabic words, which GA typically attempted to self-correct. There was a significant proportion (49%) of repeated attempts at multisyllabic word production which were ultimately unsuccessful.

2.2. Treatment design and treatment probes

Treatment consisted of structured oral reading of text, with the goal of providing a framework for systematic rehearsal of multisyllabic word production in sentence context. During treatment sessions, GA was trained in self-detection and correction of speech errors while reading text aloud. Weekly treatment sessions were supplemented by oral reading practice at home. The treatment approach involved the following steps:

Table 1
Pre- and post-treatment assessments

	Pre-Tx	Post-Tx	3 mos. post	6 mos. post	1 year post
Mini Mental State Exam (30)	29	26	29	29	30
Western Aphasia Battery					
Information content (10)	10	10	10	10	10
Fluency (10)	9	9	9	9	6
Comprehension (10)	9.75	10	10	9.8	9.75
Repetition (10)	9.4	9.4	9.2	9.5	8.9
Naming (10)	9.4	9.4	9.8	9.8	10
Aphasia Quotient	95.1	95.6	96	96.2	89.3
Motor Speech Evaluation- apraxia rating (0–7)	1	1	2	2	3
Motor Speech Evaluation- dysarthria rating (0–7)	0	0	1	1	1
UCSF sentence production (16)	16	16	16	16	16
UCSF sentence comprehension (24 or 48)	48	24/24	24/24	45/48	45/48
Pyramids and Palm Trees Test- pictures (52)	52	52			
Boston Naming Test (60)	51	53			
Boston Naming Test (15)			15	15	15
Reading words					
Regular high frequency (20 or 10)	20	20	10 /10	10/10	10/10
Regular low frequency (20 or 10)	20	20	10/10	10/10	10/10
Irregular high frequency (20 or 10)	20	20	10/10	10/10	10/10
Irregular low frequency (20 or 10)	19	20	9/10	10/10	9/10
Nonwords (20 or 10)	20	20	10/10	10/10	10/10
Spelling words					
Regular high frequency (20 or 10)	20	20	10/10	10/10	10/10
Regular low frequency (20 or 10)	20	20	10/10	10/10	10/10
Irregular high frequency (20 or 10)	20	19	10/10	10/10	10/10
Irregular low frequency (20 or 10)	20	18	10/10	10/10	10/10
Nonwords (20 or 10)	20	19	10/10	10/10	10/10
Word repetition x5 (correct repetition attempts)					
Monosyllabic (120 or 60)	120	120	60/60	60/60	60/60
Trisyllabic (120 or 60)	96	117	57/60	59/60	59/60
Sentence repetition (syllables correctly repeated)					
Short sentences (60)	59	60	60	60	
Long sentences (135)	106	121	116	111	

Note that shortened versions of some assessments were used at follow-up testing.

1. Text was read aloud until GA produced a word incorrectly. Incorrect production was specified as inability to produce a word in its entirety or a production with one or more "major" speech sound errors. We defined major errors as follows: sound deletion, insertion, transposition, substitution, or distorted substitution/insertion.
2. If the target was a multisyllabic word, it was underlined in the text and lines were drawn dividing the word into constituent syllables. The word was then produced syllable-by-syllable until each syllable was produced correctly, at which point the whole word was repeated in a non-syllabified manner. Single-syllable words were simply repeated (typically once) until produced correctly in isolation.
3. Once the word was mastered in isolation, GA returned to the beginning of the sentence and attempted to produce the word correctly in sentence context. If the word was again produced in error,

she returned to rehearsal of the word in isolation (see step 2, above) and again attempted the word in sentence context, until the entire sentence was produced correctly.

Treatment was focused on detection and correction of major speech sound errors or incomplete productions in multisyllabic words. Minor distortions (phonetic alterations that did not result in perception of a different phoneme, deletion/transposition/addition of a phoneme, or inability to produce a word in its entirety) were not targeted during training sessions because they did not disrupt intelligibility of speech to the same degree as major sound errors. Further, the participant could not be expected to reliably detect gradient phonetic changes to speech sounds. Sound prolongations and increased intersegment durations were also not targeted for treatment.

Treatment sessions were conducted by a licensed speech-language pathologist (M.H.) and lasted for one hour, once per week, for 12 weeks. During treatment sessions, one randomly-selected paragraph from the previous week's homework was read aloud in order to assess pronunciation of words therein. Treatment probe data were collected from these samples. Major sound errors were recorded on-line and total number of multisyllabic words with major sound errors was recorded for each session. In addition, all underlined words in the text (those that required rehearsal in isolation) were elicited in sentence context in order to provide additional accountability for homework practice. Words produced in error were practiced using steps 1–3 above. Subsequently, new text was trained using the above procedure (for a minimum of 30 minutes of oral reading). During each session, GA was asked to provide a spoken summary of the previous week's reading in order to encourage reading for comprehension at home. The purpose of sessions with the clinician was twofold: 1) to provide practice of multisyllabic words using the training procedure described above and 2) to check correct implementation of the training procedure in order to guarantee that home reading practice was conducted correctly.

Oral reading homework was completed at least five times per week for 30–45 minutes per day. The same text (typically 2–3 paragraphs) was reread several times per homework session, using steps 1–3 above, until the entire section was reliably produced without error. A book was selected by the clinician whose subject matter was of interest to the participant and which contained frequent multisyllabic words. The same text was used throughout. A representative sample of this text is included below:

A shrinking minority of unreconstructed apologists for Leninism clung to the past; but from Berlin to Paris a new generation of Western progressives sought solace and example outside of Europe altogether, in the aspirations and upheavals of what was not yet called the "Third World'.

–Post War: A History of Europe since 1945 by Tony Judt

In the initial treatment session, it was observed that GA detected words produced in error (as defined above) during oral reading with 100% accuracy, and in subsequent treatment sessions, she maintained this ability to self-detect major speech errors with a very high degree of accuracy. On the rare occasion that GA produced an error and did not detect it, reading was stopped by the clinician and the word was rehearsed until correct production was achieved.

GA was encouraged to continue her home reading practice after weekly sessions (i.e., the active treatment

phase) with the clinician were concluded. At each of the follow-up assessments, she confirmed that she had continued her reading practice at least 4–5 times per week since the conclusion of sessions with the clinician. We will refer to follow-up assessments as "post-treatment" time points because they were conducted after the conclusion of sessions with the clinician and because there was no longer any direct accountability for home practice. However, it should be noted that home practice did continue in the interim.

2.3. Assessment of treatment effects

Production of multisyllabic words during reading of novel texts was examined pre- and post-treatment and at follow-up assessments using the Gray Oral Reading Test-4 [30], which comprises passages of increasing difficulty and has two formats, which were used alternately. Each word was coded on-line as correctly produced on first attempt or incorrectly produced. Words that were not produced correctly were further sub-classified into those that were produced correctly after at least one repeated attempt and those that were not ultimately produced correctly (either after repeated attempts or not). Incorrect productions included incomplete attempts (i.e., partial productions) or those with speech sound errors (substitutions, additions, deletions or transpositions of sounds as well as distorted substitutions/additions). Minor sound distortions (gradient phonetic errors that did not result in perceived production of a different phoneme) were not counted as frank speech errors, but were coded. Samples were audiotaped and re-coded by the clinician after each session. For all reading probes, videotaped samples were also independently coded by another speech-language pathologist (S.T or M.M). Overall interrater reliability (percent agreement) for error coding was 93% and inconsistencies were resolved via consensus by reviewing videotaped samples. Speech errors were examined in connected speech via analysis of the WAB picture description using the same procedures.

The speech and language battery was repeated at post-treatment and follow-up sessions, using abbreviated versions of certain tests. Changes in performance on reading probes were examined using Wilcoxon signed rank tests. Performance on the Motor Speech Examination (MSE) was rated by a speech-language pathologist who did not see the patient for treatment (M.B.). The MSE was videotaped at each time point and the videos were reviewed and rated in a randomized order. Finally, we used a post-treatment survey, administered remotely via the internet, in order to gauge GA's perception of functional changes brought about by treatment.

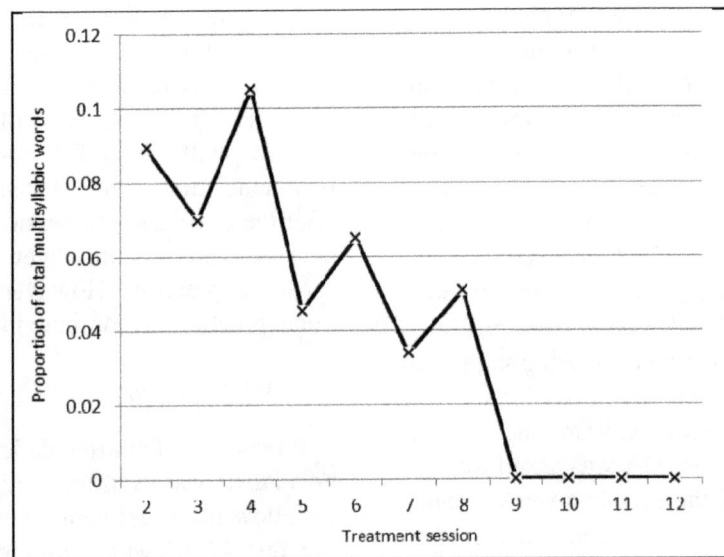

Fig. 2. Proportion of multisyllabic words produced with major speech errors in probes of trained homework text during treatment sessions.

3. Results

3.1. Multisyllabic word production during reading probes from trained homework text

Reading performance was probed in weekly sessions using a randomly-selected paragraph from text trained as homework the previous week. Performance on these probes (proportion of multisyllabic words with major speech sound errors) is depicted in Fig. 2. The figure shows that multisyllabic word production in trained text became more accurate and stable over the course of treatment and was error-free over the last four treatment sessions.

3.2. Multisyllabic word production during oral reading of untrained text

In order to assess whether our oral reading treatment could improve production of multisyllabic words during oral reading of difficult, untrained text and to examine the long-term effects of treatment, we administered the GORT-4 at post-treatment and follow-up assessments. Figure 3 depicts the proportion of multisyllabic words that were produced in error (excluding minor distortions) during reading probes. Wilcoxon signed rank tests (one-tailed) confirmed a significant reduction in speech errors on multisyllabic words at post treatment ($Z = -2.02$, $p = 0.02$), three months post-treatment ($Z = -2.02$, $p = 0.02$), six months post-treatment $Z = -2.02$, $p = 0.02$) and one year post-treatment ($Z = -1.75$, $p = 0.04$). When exam-

ining all word types together (single and multisyllable), very similar results were observed (post-treatment ($Z = -1.75$, $p = 0.04$), three months post treatment ($Z = -2.02$, $p = 0.02$), six months post-treatment treatment ($Z = -1.6$, $p = 0.05$), one year post-treatment treatment ($Z = -2.02$, $p = 0.02$)). These results confirm that oral reading treatment significantly improved production of multisyllabic words during text reading and that this pattern held when examining all word types combined. Figure 3 also shows the proportion of multisyllabic words produced in error that were self-corrected versus those that were not. There was a significant increase in the proportion of speech errors that were self-corrected at post treatment ($Z = -1.75$, $p = 0.04$) and at the three month follow-up assessment ($Z = -1.86$, $p = 0.03$). Six-month ($p = 0.17$) and one-year ($p = 0.24$) follow-up assessments were not significantly different from pre-treatment with regard to proportion of speech errors that were self-corrected.

Minor distortions (phonetic alterations that did not result in production of an incorrect speech sound or inability to produce a word in its entirety) were not targeted during training sessions; however, they were coded and analyzed for GORT-4 passages. Figure 4 shows the proportion of multisyllabic words that were produced with at least one minor distortion. The prevalence of minor distortions during oral reading of multisyllabic words did not change significantly from pre-treatment to post-treatment (two-tailed $p = 0.50$) or at the three or six month follow-up evaluations ($p = 0.69$ and $p = 0.14$, respectively). However, at one year post-treatment, there was a significant increase in the proportion of multisyllabic words produced with at

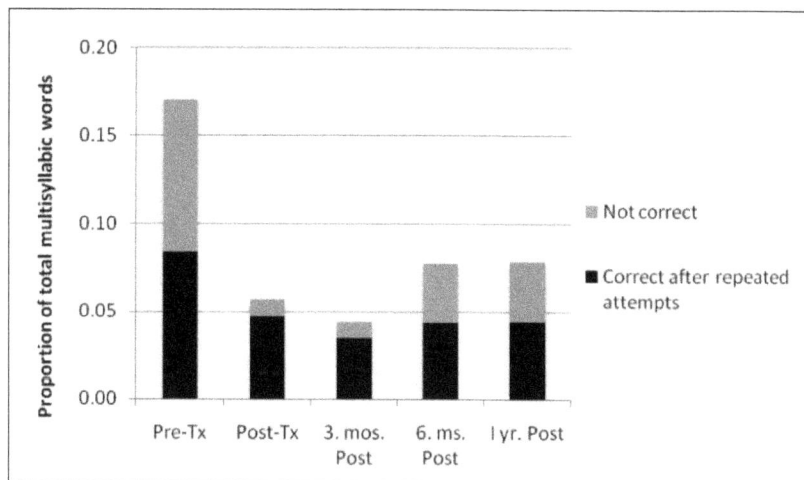

Fig. 3. Proportion of multisyllabic words with major speech errors on the Gray Oral Reading Test (GORT-4, passages 10–14).

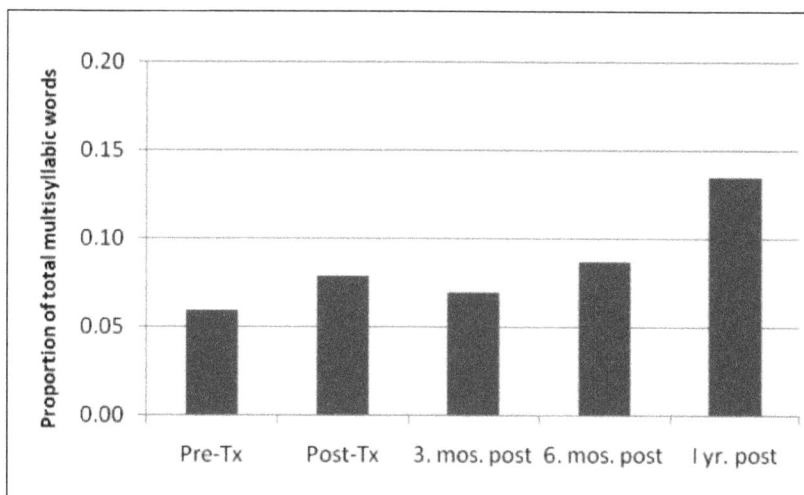

Fig. 4. Proportion of multisyllabic words with minor distortions (GORT-4).

least one minor distortion ($Z = -2.02, p = 0.04$). The same pattern was observed when all words were evaluated together (post-treatment, $p = 0.69$; three months post, $p = 0.69$; six months post, $p = 0.23$; one year post-treatment ($Z = -2.02, p = 0.04$)). These findings indicate that the rate of occurrence of minor distortions did not increase or decrease as a result of treatment and that these behaviors remained stable until one year post-treatment, at which point their frequency increased. Figure 5 depicts reading rate in words per minute, averaged across the five GORT passages at each time point. Reading of novel text showed a gradual slowing over time. Reading rate was not significantly slower at post-treatment (one-tailed $p = 0.25$) or three months post-treatment ($p = 0.11$), but was significantly slower at six-month ($Z = -2.02, p = 0.02$), and one year ($Z = -1.76, p = 0.04$) follow-up assessments.

In order to examine generalization of treatment effects to untrained tasks and contexts, GA's speech production was assessed during repeated production of mono- and trisyllabic words and during sentence repetition (Table 1). Repetition of monosyllabic words (x5) and short sentences remained stable across time points. Tri-syllabic word repetition improved considerably from pre- to post-treatment, with maintenance at three months, six months, and one year post-treatment. Repetition of long sentences was improved post-treatment, with some degree of maintenance at three and six months post-treatment. GA's speech production was also examined during connected speech in a picture description task from the Western Aphasia Battery (Fig. 6). The frequency of major speech sound errors and minor distortions in connected speech did not change considerably from pre-treatment to any of the post-treatment time points.

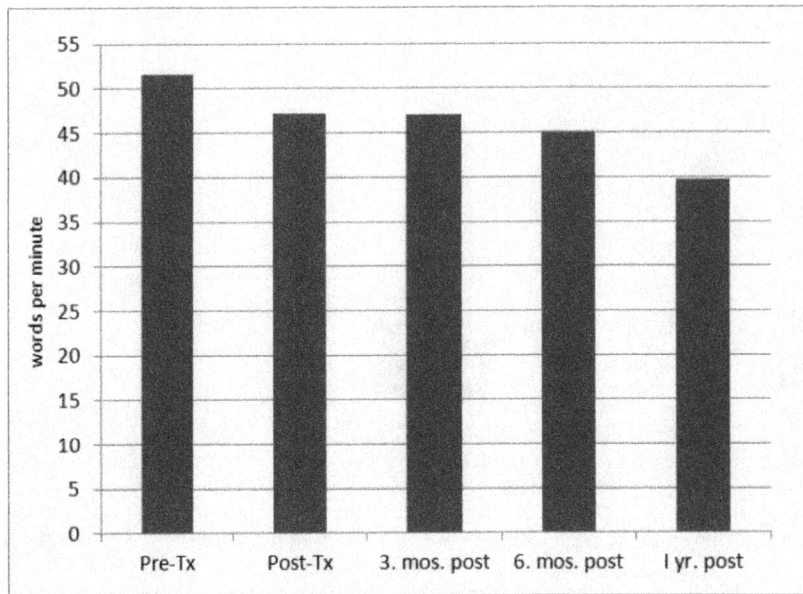

Fig. 5. Reading Rate for GORT-4 passages.

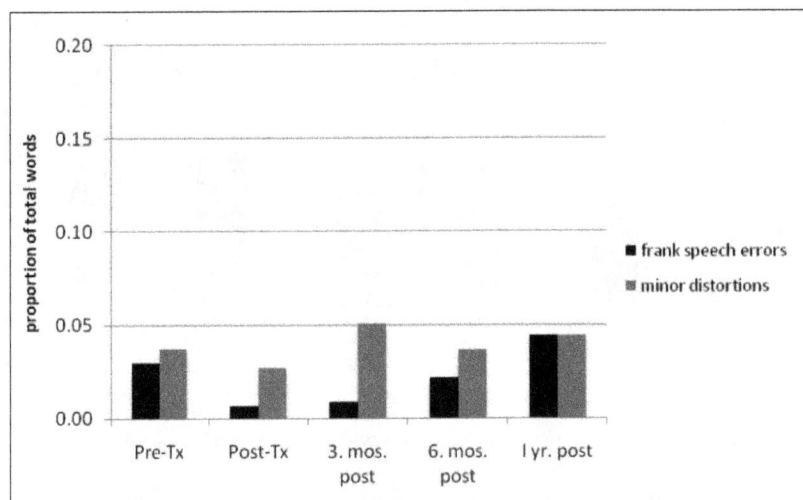

Fig. 6. Speech errors during picture description from the WAB.

3.3. Post-treatment and follow-up speech and language evaluations

Scores on the WAB remained relatively constant across treatment and follow-up assessments up to the six month follow-up, as reflected by little change in the Aphasia Quotient (Table 1). At the one year follow-up assessment, WAB AQ dropped nearly seven points. This change was due to a reduction in the fluency rating brought about by impaired speech production. AOS rating on the Motor Speech Evaluation did not change from pre-to post-treatment. At three months post-treatment, AOS severity was noted to have worsened. Changes in voice quality (harshness and breath-ened. Changes in voice quality (harshness and breath-

iness) and decreased pitch and loudness were also observed. At one year post-treatment, AOS severity was again noted to have worsened. Changes in AOS severity at 3 months and one year were largely due to an increase in what we have termed "minor distortions" as well as a slower rate of speech, increased frequency of pauses within and between words, and further reduction in prosody. Syntactic and semantic assessments and single-word reading/spelling showed little change over time.

3.4. Post-treatment survey

Table 2 shows results of a post-treatment survey examining GA's self-ratings of treatment effects. GA in-

Table 2
GA's self-ratings of treatment effects

Since you began oral reading treatment, how would you rate your	a lot worse (1)	worse (2)	some-what worse (3)	un-changed (4)	some-what better (5)	better (6)	a lot better (7)
—Reading fluency (ability to read smoothly and without errors)						X	
—Speaking fluency (ability to speak smoothly and without errors)					X		
—Comfort level while reading aloud							X
—Comfort level while speaking					X		
—Reading comprehension (ability to understand written passages)				X			
—Word production (ability to produce single words with several syllables)						X	
—Sentence production (ability to speak in complete sentences without errors)						X	
—Ability to detect any errors in your speech				X			
—Ability to correct your own speech errors when they occur				X			
—Ability to assign proper stress to words when reading or speaking						X	
—Confidence in communication with your primary communication partner (e.g., spouse)				X			
—Confidence in communication with familiar people						X	
—Confidence in communication with unfamiliar people					X		
—Frustration level during communication exchanges with primary communication partner					X		
—Frustration level during communication exchanges with familiar people						X	
—Frustration level during communication exchanges with unfamiliar people					X		

dicated that she perceived improved performance and comfort level in reading aloud and speaking (fluency), as well as improvements in multisyllabic word production, sentence production, and stress assignment in words post-treatment. She also indicated improved confidence and reduced frustration in communication with both familiar and unfamiliar people as a result of treatment.

4. Discussion

Individuals with the nonfluent variant of PPA often face a slow decline in motor programming ability for speech, or AOS, in the relative absence of other linguistic and cognitive deficits [16,23]. These patients ultimately become mute and reliant on augmentative and alternative communication (AAC) strategies/devices. Whereas AAC approaches provide an important substitute for or complement to spoken communication in many individuals, the loss of spoken language is devastating and debilitating and patients frequently express a desire for behavioral treatment options to help manage motor speech deficits.

Individuals with PPA may benefit from strategies to improve speech production when their impairments are still mild and, potentially, slow the inevitable progression of their difficulties. Despite the need for rehabilitation strategies addressing the motor speech deficits observed in nonfluent variant PPA, there have been virtually no investigations of such treatments that we are aware of to-date. Attempts to rehabilitate AOS in stroke patients, while promising, are often not appropriate in patients with mild AOS due to progressive disease. These treatments are typically designed to address severe motor speech planning deficits, with single sound, syllable, or monosyllabic word targets that are not appropriate for mild cases.

We attempted to address the need for treatment research in this area by implementing a novel treatment approach with an individual with mild AOS associated with nonfluent PPA. The treatment was designed to provide a context within which to rehearse self-detection and correction of speech sound errors due to AOS, with the specific goal of improving multisyllabic word production during oral reading. We sought to determine whether structured oral reading practice can improve production of multisyllabic words during text reading, whether treatment effects generalize to untrained behaviors, and also to examine the long-term effects of treatment.

Over the course of this intervention, GA showed a decrease in major speech errors on multisyllabic words in trained text, with error-free reading of these words over the last few treatment sessions. She also showed a decrease in major speech errors on multisyllabic words (and all words) when reading difficult untrained text (GORT-4 passages 10–14) as well as an increase in successful self-corrections post-treatment. This improvement was maintained up to 1 year following the completion of treatment with the clinician, with continued home practice. The frequency of speech sounds with minor distortions did not change from pre- to post-treatment, but did remain stable until at least six months after treatment with the clinician was completed. With regard to generalization, we observed improved speech production during repetition of long sentences at post-treatment and improvement on repeated production of trisyllabic words up to one year post-treatment, suggesting that treatment effects generalized to untrained tasks.

In addition, we observed little change in the frequency of major speech sound errors during connected speech probes up to one year post-treatment, suggesting that treatment may have helped to stabilize speech production in non-reading contexts. However, an increase in phonetic distortions on consonants and vowels, slowed speech rate, and an increase in the number of pauses within and between words resulted in a greater AOS severity rating on the MSE, a test that is designed to elicit motor speech errors in AOS and dysarthria by taxing the speech production system with a variety of tasks. This worsening of the AOS severity rating reflects a continuing decline in certain aspects of motor programming for speech that was not captured by oral reading and connected speech probes. For example, diadochokinetic productions were increasingly slow and irregular over time. In addition, the MSE rating is a subjective measure that likely takes into account the overall effortfulness of speech production and visually observable behaviors, such as groping of the articulators, which were not reflected in our treatment outcome measures.

In addition to our observations that speech error rates declined as a result of treatment, GA indicated that she perceived improvement in her own speaking and reading, as well as increased confidence and decreased frustration when communicating with others. She also reported that friends and family who were unaware of her participation in this study indicated that her speech intelligibility was improved after treatment.

Oral reading of text provides a context within which to rehearse production of multisyllabic words in connected speech. Treatment techniques for AOS have incorporated written word forms, but no previous treat-

ment paradigm has focused on use of the written word as a primary cue for speech production. Our method, wherein GA broke the written word down into constituent syllables and produced the word syllable-by-syllable, may have provided visual cues via orthography that helped to guide implementation of the correct speech motor program. Short words are typically produced with less difficulty in individuals with AOS, likely because of reduced complexity of motor programming. By breaking multisyllabic words into constituent syllables, the motor programming demands are reduced to syllable-sized chunks. Application of this technique in the context of reading aloud enables the visual word form to serve as a guide to correct production of each sound and syllable in the proper sequence.

It is our conclusion that changes in GA's oral reading and speech performance reflected improvements in motor planning for multisyllabic words. However, we acknowledge that our classification scheme for speech sound errors in this study assumed that all errors were motor, rather than phonological, in nature, even when sounds were not produced in a distorted manner. Major sound errors, which were the object of treatment, were defined as distorted or non-distorted productions that resulted in perception of a substituted, deleted, transposed, or added phoneme or in an incompletely produced target. We cannot rule out the possibility that some portion of these errors arose at a phonological level. However, GA's overall pattern of speech impairment was highly consistent with AOS, she was classified as non-aphasic by the WAB (AQ of 93.8 or higher), and she performed within the normal range on measures of naming, reading, and writing, all of which reflect a relative sparing of phonological processing. Therefore, we are confident that the majority of errors targeted in treatment and quantified by our outcome measures arose at the level of motor planning and that this is the level at which change was brought about by treatment.

Our preliminary findings in this case suggest that structured oral reading treatment for multisyllabic words may hold promise as a feasible, cost-effective, and efficient means of delivering therapy for patients with nonfluent variant PPA. First, it is simple to implement and can be tailored to any difficulty level, from very complex text, as was used with GA, to simple passages conveying personal information that may serve as material for script training in more severely apraxic individuals. Our participant, GA, was very accurate at self-detection of major speech sound errors and failed attempts at word production. This skill is critical to the implementation of this procedure outside the clinic.

Once it is ascertained that the participant can reliably detect speech sound errors, however, it is possible to complement treatment sessions with the clinician with homework practice, allowing the individual to receive therapeutic stimulation daily. It is quite likely that GA's maintenance of treatment effects after cessation of sessions with the clinician was due to her continued oral reading practice at home.

Finally, the treatment has the potential to stimulate and even improve grammatical processing in agrammatic patients, as has been shown with other oral reading treatments in aphasia resulting from stroke [20]. This is important given that many individuals with nonfluent PPA will ultimately develop impairments of syntactic comprehension and production with disease progression. Thus, oral reading treatment may prove beneficial for both motor speech and, ultimately, syntactic impairments observed in nonfluent variant PPA. Because GA was still near ceiling on measures of syntactic processing post-treatment, the latter will require systematic examination in future patients.

We have presented a novel approach to treatment of motor speech impairment in nonfluent variant PPA. This structured oral reading treatment, designed to facilitate self-detection and correction of speech errors on multisyllabic words, resulted in a reduction of speech errors on trained and untrained tasks and behaviors that was maintained for one year after the end of treatment with the clinician. This study provides an initial account of the utility of this type of treatment in mild AOS, which will need to be explored further and replicated with a larger group of individuals.

Acknowledgements

We wish to thank our research participant for all of her hard work and dedication. This work was supported by the NIH (NIDCD F32DC010945, NIA P01 AG019724, and NINDS R01 NS050915).

References

[1] M.L. Gorno-Tempini, A.E. Hillis, S. Weintraub, A. Kertesz, M. Mendez, S.F. Cappa et al., Classification of primary progressive aphasia and its variants, *Neurology* **76**(11) (2011), 1006–1014.

[2] M.L. Gorno-Tempini, N.F. Dronkers, K.P. Rankin, J.M. Ogar, L. Phengrasamy, H.J. Rosen et al., Cognition and anatomy in three variants of primary progressive aphasia, *Ann Neurol* **55**(3) (2004), 335–346.

[3] M. Mesulam, A. Wicklund, N. Johnson, E. Rogalski, G.C. Leger, A. Rademaker et al., Alzheimer and frontotemporal pathology in subsets of primary progressive aphasia, *Ann Neurol* **63**(6) (2008), 709–719.

[4] K.A. Josephs, J.R. Duffy, E.A. Strand, J.L. Whitwell, K.F. Layton, J.E. Parisi et al., Clinicopathological and imaging correlates of progressive aphasia and apraxia of speech, *Brain* **129** (2006), 1385–1398.

[5] E. Ratnavalli, C. Brayne, K. Dawson and J.R. Hodges, The prevalence of frontotemporal dementia, *Neurology* **58**(11) (2002), 1615–1621.

[6] D. Knopman, R. Petersen, S. Edland, R. Cha and W. Rocca, The incidence of frontotemporal lobar degeneration in Rochester, Minnesota, 1990 through 1994, *Neurology* **62**(3) (2004), 506–508.

[7] C. Taylor, R.M. Kingma, K. Croot and L. Nickels, Speech pathology services for primary progressive aphasia: Exploring an emerging area of practice, *Aphasiology* **23**(2) (2009), 161–174.

[8] M. Henry, Treatment for Progressive Impairments of Language, *Perspectives on Neurophysiology and Neurogenic Speech and Language Disorders* **20**(1) (2010), 13–20.

[9] K. Croot, L. Nickels, F. Laurence and M. Manning, Impairment-and activity/participation-directed interventions in progressive language impairment: Clinical and theoretical issues, *Aphasiology* **23**(2) (2008), 125–160.

[10] S.L. Schneider, C.K. Thompson and B. Luring, Effects of verbal plus gestural matrix training on sentence production in a patient with primary progressive aphasia, *Aphasiology* **10**(3) (1996), 297–317.

[11] B. Rapp and B. Glucroft, The benefits and protective effects of behavioural treatment for dysgraphia in a case of primary progressive aphasia, *Aphasiology* **23**(2) (2009), 236–265.

[12] R. Jokel, E. Rochon and C. Leonard, Treating anomia in semantic dementia: improvement, maintenance, or both? *Neuropsychol Rehabil* **16**(3) (2006), 241–256.

[13] S.L. Schneider and C.K. Thompson, Verb production in agrammatic aphasia: The influence of semantic class and argument structure properties on generalisation, *Aphasiology* **17**(3) (2003), 213–241.

[14] M. Louis, R. Espesser, V. Rey, V. Daffaure, A.D. Cristo and M. Habib, Intensive training of phonological skills in progressive aphasia: a model of brain plasticity in neurodegenerative disease, *Brain Cogn* **46**(1–2) (2001), 197–201.

[15] R. Jokel, J. Cupit, E. Rochon and C. Leonard, Relearning lost vocabulary in nonfluent progressive aphasia with MossTalk Words®, *Aphasiology* **23**(2) (2009), 175–191.

[16] K.A. Josephs, J.R. Duffy, E.A. Strand, M.M. Machulda, M.L. Senjem, A.V. Master et al., Characterizing a neurodegenerative syndrome: primary progressive apraxia of speech. Brain in press.

[17] J. Wambaugh, J. Duffy, M. McNeil, D. Robin and M. Rogers, Treatment guidelines for acquired apraxia of speech: A synthesis and evaluation of the evidence, *Journal of Medical Speech Language Pathology* **14**(2) (2006).

[18] J.R. Duffy, Motor speech disorders. St. Louis: Mosby, Incorporated, 1995.

[19] L. Cherney, Efficacy of oral reading in the treatment of two patients with chronic Broca's aphasia, *Topics in Stroke Rehabilitation* **2**(1) (1995), 57–67.

[20] S. Orjada and P. Beeson, Concurrent treatment for reading and spelling in aphasia, *Aphasiology* **3**(5) (19 2005), 341–351.

[21] M.M. Mesulam, Primary progressive aphasia, *Ann Neurol* **49**(4) (2001), 425–432.

[22] R.T. Wertz, L.L. LaPointe and J.C. Rosenbek, Apraxia of speech in adults: The disorder and its management, New York: Grune and Stratton; 1984.

[23] J.M. Ogar, N.F. Dronkers, S.M. Brambati, B.L. Miller and M.L. Gorno-Tempini, Progressive nonfluent aphasia and its characteristic motor speech deficits, *Alzheimer Disease and Associated Disorders* **21**(4) (2007), S23–S30.

[24] S.M. Wilson, N.F. Dronkers, J.M. Ogar, J. Jang, M.E. Growdon, F. Agosta et al., Neural Correlates of Syntactic Processing in the Nonfluent Variant of Primary Progressive Aphasia, *The Journal of Neuroscience* **30**(50) (2010), 16845–16854.

[25] D. Howard and K. Patterson, Pyramids and palm trees: A test of semantic access from pictures and words, Bury St.Edmunds, UK: Thames Valley Test Company 1992.

[26] E. Kaplan, H. Goodglass and S. Weintraub, Boston Naming Test. Philadelphia: Lippincott, Williams and Wilkins, 2001.

[27] P.M. Beeson, K. Rising, E.S. Kim and S.Z. Rapcsak, A treatment sequence for phonological alexia/agraphia, *Journal of Speech, Language, and Hearing Research* **53**(2) (2010), 450–468.

[28] J.V. Baldo, D.P. Wilkins, J. Ogar, S. Willock and N.F. Dronkers, Role of the precentral gyrus of the insula in complex articulation, *Cortex* **47**(7) (2010), 800–807.

[29] K.A. Bayles, C.K. Tomoeda and J.A. Rein, Phrase repetition in Alzheimer's disease: effect of meaning and length, *Brain Lang* **54**(2) (1996), 246–261.

[30] J.L. Wiederholt and B.R. Bryant, Gray oral reading tests-(GORT-4). Austin, TX: Pro-Ed 2001.

15

Change of accent as an atypical onset of non fluent primary progressive aphasia

Susy Paolini[a,*], Lucia Paciaroni[a], Antonio Manca[b], Roberto Rossi[b], Daniela Fornarelli[b], Stefano F. Cappa[c], Angela M. Abbatecola[d] and Osvaldo Scarpino[a]

[a] Unit of Neurology, Italian National Research Center on Aging, Via della Montagnola, Ancona, Italy
[b] Unit of Radiology, Italian National Research Center on Aging, Ancona, Italy
[c] Vita-Salute University and Division of Neuroscience, San Raffaele Scientific Institute, Milan, Italy
[d] Scientific Direction, Italian National Research Center on Aging, Ancona, Italy

Abstract. Language disorders can be the first symptom of many neurodegenerative diseases, including Alzheimer's disease (AD) and primary progressive aphasia (PPA). The main variants of PPA are: the non-fluent/agrammatic variant, the semantic variant and the logopenic variant.
Several additional variants of PPA, however, have been described and are considered as atypical presentations.
We describe the case of a woman presenting a progressive isolated language disturbance, characterized by an early dysprosodia, phonological and semantic paraphasias, agrammatism, impairment in repetition, writing of non-words and sentence comprehension. This clinical picture pointed to an atypical presentation of the non-fluent variety. The frequent symptom overlap between the different variants of PPA, most likely reflecting differences in the topography of the pathological changes, needs to be considered in the definition of diagnostic criteria.

Keywords: Dementia, primary progressive aphasia, progressive non fluent aphasia, dysprosodic disorder, foreign accent syndrome

1. Introduction

Isolated language disturbances can be the first symptoms of fronto-temporal lobar degeneration (FTLD). In 1982, Mesulam first introduced Primary Progressive Aphasia (PPA) [1,2] to describe an isolated language impairment that manifests in an insidious manner, remains isolated for at least two years and then evolves into dementia. Subsequent studies identified different clinical presentations of PPA and at the present, three main variants of PPA have been described as: progressive non fluent aphasia, semantic dementia, and logopenic progressive aphasia [3–5].

In 2011, the International Consensus Criteria [6] adopted the following three clinical subtypes for the classification of PPA: nonfluent/agrammatic variant PPA (PPA-NFV), semantic variant PPA (PPA-SV) and logopenic variant PPA (PPA-LV) (Table 1). PPA-NFV is characterized by an effortfull and halting speech with agrammatism, possible anomias and phonologic paraphasias [3,5,7]. Patient comprehension is preserved for single words, while it is slightly impaired for sentences, especially for difficult morphosyntactic constructions [8]. In this variant, apraxia of speech, dysarthria, stuttering, impaired repetition, alexia and agraphia can be found without severe amnesia and/or perceptuo-spatial disorder [5]. Studies of structural and functional imaging suggest an involvement of left inferior frontal region and left anterior insular cortex [7, 9,10]. Clinical presentation of the PPA-SV is associ-

*Corresponding author: S. Paolini, Unit of Neurology, INRCA, Via della Montagnola 81, 60125, Ancona, Italy.
E-mail: paosusy@yahoo.it.

Table 1
Addendum criteria for subtypes of PPA [6]

Clinical diagnosis of nfvPPA
  At least one of the following core features must be present:
    1- Agrammatism in language production
    2- Effortful, halting speech with inconsistent speech sound errors and distortions (apraxia of speech)
  At least 2 of the 3 following other features must be present:
    1- Impaired comprehension of syntactically complex sentences
    2- Spared single-word comprehension
    3- Spared object knowledge

Clinical diagnosis for svPPA
  Both of the following core features must be present:
    1- Impaired confrontation naming
    2- Impaired single-word comprehension
  At least 3 of the following other diagnostic features must be present:
    1- Impaired object knowledge, particularly for low-frequency or low-familiarity items
    2- Surface dyslexia or dysgraphia
    3- Spared repetition
    4- Spared speech production (grammar and motor speech)

Clinical diagnosis for lvPPA
  Both of the following core features must be present:
    1- Impaired single-word retrieval in spontaneous speech and naming
    2- Impaired repetition of sentences and phrases
  At least 3 of the following other features must be present:
    1- Speech (phonologic) errors in spontaneous speech and naming
    2- Spared single-word comprehension and object knowledge
    3- Spared motor speech
    4- Absence of frank agrammatism

ated with normal fluency, as well as an impairment of object naming, deficit of single words comprehension and surface dyslexia, all explained by the disruption of semantic knowledge [8,11–14]. Generally, patients with PPA-SV have a bilateral atrophy of anterior and inferior temporal lobes that is more extensive in the left hemisphere [15–17]. Finally, PPA-LV patients exhibit word finding difficulties and decreased output, impaired naming and repetition in the context of spared semantic and syntactic abilities, while mantaining syntactically simple correct language output [3, 18]. Phonemic paraphasias are also frequent, as well as an impairment in sentence comprehension especially for long sentences, whereas single word comprehension and semantic memory are preserved [18,19]. In these patients, atrophy is localized in the posterior temporal and inferior parietal regions of dominant hemisphere [16,18,19].

In the literature, diverse clinical presentations of language progressive disorders that do not fit the recent criteria have been described, including progressive anarthria [20–23] and progressive jargon aphasia [24]. Some authors have hypothesized that some of these clinical variants could represent different stages of the same disease or an atypical presentation due to variations in specific areas of cerebral degeneration [25].

Regarding the PPA-NFV, a recent study by Luzzi et al. [26] reported an atypical onset of the foreign accent syndrome (FAS). These authors reported a case of an Italian woman presenting a progressive change in her accent, so that listeners perceived her as a foreigner. No other linguistic or cognitive disorders were observed at onset and after one year, a PPA-NFV was diagnosed.

In this report, we also describe an atypical onset of PPA-NFV in a woman presenting as first symptom a prosodic change perceived as a regional accent change rather than as a foreign accent. The change of regional accent has been already described in different diseases and is considered as a variant of FAS [27,28]. We suggest that it may represent an atypical feature of PPA-NFV presentation.

2. Case report

2.1. Clinical details

A 78-year right-handed Italian woman with 8 years of formal education came to our attention in March 2008 for a language disorder characterized by dysprosodia, with sporadic phonologic and semantic paraphasias that had been evolving over the last two years.

Her family members claimed that her symptoms began with a progressive change in the loudness and pitch

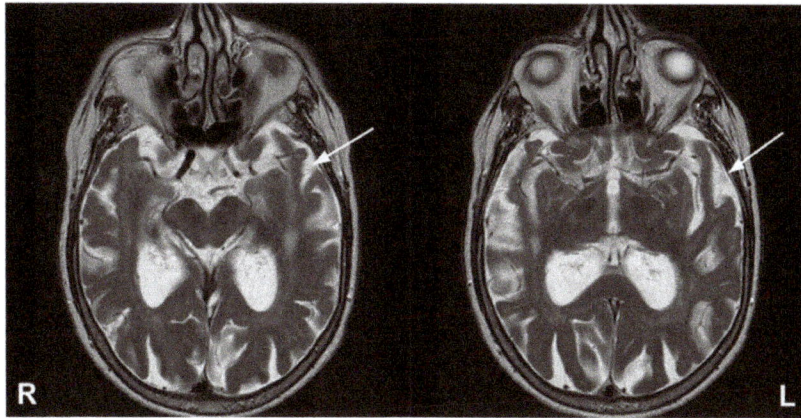

Fig. 1. MRI-scan: Spin Echo sequences T2-weighted, parallel to the long axis of the temporal lobe, showed cortical atrophy more evident in the left side.

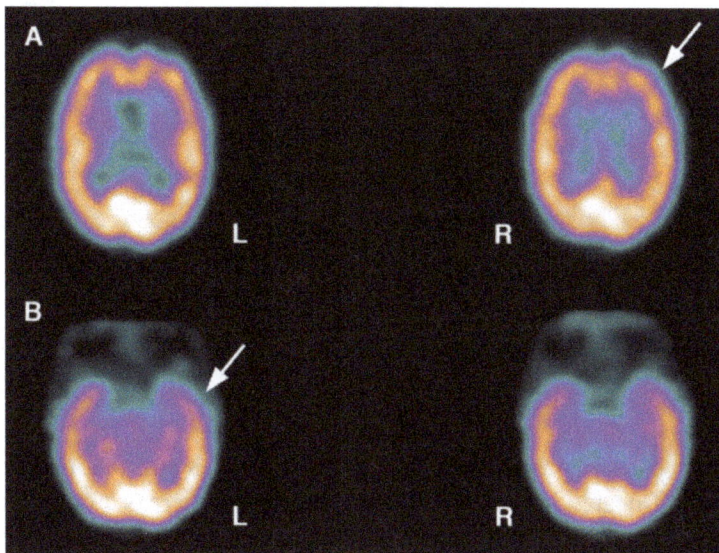

Fig. 2. 99m-Tc-ECD-SPECT evidenced hypoperfusion in the lateral frontal regions (A) and in the surface and mesial temporal lobes, especially in the left side (B).

of the voice. Her speech was perceived as having undergone a regional accent change.

She lived alone and she was entirely independent in activities of daily living. Minimal behavioural changes were also reported (disinhibition, impulsiveness, euphoria and irritability). Her past medical or psychiatric history was unremarkable and her neurological examination was normal.

2.2. Neuroimaging

During the first clinical examination, she underwent a MRI brain scan showing cortical atrophy, especially in the left temporal hemisphere (Fig. 1). A 99m-Tc-ECD-SPECT was also performed and evidenced hypoperfusion of the lateral frontal regions especially in

the left hemisphere, as well as in lateral and medial temporal lobes (Fig. 2).

2.3. Neuropsychological evaluation

A comprehensive neuropsychological testing battery, including attention, executive functions, memory, praxis and visuo-spatial abilities was performed, and the results are shown in Table 2.

A mild frontal executive dysfunction was evident, while there were no deficits in visual and verbal episodic memory, visuo-spatial abilities and object/people knowledge. An impairment in short-term memory was found with a low performance in the Digit Span test. She also showed a mild bucco-linguo-facial apraxia.

A detailed language evaluation showed agrammatic, dysprosodic, anomic spontaneous speech with phono-

Table 2
Neuropsychological testing (scores adjusted for age and education according to published norms)

Tests	Baseline	Follow-up (12 month)	Normal values
Mini mental state examination	26	9.7	> 24
Attention and executive functioning			
Attentional matrices	47.5	43	> 31
Trail making test			
Part A	29	40	< 93
Part B	232		< 282
Weigl's sorting test	7.25	4.5	> 4.25
FAB	5.9*	4.2*	> 13.4
Stroop test (Time)	22.25		< 36.92
Memory			
Corsi test	5.25		> 3.5
Digit span	3.25*	2.5*	> 3.5
Rey AVLT (Immediate recall)	35.9		> 28.52
Rey AVLT (Delayed recall)	9.6		> 4.68
Visuospatial and constructional skill			
Rey complex figure copy	30	28.7	> 23.76
Praxis			
Ideomotor praxis	20		> 16
Bucco-linguo-facial praxis	12,25*		> 16
Language			
Noun naming (ENPA)	8/10*	1/10*	> 8.2
Verb naming (ENPA)	6.5/10	5.5/10*	> 6.1
Token test	18.25*	10.75*	> 26.25
Oral words comprehension (ENPA)	20/20	15.6/20*	> 18.4
Animal fluency	12.5	8*	> 9
Phonemic fluency	1.9*	0*	> 5.8
Pyramids and palms test	45,78		> 40.15

*Pathological score. Abbreviations: FAB = Frontal Assessment Battery; Rey AVLT = Rey Auditory Verbal Learning Test; ENPA = Esame Neuropsicologico per l'Afasia (Capasso R., Miceli G. Esame Neuropsicologico per l'Afasia. Milano: Springer; 2001).

logic errors and rare semantic paraphasias. Although she was born in Marche region (located in the central Italy), where she permanently lived, she gradually began to present a change in her native accent over the last two years. Her accent change was evaluated by 6 native speaking Italians that listened to her speech and all of them judged her accent as similiar to that of the Veneto region (located in the north-east of Italy).

In addition, her prosodic comprehension was impaired for both linguistic (question, command, statement) and affective prosody (angry, sad, surprised, happy, sarcastic). For example, she was unable to distinguish if pairs of sentences were identical or if they differed in terms of intonation or location of stress. During the examination she was not troubled and was unaware of her dysprosody.

Results of formal language testing are reported in Fig. 3 and Table 2. The production tasks showed a mild to moderate naming impairment (more severe for verbs compared to nouns), low phonemic fluency and normal semantic fluency. Single word comprehension was good for nouns and slightly impaired for verbs. Sentence comprehension was severely affected.

Repetition and writing of non-words were seriously impaired, whereas a mild deficit was found for words. Her reading ability was good for both words and nonwords.

A brief neuropsychological evaluation was performed at the 12-month of follow up and results underlined a severe worsening on oral production and comprehension, with a relative preservation of time and space orientation, memory in daily living, visuospatial abilities and selective attention. A mild executive deficit was also confirmed.

At the 24-month of follow-up she was almost mutacic and oral comprehension was severely impaired, but was able to read and to recognize familiar faces. Her family members confirmed an overall worsening of her behaviour with impulsivity, aggression and disinhibition.

3. Discussion

Neurodegenerative diseases that manifest with language disorders include an overlapping of diverse neu-

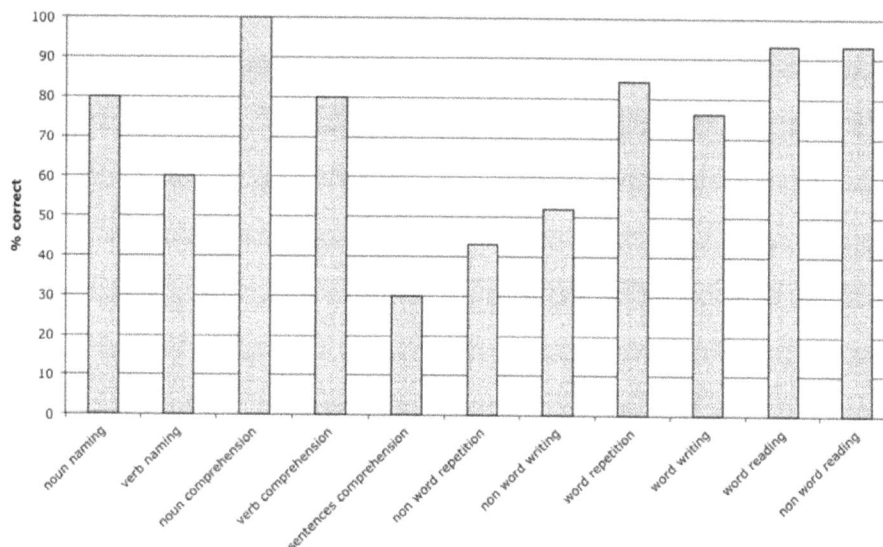

Fig. 3. Performances on BADA Aphasia Examination. BADA = Batteria per l'Analisi del Deficit Afasico (Miceli G. et al. B.A.D.A. Batteria per l'Analisi dei Deficit Afasici. Roma: CEPSAG; 1994).

ropsychological patterns, which may be problematic for a differential diagnosis between an atypical form of Alzheimer's disease (AD), PPA-NFV, PPA-SV and PPA-LV. Indeed, a correct differential diagnosis is extremely important because different clinical patterns may be correlated to distinct neuropathological substrates [29]. In general PPA-NFV is highly associated with tauopathies [24,30,31], while PPA-SV is often due to progranulin/TDP43 pathologies [32–34] and PPA-LV to AD pathology [18,31,33].

Our patient presented with a prominent language disorder, accompanied by an integrity of episodic memory, attention and visuo-spatial abilities. The clinical history of the patient, as reported by her relatives, confirmed an isolated language impairment that had been progressing over the last two years, thus fulfilling the criteria for PPA.

The patient presented frequent anomias and sporadic semantic paraphasias. This could raise the suspicion of the PPA-SV form, given also the cortical atrophy in temporal lobes shown by MRI. However, she had excellent single word comprehension, preserved semantic knowledge and agrammatism, which are incompatible with PPA-SV. The patient also showed moderate difficulties in naming (Table 2; Fig. 3). A qualitative analysis of the errors was performed, and showed that different types of errors were made in response to object and action pictures. Regarding object nouns, the patient presented prevalently phonological errors, whereas for action pictures (verbs) we observed predominantly anomias, circonlocutions and semantic paraphasias, substituting nouns for the target verbs.

This finding is atypical for PPA-SV [35]. Furthermore, during her first clinical evaluation, we found difficulties in repetition, which is typically intact in early PPA-SV. Despite the MRI findings of temporal atrophy, this linguistic pattern excluded a PPA-SV.

Patients with PPA-LV usually show a pattern of speech output that is slow, syntactically simple but correct, with frequent word-finding pauses, naming difficulties, phonemic paraphasias and impaired repetition [18,19]. In this variant, the core problem is a deficit in phonological short-term memory [3,19,36], which is related to involvement of the inferior parietal lobule [36–38]. Our patient presented a phonological short-term memory impairment. Furthermore, her difficulty in single word retrieval, in repetition and the speech phonological errors were similar to PPA-LV. Nevertheless, the presence of agrammatism in production, the presence of dysprosodia/regional accent syndrome and the bucco-faccial apraxia are atypical for this variant.

The patient shared many of the diagnostic features of PPA-NFV [6], such as agrammatism in language production, impaired comprehension of syntactically complex sentences, preservation of single word comprehension and object knowledge. Over time her clinical symptoms evolved toward mutism, as expected in PPA-NFV.

Her dysprosodic disorder was an additional clinical sign for PPA-NFV. Disrupted prosody is often found in advanced PPA-NFV as the consequence of articulation disturbances. Only one case of an Italian patient showing dysprosody as early onset of PPA-NFV has been reported [26]. Three years before the onset of PPA-NFV, this patient presented a speech disorder characterized by the foreign accent syndrome (FAS), that is a linguistic prosody disorder in which a new accent is perceived by listeners as foreign. This prosodic disorder is distinct from apraxia of speech, dysathria and aphasic output disorder, but it can occur at the same time [39]. Generally, FAS emerges as consequence of damage to the language dominant frontal systems underlying speech. The main areas affected are the primary motor cortex, cortico-cortical connections and cortico-subcortical projections [39–41]. FAS is also distinct from emotional or affective dysprosody, which has been conceptualised as a dominant and lateralized function of the right hemisphere [40]. Thus, both hemispheres are necessary for successful prosodic performances.

In comparison to the case reported by Luzzi et al. [26], our patient was perceived as a native Italian, but with a significant change in her regional accent. It is often acknowledged that regional and foreign accents share the same mechanisms in production and comprehension. A recent report [42] suggests a continuum between regional and foreign conditions. The damage within the motor speech network can give rise to specific phonological changes, resulting in a different accent, including ones that sound like a regional change, rather than a FAS [42]. Both regional and foreign accents show the same pattern in comprehensibility and intelligibility of the listener [43]. Furthermore, the close relationship between the two conditions is supported by the linguistic theory, confirming that a dialect is a language, as reported in the statement by Max Weinreich [44]: "A language is a dialect with an army and a navy". For these reasons, our patient may be considered as having a variant of FAS.

In addition, she showed a more severe aphasic picture than the case reported by Luzzi [26], probably because she came to our observation later. She also presented an affective dysprosodia, either in production or in comprehension. Thus, her dysprosodic disorder was characterized by both a linguistic and affective dysprosody, probably because the atrophy interested not only the left linguistic areas, but also the corresponding right ones.

We suggest that the pattern of dysprosodic disorder as the onset of PPA-NFV can vary in function of the prevalent atrophy. If the damage is more evident in the left side, the dysprosodic disorder is characterised by linguistic dysprosodia as in FAS. If atrophy is bilateral then a disorder of affective aspects of prosody will also be associated with linguistic dysprosodia.

Taken together the linguistic findings of our patient were consistent with a probable diagnosis of PPA-NFV, with some atypical features (semantic pharaphasias and the early severe impairment of syntactic comprehension, as well as the cortical atrophy of temporal lobes).

References

[1] Mesulam MM. Slowly progressive aphasia without generalized dementia. Ann Neurol. 1982; 11: 592-8.

[2] Mesulam MM. Primary Progressive Aphasia. Ann Neurol. 2001; 49: 425-32.

[3] Gorno-Tempini ML, Dronkers NF, Rankin KP, Ogar JM, Phengrasamy L, Rosen HJ, et al. Cognition and anatomy in three variants of primary progressive aphasia. Ann Neurol. 2004; 55: 335-46.

[4] Mesulam MM. Primary progressive aphasia – A 25-year retrospective. Alzheimer Dis Assoc Disord. 2007; 21: S8–S11.

[5] Neary D, Snowden JS, Gustafson L, Passant U, Stuss D, Black S, et al. Frontotemporal lobar degeneration: a consensus on clinical diagnostic criteria. Neurology. 1998; 51: 1546-54.

[6] Gorno-Tempini ML, Hillis AE, Weintraub S, Kertesz A, Mendez M, Cappa SF, et al. Classification of primary progressive aphasia and its variants. Neurology. 2011; 76: 1006-14.

[7] Ogar JM, Dronkers NF, Brambati SM, Miller BL, Gorno-Tempini ML. Progressive nonfluent aphasia and its characteristic motor speech deficits. Alzheimer Dis Assoc Disord. 2007; 21: S23–S30.

[8] Hodges JR, Patterson K. Nonfluent progressive aphasia and semantic dementia: A comparative neuropsychological study. J Int Neuropsychol Soc. 1996; 2: 511-24.

[9] Nestor PJ, Graham NL, Fryer TD, Williams GB, Patterson K, Hodges JR. Progressive non-fluent aphasia is associated with hypometabolism centred on the left anterior insula. Brain. 2003; 126: 2406-18.

[10] Rosen HJ, Kramer JH, Gorno-Tempini ML, Schuff N, Weiner M, Miller BL. Patterns of cerebral atrophy in primary progressive aphasia. American J Geriatr Psychiatry. 2002; 10: 89-97.

[11] Grossman M, Ash S. Primary progressive aphasia: A review. Neurocase. 2004; 10: 3-18.

[12] Hodges JR, Patterson K, Oxbury S, Funnell E. Semantic dementia. Progressive fluent aphasia with temporal lobe atrophy. Brain. 1992; 115: 1783-806.

[13] Jefferies E, Patterson K, Lambon Ralph MA. The natural history of late-stage "pure" semantic dementia. Neurocase. 2006; 12: 1-14.

[14] Knibb J, Hodges J. Semantic dementia and primary progressive aphasia: A problem of categorization? Alzheimer Dis Assoc Disord. 2005; 19: S7-S14.

[15] Garrard P, Hodges JR. Semantic dementia: Clinical, radiological and pathological perspectives. J Neurol. 2000; 247: 409-22.

[16] Rohrer JD, Ridgway GR, Crutch SJ, Hailstone J, Goll JC, Clarkson MJ, et al. Progressive logopenic/phonological aphasia: erosion of the language network. Neuroimage. 2010; 49: 984-93.

[17] Rosen HJ, Gorno-Tempini ML, Goldman WP, Perry RJ, Schuff N, Weiner M, et al. Patterns of brain atrophy in frontotemporal dementia and semantic dementia. Neurology. 2002; 58: 198-208.

[18] Gorno-Tempini ML, Brambati S, Ginex V, Ogar J, Dronkers NF, Marcone A, et al. The logopenic/phonological variant of primary progressive aphasia. Neurology. 2008; 71: 1227-34.

[19] Amici S, Gorno-Tempini ML, Ogar JM, Dronkers NF, Miller BL. An overview on Primary Progressive Aphasia and its variants. Behav Neurol. 2006; 17: 77-87.

[20] Lucchelli F, Papagno C. Is slowly progressive anarthria a "pure" motor-speech disorder? Evidence from writing performance. Neurocase. 2005; 11: 234-41.

[21] Silveri MC, Cappa A, Salvigni BL. Speech and language in primary progressive anarthria. Neurocase. 2003; 9: 213-20.

[22] Hachisuka K, Uchida M, Nozaki Y, Hashiguchi S, Sasaki M. Primary progressive aphasia presenting as conduction aphasia. J Neurol Sci. 1999; 167: 137-41.

[23] Kimura N, Kumamoto T, Hanaoka T, Hazama Y, Nakamura K, Arakawa R. Cortical basal degeneration presenting with progressive conduction aphasia. J Neurol Sci. 2008; 269: 1638.

[24] Deramecourt V, Lebert F, Debachy B, Mackowiak-Cordoliani MA, Bombois S, Kerdraon O, et al. Prediction of pathology in primary progressive language and speech disorders. Neurology. 2010; 74: 42-9.

[25] Kertesz A, Davidson W, McCabe P, Takagi K, Munoz D. Primary progressive aphasia: Diagnosis, varieties, evolution. J Int Neuropsychol Soc. 2003; 9: 710-9.

[26] Luzzi S, Viticchi G, Piccirilli M, Fabi K, Pesallaccia M, Bartolini M, et al. Foreign accent syndrome as the initial sign of primary progressive aphasia. J Neurol Neurosurg Psychiatry. 2008; 79: 79-81.

[27] Kwon M, Kim JS. Change of dialect after stroke: A variant of foreignaccent syndrome. Eur Neurol. 2006; 56: 249-52.

[28] Verhoeven J, Marien P. Change of dialect after stroke: A variant of foreign accent syndrome. Eur Neurol. 2007; 58: 191.

[29] Hillis AE. Lost for words. Neurology. 2008; 71: 1218-9.

[30] Josephs KA, Petersen RC, Knopman DS, Boeve BF, Whitwell JL, Duffy JR, et al. Clinicopathologic analysis of frontotemporal and corticobasal degenerations and PSP. Neurology. 2006; 66: 41-8.

[31] Mesulam M, Wicklund A, Johnson N, Rogalski E, Léger GC, Rademaker A, et al. Alzheimer and frontotemporal pathology in subsets of primary progressive aphasia. Ann of Neurol. 2008; 63: 709-19.

[32] Davies RR, Hodges JR, Kril JJ, Patterson K, Halliday GM, Xuereb JH. The pathological basis of semantic dementia. Brain. 2005; 128: 1984-95.

[33] Josephs KA., Whitwell JL, Duffy JR, Vanvoorst WA, Strand EA, Hu WT, et al. Progressive aphasia secondary to Alzheimer disease vs FTLD pathology. Neurology. 2008; 70: 25-34.

[34] Kertesz A, McMonagle P, Blair M, Davidson W, Munoz DG. The evolution and pathology of frontotemporal dementia. Brain. 2005; 128: 1996-2005.

[35] Hillis AE, Oh S, Ken L. Deterioration of naming nouns versus verbs in primary progressive aphasia. Ann Neurol. 2004; 55: 268-75.

[36] Vallar G, Di Betta AM, Silveri MC. The phonological short-term store-rehearsal system: patterns of impairment and neural correlates. Neuropsychologia. 1997; 35: 795-812.

[37] Damasio H, Damasio AR. The anatomical basis of conduction aphasia. Brain. 1980; 103: 337-50.

[38] Paulesu E, Frith CD, Frackowiak RS. The neural correlates of the verbal component of working memory. Nature. 1993; 362, 342-5.

[39] Blumstein S, Kurowsky K. The foreign accent syndrome: A perspective. Journal of neurolinguistics. 2006; 19: 346-55.

[40] Ross E, Monnot M Neurology of affective prosody and its functional-anatomic organization in right hemisphere. Brain Lang. 2008: 104; 51-74.

[41] Van Lancker Sidtis D, Pachana N, Cummings JL., Sidtis JJ. Dysprosodic speech following basal ganglia insult: toward a conceptual framework for the study of the cerebral representation of prosody. Brain Lang. 2006; 97: 135-53.

[42] Naidoo R, Warriner EM, Oczkowski WJ, Sevigny A, Humphreys KR. A case of foreign accent resulting in regional dialect. Can J Neurol Sci. 2008; 35: 360-5.

[43] Floccia C, Butler J, Goslin J, Ellis L. Regional and foreign accent processing in english: Can listeners adapt? J Psycholinguistic Res. 2009; 38: 379-412.

[44] Chomsky N. Knowledge of language: its nature, origin and use. New York: Praeger, 1986.

16

Syntactic and morphosyntactic processing in stroke-induced and primary progressive aphasia

Cynthia K. Thompson[a,b,c], Aya Meltzer-Asscher[a,*], Soojin Cho[a,c], Jiyeon Lee[a], Christina Wieneke[c], Sandra Weintraub[b,c,d] and M.-Marsel Mesulam[b,c]

[a]*Department of Communication Sciences and Disorders, Northwestern University, Evanston, IL, USA*
[b]*Department of Neurology, Northwestern University, Evanston, IL, USA*
[c]*Cognitive Neurology and Alzheimer's Disease Center, Northwestern University, Evanston, IL, USA*
[d]*Department of Psychiatry and Behavioral Sciences, Northwestern University, Evanston, IL, USA*

Abstract. The paper reports findings derived from three experiments examining syntactic and morphosyntactic processing in individuals with agrammatic and logopenic variants of primary progressive aphasia (PPA-G and PPA-L, respectively) and stroke-induced agrammatic and anomic aphasia (StRAg and StRAn, respectively). We examined comprehension and production of canonical and noncanonical sentence structures and production of tensed and nontensed verb forms using constrained tasks in experiments 1 and 2, using the Northwestern Assessment of Verbs and Sentences (NAVS [57]) and the Northwestern Assessment of Verb Inflection (NAVI, Thompson and Lee, experimental version) test batteries, respectively. Experiment 3 examined free narrative samples, focusing on syntactic and morphosyntactic measures, i.e. production of grammatical sentences, noun to verb ratio, open-class to closed-class word production ratio, and the production of correctly inflected verbs. Results indicate that the two agrammatic groups (i.e., PPA-G and StRAg) pattern alike on syntactic and morphosyntactic measures, showing more impaired noncanonical compared to canonical sentence comprehension and production and greater difficulties producing tensed compared to nontensed verb forms. Their spontaneous speech also contained significantly fewer grammatical sentences and correctly inflected verbs, and they produced a greater proportion of nouns compared to verbs, than healthy speakers. In contrast, PPA-L and StRAn individuals did not display these deficits, and performed significantly better than the agrammatic groups on these measures. The findings suggest that agrammatism, whether induced by degenerative disease or stroke, is associated with characteristic deficits in syntactic and morphosyntactic processing. We therefore recommend that linguistically sophisticated tests and narrative analysis procedures be used to systematically evaluate the linguistic ability of individuals with PPA, contributing to our understanding of the language impairments of different PPA variants.

Keywords: Aphasia, primary progressive aphasia, agrammatism, syntactic processing, narrative speech

1. Introduction

A large body of literature exists, which describes the linguistic deficits associated with different types of aphasia caused by stroke (StRAph). Many individuals with stroke-induced agrammatic aphasia (StRAg) of Broca's type present a characteristic pattern of nonfluent speech, as well as grammatical, or (morpho)syntactic, deficits. The latter are exhibited by impaired comprehension and production of sentences with complex syntactic structures, in particular semantically reversible noncanonical sentences involving syntactic movement (e.g. [9,11,31,62]), impaired production of grammatical morphemes, in particular tense inflec-

*Corresponding author: Aya Meltzer-Asscher, Aphasia and Neurolinguistics Research Laboratory, Frances Searle Building, 2240 Campus Drive, Evanston, IL, 60208, USA.
E-mail: a-meltzer-asscher@northwestern.edu.

tion (e.g. [1,22,58]), and greater difficulty producing verbs as compared to nouns (e.g. [44,69]). In contrast, stroke-induced anomic aphasic (StrAn) individuals speak fluently and present with intact syntactic abilities, but evince significant naming difficulties, primarily for nouns [24–26,44,69].

Language deficits have also been reported for individuals with primary progressive aphasia (PPA), a language impairment caused by a neurodegenerative disease [39,40]. According to current guidelines, PPA can be subdivided into three variants: agrammatic/ nonfluent (PPA-G), logopenic (PPA-L), and semantic (PPA-S) [27,29,42]. Individuals with the PPA-G variant present with nonfluent speech, verb production deficits, and difficulties with comprehension and production of syntactically complex sentences [13,32,34, 48,55,64,67]. Conversely, PPA-L is associated with fluctuating fluency, difficulties with word retrieval, and impaired repetition, with relatively spared syntax and word comprehension [28], and individuals with PPA-S show relatively fluent patterns of speech production, but have problems with naming and comprehension of single words [35,41,42]. The term progressive nonfluent aphasia (PNFA) used in the earlier literature has inconsistently included what is now known as PPA-G and PPA-L patients without making a distinction between the two groups.

Importantly, the underlying neurological deficits of the PPA and StrAph clinical populations are distinctly different. Areas of the brain impaired by stroke follow the territory of the cerebral vascular system, whereas those associated with PPA do not. In addition, neurodegenerative disease, as in PPA, affects only particular groups and layers of cells, leaving others relatively intact. Hence, affected regions of the brain can remain active during language task performance [52]. Nevertheless, in general, PPA-G and StrAg are associated with necrosed or atrophied tissue in the left frontal region, although tissue atrophy in PPA-G also may involve the temporo-parietal junction (TPJ) and lesions in StrAg can include both anterior and posterior perisylvian brain regions [44,56,65]. Conversely, PPA-L and StrAn typically result from compromised tissue in the temporo-parietal region. PPA-L is correlated with atrophy in the left TPJ, and the adjacent parts of the lateral temporal cortex [27,42] and classic StrAn often results from damage to posterior temporal and parietal regions, which tends to spare the superior temporal gyrus [36], although some anomic aphasic individuals present with left anterior temporal lobe lesions, including the temporal pole and inferior temporal gyrus [15].

Finally, PPA-S results from anterior temporal atrophy, more pronounced in the left hemisphere [27,42].

Despite these neuropathophysiological differences between PPA and StrAph there is some evidence, at least for the two agrammatic groups, i.e., PPA-G and StrAg, that they present with similar behavioral deficits. For example, Thompson et al. [60] examined production and comprehension of nouns and verbs in PPA and StrAph individuals, using the Northwestern Naming Battery [63] and found similar behavioral patterns for PPA-G and StrAg participants. Both groups had greater difficulty naming verbs compared to nouns, and showed effects of argument structure complexity on verb production. However, it is still unclear whether the grammatical impairment in PPA-G is parallel to that in StrAg. For example, Graham et al. [30] argue that PNFA is not characterized by agrammatism, as the speech of individuals with this PPA subtype includes normal proportions of content and function words as well as nouns and verbs, unlike that of StrAg speakers. This conclusion is difficult to interpret since their PNFA group may have included a mixture of PPA-G and PPA-L. Furthermore, to our knowledge, syntactic and morphosyntactic impairments associated with PPA and StrAph have not been examined systematically and no studies have compared language deficit patterns in other types of stroke-induced aphasia (e.g., StrAn) with those found in other PPA variants (e.g., PPA-L).

The aim of the present study is to explore (morpho)syntactic impairment patterns in individuals with PPA-G and PPA-L and to compare them with individuals with StrAg and StrAn. We examined comprehension and production of canonical and noncanonical sentences, production of verb inflection and other syntactic and morphosyntactic variables in three experiments. As detailed below, in Experiments 1 and 2 constrained tasks were used to evaluate sentence comprehension and production abilities as well as production of grammatical morphemes, i.e., the Northwestern Assessment of Verbs and Sentences (NAVS [54]) and the Northwestern Assessment of Verb Inflection (NAVI; Lee and Thompson, experimental version), respectively. Experiment 3 included analysis of free narrative speech samples obtained from participants.

2. Experiment 1. Patterns of sentence comprehension and production

Whereas canonical sentences in English display the subject-verb-object order typical of this language (e.g.

Table 1
Demographic data for paticipants in Experiments 1, 2, and 3

Participants	N	Males	Handedness (left/right)	Age	Education	Duration of symptoms (years)
Experiment 1						
Primary Progressive Aphasia (PPA)						
PPA-G	11	6	1/10	63.8	16.3	3.3
PPA-L	15	9	2/13	62.9	16.1	3.9
Stroke Aphasia (StrAph)						
StrAg	22	16	2/20	53.7	16.7	5.8
StrAn	18	10	4/14	59.8	15.6	4.9
Experiment 2						
Primary Progressive Aphasia (PPA)						
PPA-G	7	2	0/7	64.1	16.0	2.7
PPA-L	10	6	0/10	66.2	16.9	2.8
Stroke Aphasia (StrAph)						
StrAg	20	14	2/18	55.3	16.7	6.5
StrAn	9	5	2/7	56.2	15.4	3.0
Experiment 3						
Primary Progressive Aphasia (PPA)						
PPA-G	9	5	1/8	63.0	16.6	3.8
PPA-L	15	9	2/13	66.5	15.9	3.7
Stroke Aphasia (StrAph)						
StrAg	8	5	1/7	50.3	16.3	4.6

'The dog chased the cat'), in noncanonical structures the object is moved across the verb and the subject, and surfaces in a clause-initial position (e.g. 'The cat was chased by the dog') (see e.g. [12]). Many studies have established that individuals with StrAg have difficulties comprehending and producing noncanonical sentences that are semantically reversible [9,11,31,62]. This pattern also has been noted in PPA-G in production, using the Northwestern Anagram Test (NAT [63, 67]). However, patterns of canonical and noncanonical sentence comprehension have not been established in PPA-G or other PPA variants and the performance of PPA and StrAph groups have not been directly compared with one another. In the present experiment we used the Sentence Comprehension Test (SCT) and Sentence Production Priming Test (SPPT) from the NAVS to compare comprehension and production of canonical and noncanonical sentences in participant groups with PPA and StrAph.

2.1. Method

2.1.1. Participants

Eleven PPA-G, 15 PPA-L, 22 StrAg and 18 StrAn volunteers, recruited from the subject pools of the Aphasia and Neurolinguistics Research Laboratory in Evanston, IL and the Cognitive Neurology and Alzheimer's Disease Center in Chicago, IL, participated in the study. All were native, monolingual English speakers, with normal or corrected-to-normal hearing and vision. Three of the PPA participants and six of the StrAph ones were left handed, and the rest were right handed. The four groups were matched for education (Kruskal Wallis, $\chi^2(3) = 2.84$, $p = 0.417$). Participants ranged in age from 35 to 79 years (mean 63.8 yrs for PPA-G; 62.9 yrs for PPA-L; 53.6 yrs for StrAg; 59.8 yrs for StrAn), with the PPA participants, in general, older than the StrAph participants (Mann-Whitney, $Z = -2.61$, $p = 0.009$). The four groups were, therefore, not completely matched for age (Kruskal Wallis, $\chi^2(3) = 9.9$, $p = 0.019$), although there was no significant difference between the PPA-G and PPA-L groups (Mann-Whitney, $Z = -1.56$, $p = 0.876$) or between the StrAg and StrAn groups (Mann-Whitney, $Z = -1.6$, $p = 0.102$) (see Table 1). All participants provided informed consent, and the study was approved by the Institutional Review Board at Northwestern University.

The diagnosis of PPA was based on neurological examination, clinical presentation, and neuropsychological test performance. None of the PPA patients showed evidence of stroke or other neurological disorder and all presented a history of progressive language deficits in the face of relatively spared performance in other cognitive domains. To rule out memory and attention deficits we administered the Mini-Mental State Examination (MMSE) [21], Wechsler Memory Scale (WMS) [66], Facial Recognition [7], and Trail Making Tests [46] (see test scores in Table 2). Twenty-two of the 26 PPA participants achieved a score of 24 or higher on the MMSE, indicating normal performance. The remaining four achieved scores between 16 and 23, suggesting mild impairment, (but importantly, scores on this measure are influenced by patients' compromised language ability [23,45]).

PPA variants were determined based on single word comprehension ability, measured by the Peabody Picture Vocabulary Test (PPVT [18]) (moderately difficult items, #157–192), and on canonical and noncanonical sentence generation, measured by the NAT (see scores in Table 3). Individuals showing relatively spared single word comprehension as well as sentence generation (a score of 60% or higher on both the PPVT and the NAT) were classified as PPA-L, whereas speakers showing spared single word comprehension (60% or higher on the PPVT) but impaired sentence generation (a score lower than 60% on the NAT) were classified as PPA-G. Accordingly, both the PPA-G and the PPA-L groups showed relatively spared word comprehension (PPA-G PPVT mean: 95.2; PPA-L PPVT mean: 92.9), with no significant difference between the groups (Mann-Whitney, $Z = -0.447$, $p = 0.655$). On the NAT, the two groups performed in a similar manner on canonical sentences (Mann-Whitney, $Z = -1.27$, $p = 0.204$), but differed significantly on noncanonical sentences (Mann-Whitney, $Z = -3.43$, $p = 0.001$), with PPA-G participants showing poorer performance, consistent with their syntactic impairment.

To further assess the linguistic impairment of the PPA participants, the Western Aphasia Battery (WAB [36]) was administered, and Aphasia Quotients (AQs) were computed based on WAB subtest scores (see Table 3). Mean WAB-AQ for the PPA-G participants was 82.95 (range: 75.3–95.2), and for the PPA-L participants was 88.5 (range: 74.4–95.8). WAB-AQs differed significantly between the two groups (Mann-Whitney $Z = -2.18$, $p = 0.027$), reflecting significant differences between the two groups on WAB fluency scores (Mann-Whitney, $Z = -3.01$, $p = 0.002$). However, the groups did not differ significantly on the auditory comprehension (Mann-Whitney, $Z = -1.2$, $p = 0.237$), repetition[1] (Mann-Whitney, $Z = -1.49$, $p = 0.148$) or naming (Mann-Whitney, $Z = -0.47$, $p = 0.646$) subtests of the WAB.

All of the StrAph participants suffered left-hemisphere strokes, on average 5.4 years prior to the study.

Aphasia type was determined by participants' performance on the WAB (also shown in Table 3) as well as clinical impression. Participants were classified as agrammatic if their spontaneous speech was nonfluent, consisting of short, simple phrases with omission of some grammatical morphemes. Conversely, participants were diagnosed as anomic if their speech was fluent, with primarily word retrieval difficulties. Accordingly, the StrAg participants in the experiment presented with mild-to-moderate aphasia (WAB-AQ mean: 77.13, range: 66–87.2) and nonfluent speech (WAB fluency mean: 4.5, range 4–5). The StrAn participants also presented with mild-to-moderate aphasia (WAB-AQ mean: 85.6, range: 69.4–92.4), but with fluent speech (WAB fluency mean: 7.6, range: 6–9) and mild-to-moderate word retrieval difficulty. WAB-AQs for the two groups differed significantly (Mann-Whitney, $Z = -3.78$, $p < 0.001$) largely because of significant differences in fluency scores (Mann-Whitney $Z = -5.08$, $p < 0.001$). The two groups also differed on the WAB repetition test (Mann-Whitney $Z = -2.26$, $p = 0.024$), but not on the auditory comprehension (Mann-Whitney $Z = -1.89$, $p = 0.058$) or naming subtests (Mann-Whitney $Z = -0.613$, $p = 0.545$).

Comparing the PPA and StrAph groups' WAB-AQ scores, there were no significant differences between the PPA-L and StrAn groups (Mann-Whitney, $Z = 1.57$, $p = 0.11$), but a significant difference was found between the PPA-G and StrAg groups (Mann-Whitney, $Z = 2.54$, $p = 0.011$), stemming from a significant difference in naming subtest scores (Mann-Whitney, $Z = 2.21$, $p = 0.027$), such that the PPA-G participants performed better on this subtest than the StrAg participants. However, there were no significant differences between the two agrammatic groups on other subtests of the WAB.

2.1.2. Materials and procedure

Participants were tested using the SCT and SPPT subtests from the NAVS, with the former always administered prior to the latter. The SCT and SPPT items included 30 sentences, five sentences for each of six sentence types: actives, subject wh-questions, subject relative clauses, passives, object wh-questions, and object relative clauses. The first three constructions are canonical, whereas, the latter three are noncanonical. All sentences were semantically reversible with world-knowledge alone insufficient for determining which participant was the agent (doer of the action) and which the theme (recipient of the action). Table 4 contains examples of the sentence types tested. Picture stim-

---

[1]Gorno-Tempini et al. [29] proposed a classification system, according to which PPA-L individuals should present with impaired repetition of sentences and phrases, consistent with the notion that these individuals have a phonological short-term memory deficit. The subtyping criteria used here are those suggested by Mesulam et al. [42], which do not include repetition.

Table 2
Mean neuropsychological scores (standard deviations) for PPA participants in Experiments 1, 2, and 3

Participants	MMSE (30)	WMS-iii		Visual perception Facial Rec (54)	Processing speed Trail making test A
		Immediate (48)	Delayed (48)		
Experiment 1					
PPA-G	27.2 (2.82)	34.0 (4.24)	35.0 (4.52)	47.9 (3.21)	58.4 (35.26)
PPA-L	25.7 (4.11)	35.8 (5.21)	38.9 (5.45)	46.6 (3.74)	44.6 (21.73)
Experiment 2					
PPA-G	27.8 (1.95)	34.0 (4.08)	34.1 (4.3)	46.9 (3.39)	59.3 (38.43)
PPA-L	28.0 (1.63)	33.6 (4.12)	35.8 (4.13)	48.8 (3.12)	32.2 (9.59)
Experiment 3					
PPA-G	27.2 (2.99)	34.4 (4.53)	36.4 (3.7)	48.9 (3.62)	48.3 (25.6)
PPA-L	25.1 (5.57)	34.6 (4.79)	38.7 (5.46)	47.5 (3.82)	53.2 (29.99)

Note: MMSE = Mini-Mental State Exam, WMS = Wechsler Memory Scale, Facial Rec. = Facial Recognition.

uli used for the SCT and the SPPT depicted reversible scenes corresponding with each sentence, such as a cat watching a dog and a dog watching a cat (see Fig. 1).

In the SCT, participants were presented with a randomly selected picture pair while a target sentence, corresponding to one of the pictures, was read aloud by the examiner. Participants were then asked to point to the picture depicting the scenario described. A 10-sec response time was allowed, and if no response occurred within the allotted time, or if requested, sentences were repeated once. Responses were counted as correct if provided within the given time, and if the chosen picture matched the target sentence.

In the SPPT, for each picture pair presented, the examiner modeled the target sentence structure, describing the picture on the participant's left. The participant was then asked to produce a sentence 'just like it' for the picture on the right. Target sentence types were tested in blocks, with five exemplars of each type presented consecutively. A 15-sec response time was provided for each trial, which was repeated once if no response or an incorrect response was produced. Grammatical sentences of the target syntactic structure produced within the allotted time were counted as correct, with any inflection or paraphasic (either phonological or semantic) errors accepted, unless phonological errors resulted in nonwords, or semantic errors reversed the agent and theme of target sentences.

2.2. Results

Percent correct production (SPPT) and comprehension (SCT) of each sentence type for the PPA and StrAph participant groups are presented in Tables 5 and 6, respectively and in Fig. 2. A 2 (group) x 2 (modality) x 2 (canonicity) ANOVA for the PPA participants revealed significant main effects of group (F (1, 23) =

5.87, $p = 0.024$), with PPA-G showing poorer performance than PPA-L, modality (F (1, 23) = 9.55, $p = 0.005$), with production more difficult than comprehension, and sentence canonicity (F (1, 23) = 39.61, $p < 0.001$), with noncanonical sentences more difficult than canonical ones. A significant two-way interaction effect also was found between modality and canonicity (F (1, 23) = 8.13, $p = 0.009$), indicating that the difference between canonical and noncanonical sentences was greater for production compared to comprehension. Additionally, there was a significant interaction between group and canonicity (F (1, 23) = 10.73, $p = 0.003$), with the canonicity effect greater for the PPA-G than for the PPA-L group. There was also a significant group x canonicity x modality interaction (F (1, 23) = 9.328, $p = 0.006$). Post-hoc analysis using the Mann-Whitney test revealed that the PPA-L group performed significantly better than the PPA-G group in production of noncanonical sentences ($Z = -2.19$, $p = 0.028$). Further, the difference between groups for comprehension of noncanonical sentences approached significance ($Z = -1.72$, $p = 0.085$). However, the two groups did not differ in production or comprehension of canonical forms ($Z = -.0784$, $p = 0.433$ and $Z = -1.28$, $p = 0.281$, respectively).

For the StrAph data, a 2 × 2 × 2 ANOVA revealed a main effect of group (F (1, 35) = 5.75, $p = 0.021$), with StrAg showing poorer performance than StrAn, as well as a main effect of modality (F (1, 35) = 14.01, $p = 0.001$) and canonicity (F (1, 35) = 54.28, $p < 0.001$) similar to those found in the PPA analysis. Significant interactions were also found between modality and canonicity (F (1, 35) = 10.99, $p = 0.002$), and between canonicity and group (F (1, 35) = 5.4, $p = 0.026$). Although we did not find a three-way group x canonicity x modality interaction, follow-up comparisons between the StrAg and StrAn groups, us-

Table 3
Mean language scores (standard deviations) for PPA and stroke-induced aphasic groups in Experiments 1, 2, and 3

Participants	Western aphasia battery					PPVT	NAT	
	AQ (100)	F (10)	Comp (10)	Rep (10)	Nam (10)	(%)	C (%)	NC (%)
Experiment 1								
Primary Progressive Aphasia (PPA)								
PPA-G	82.9 (5.8)	5.6 (1.7)	9.3 (0.6)	8.0 (1.0)	9.1 (0.4)	95.2 (4.3)	86.6 (17.0)	41.5 (14.1)
PPA-L	88.5 (6.1)	8.0 (1.3)	9.5 (0.6)	8.6 (1.0)	8.7 (1.5)	92.9 (8.3)	95.6 (6.5)	78.3 (18.2)
Stroke Aphasia (StrAph)								
StrAg	77.1 (5.8)	4.5 (0.5)	8.8 (1.0)	8.1 (1.2)	8.4 (1.1)			
StrAn	85.6 (6.4)	7.6 (1.6)	9.4 (0.6)	9.0 (0.8)	8.1 (1.3)			
Experiment 2								
Primary Progressive Aphasia (PPA)								
PPA-G	84.2 (7.1)	6.0 (1.9)	9.4 (0.7)	8.5 (0.8)	9.1 (0.3)	95.2 (4.5)	85.7 (18.6)	43.8 (15.3)
PPA-L	91.5 (4.7)	8.5 (1.4)	9.7 (0.5)	9.1 (0.9)	8.7 (1.5)	92.8 (8.6)	95.3 (6.30)	90 (12.3)
Stroke Aphasia (StrAph)								
StrAg	78.3 (6.7)	4.5 (0.5)	9.1 (0.9)	8.0 (1.3)	8.5 (0.9)			
StrAn	87.4 (7.5)	8.0 (1.3)	9.5 (0.7)	8.7 (0.8)	8.5 (1.9)			
Experiment 3								
Primary Progressive Aphasia (PPA)								
PPA-G	79.4 (3.4)	5.0 (1.0)	9.0 (0.7)	7.4 (1.2)	9.1 (0.5)	94.8 (4.3)	76.2 (26.3)	30.5 (18.0)
PPA-L	88.4 (5.4)	8.1 (1.2)	9.6 (0.5)	8.5 (1.0)	8.6 (1.5)	94.0 (7.8)	94.5 (6.5)	78.2 (16.4)
Stroke Aphasia (StrAph)								
StrAg	75.3 (6.9)	4.4 (0.7)	8.6 (1.0)	7.7 (1.0)	8.0 (1.6)			

Note: AQ = Aphasia Quotient, F = Fluency, Comp = Auditory Comprehension, Rep = Repetition, Nam = Naming, PPVT = Peabody Picture Vocabulary Test, NAT = Northwestern Anagram Test, C = Canonical, NC = Noncanonical.

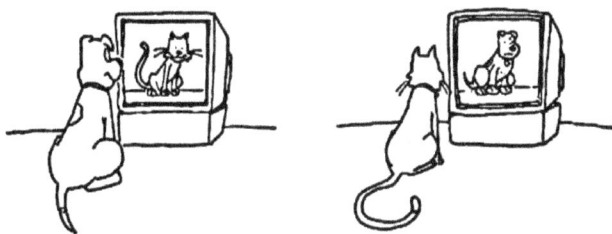

Fig. 3. Example of a picture stimulus pair used in the NAVS-SCT and NAVS-SPPT in Experiment 1.

ing the Mann-Whitney test, were performed. These analyses revealed that the StrAg group's performance was significantly poorer than that of the StrAn group for production of noncanonical sentences ($Z = -2.78$, $p = 0.005$) and the difference in comprehension of noncanonical sentences approached significance ($Z = -1.91$, $p = 0.056$). However, the two groups did not differ significantly in the comprehension ($Z = -1.53$, $p = 0.125$) or production ($Z = -1.1$, $p = 0.272$) of canonical sentences.

Statistical comparison between the two agrammatic groups, namely PPA-G and StrAg, yielded no main effect of aphasia type ($F (1, 31) = 0.078$, $p = 0.782$) (see Fig. 2). There was a significant effect of modality ($F (1, 31) = 16.03$, $p < 0.001$), with production more impaired than comprehension, and of canonicity ($F (1, 31) = 49.85$, $p < 0.001$), with noncanonical sentences more difficult than canonical ones. There was also a significant two-way interaction between modality and canonicity ($F (1, 31) = 13.35$, $p = 0.001$), with the canonicity effect larger for production than for comprehension.

2.3. Discussion

This experiment revealed considerable similarities between PPA and StrAph. In both groups, individuals with agrammatic deficits (namely, PPA-G and StrAg) were significantly more impaired in production of noncanonical sentences than participants with the logopenic variant of PPA or stroke-induced anomic aphasia. Likewise, there was a trend toward impaired comprehension of noncanonical sentences in the two agrammatic groups, compared to the other two groups. Interestingly, the deficits did not extend to canonical sentences, on which production and comprehension for the agrammatic participants was comparable to that of the logopenic and anomic groups. The selective deficit in noncanonical sentences for agrammatic speakers indicates a syntactically related impairment. It is important to point out that deficits in comprehension of noncanonical sentence comprehension may be related to general impairments in verbal working memory (e.g., [10]; but see [51] for arguments against this view). However, we find that a working memory account does not completely explain the deficit patterns

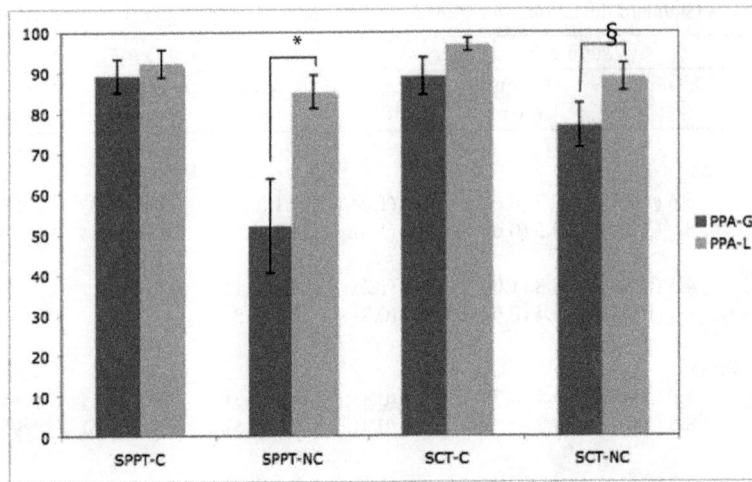

(a)

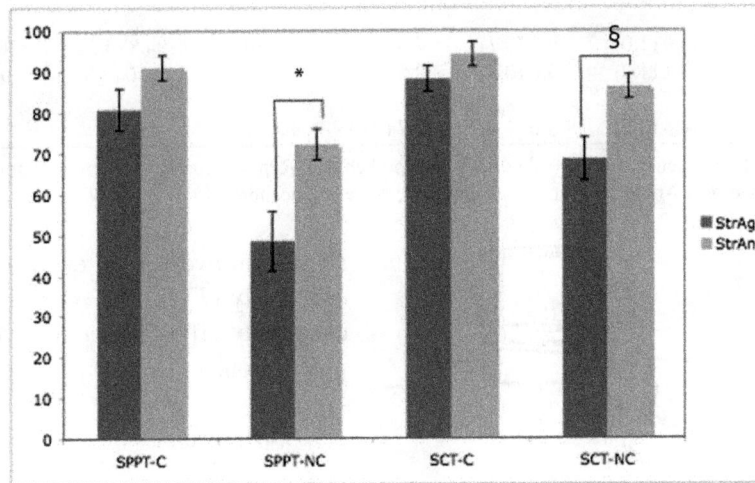

(b)

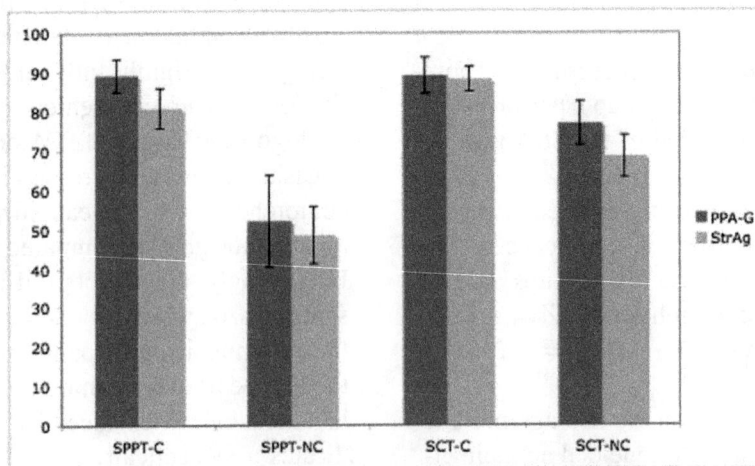

(c)

Fig. 2. Percent correct responses (and standard error), Experiment 1: NAVS Sentence Production Priming Test (SPPT) and Sentence Comprehension Test (SCT) for (a) PPA and (b) StrAph participants for canonical (C) and noncanonical sentences (NC) sentences; (c) depicts results for the two agrammatic groups. $\S p < 0.1$; $*p < 0.05$, Mann-Whitney test, two-tailed.

Table 4

Sentence class	Sentence type	Example
Canonical	Active	The dog was watching the cat
	Subject relative	Pete saw the dog who was watching the cat
	Subject Wh-question	Who was watching the cat?
Non-canonical	Passive	The cat was watched by the dog
	Object relative	Pete saw the cat who the dog was watching
	Object Wh-question	Who was the dog watching?

Table 5
Percent correct responses (standard deviation) for PPA participants in Experiment 1

Test	Participants	Active	SWQ	SR	Passive	OWQ	OR
SPPT	PPA-G	100 (0.0)	88.0 (25.3)	80.0 (35.3)	54.0 (47.2)	70.0 (38.0)	32.0 (42.4)
	PPA-L	97.3 (10.3)	93.3 (12.3)	86.7 (27.9)	92.0 (16.6)	96.0 (15.5)	68.0 (32.8)
SCT	PPA-G	94.5 (9.3)	87.3 (20.5)	85.4 (23.8)	70.9 (35.1)	83.6 (17.5)	74.5 (20.2)
	PPA-L	97.3 (7.0)	94.7 (11.9)	98.7 (5.20)	93.3 (12.3)	86.7 (19.5)	86.7 (16.3)

Note: SPPT = Sentence Production Priming Test, SCT = Sentence Comprehension Test, SWQ = Subject Wh-Questions, OWQ = Object Wh-Questions, SR = Subject Relatives, OR = Object Relatives.

Table 6
Percent correct responses (standard deviation) for StrAph participants in Experiment 1

Test	Participants	Active	SWQ	SR	Passive	OWQ	OR
SPPT	StrAg	94.5 (17.6)	74.5 (33.3)	73.6 (38.2)	50.9 (44.0)	65.4 (41.5)	29.1 (36.4)
	StrAn	97.8 (6.5)	86.7 (25.7)	88.9 (18.4)	85.6 (22.5)	90.0 (20.9)	41.0 (38.5)
SCT	StrAg	90.9 (16.0)	83.6 (24.4)	90.0 (17.2)	67.3 (34.7)	77.7 (21.6)	60.9 (33.5)
	StrAn	100 (0.0)	86.7 (28.9)	96.0 (11.2)	89.3 (18.3)	88.0 (22.4)	81.3 (22.0)

Note: SPPT = Sentence Production Priming Test, SCT = Sentence Comprehension Test, SWQ = Subject Wh-Questions, OWQ = Object Wh-Questions, SR = Subject Relatives, OR = Object Relatives.

found here. Notably, comprehension of subject-relative constructions, which are canonical and similar in length to object relative constructions, was superior to object-relative structures (85.4% correct for subject relatives, 74.5% correct for object relatives for PPA-G; 90% for subject relatives compared to 60.9% for object relatives for StrAg).

Another interesting result of the experiment is that the PPA-G and the StrAg groups performed very similarly, with no significant differences found for any tasks or condition. This indicates that PPA-G individuals indeed exhibit noncanonical sentence deficits in line with those seen in stroke-induced agrammatic speakers.

3. Experiment 2. Production of verb inflections

A large number of studies have shown that StrAg aphasic individuals have difficulty with inflectional morphology, shown by a tendency to omit or substitute grammatical morphemes that mark tense, aspect and agreement [1,4,22,37,58]. In particular, finite verb forms, inflected for tense (e.g., the past-tense form 'fixed'), are especially vulnerable to disruption in stroke-induced agrammatism, whereas non-

finite verb forms (e.g. the infinitive 'to fix') are generally spared [5,17,19,20]; also see Thompson et al. [59] for review. However, to our knowledge no studies have systematically investigated grammatical morphology deficits related to tense in individuals with PPA. Because difficulty producing grammatical morphemes, particularly those marking verb tense, is one of the major deficits seen in StrAg, investigation of inflectional morphology is important for detailing morphosyntactic deficits in PPA-G. Further, detailing patterns of impaired/spared grammatical morphology across PPA subtypes will help to distinguish between them. In this experiment, we therefore compared PPA and StrAph participant groups on verb inflection production, using the NAVI, a test designed to evaluate production of nonfinite and finite verb forms.

3.1. Participants

Participants included 7 PPA-G, 10 PPA-L, 20 StrAg and 9 StrAn individuals, recruited from the subject pools of the Aphasia and Neurolinguistics Research Laboratory in Evanston, IL and the Cognitive Neurology and Alzheimer's Disease Center in Chicago, IL. The participants met the same selection criteria as in

Experiment 1. All 17 PPA participants, and 25 of the 29 StrAph participants, were right handed. The groups were matched for education (Kruskal Wallis, $\chi^2(3) = 3.36$, $p = 0.339$) and age (Kruskal-Wallis, $\chi^2(3) = 7.64$, $p = 0.054$) (see Table 1).

The PPA participants recruited for the study showed no evidence of stroke or other neurological disorder and all presented a history of progressive language deficits with relatively spared performance in other cognitive domains. As in Experiment 1, the MMSE, WMS, Facial Recognition and Trail Making Tests were administered to rule out possible memory, visual perceptual, and attention deficits (see scores in Table 2). All participants scored 24 or higher on the MMSE.

As in Experiment 1, PPA variants were determined based on scores in the PPVT and the NAT. Both the PPA-G and the PPA-L groups showed relatively spared word comprehension, with no significant difference between groups (PPA-G PPVT mean: 95.2; PPA-L PPVT mean: 92.8, Mann-Whitney, $Z = -0.453$, $p = 0.650$). Further, on the NAT, the two groups did not differ significantly on canonical sentences (PPA-G mean: 85.7, PPA-L mean: 95.3, Mann-Whitney, $Z = -0.959$, $p = 0.338$). However, the PPA-G group was significantly more impaired than the PPA-L group on noncanonical sentences (PPA-G mean: 43.8, PPA-L mean: 90.0, Mann-Whitney, $Z = -3.45$, $p = 0.001$).

We also administered the WAB to all PPA participants, with mean AQs of 84.2 (range: 75.3–95.2) and 91.5 (range: 83.2–97.2), for the PPA-G and PPA-L participants, respectively, which again differed significantly between groups (Mann-Whitney, $Z = -2.0$, $p = 0.045$) due to significant differences in WAB fluency scores (Mann-Whitney, $Z = -2.39$, $p = 0.017$). However, the groups did not differ significantly on the auditory comprehension (Mann-Whitney, $Z = -0.86$, $p = 0.389$), repetition (Mann-Whitney, $Z = -1.468$, $p = 0.142$) or naming (Mann-Whitney, $Z = -0.245$, $p = 0.806$) subtests of the WAB.

The stroke aphasic participants all suffered a left hemisphere stroke, with the exception of one, who presented with a right hemisphere lesion and crossed aphasia, with an average of 5.6 years post onset. Aphasia type was determined as in Experiment 1. All participants presented with mild-to-moderate aphasia (WAB-AQ mean: StrAg: 78.3, range 65.5–87.6; StrAn: 87.4, range: 69.4–93.3), with WAB fluency scores ranging from 4 to 5 (mean = 4.5) for the former group and from 6 to 9 (mean = 8.0) for the latter. As in Experiment 1, statistical analyses comparing the two groups indicated significant differences in WAB-AQ (Mann-

Whitney, $Z = -3.39$, $p = 0.001$) and fluency scores (Mann-Whitney, $Z = -4.44$, $p < 0.001$), but the two groups did not differ significantly on the auditory comprehension (Mann-Whitney, $Z = -0.33$, $p = 0.74$), repetition (Mann-Whitney, $Z = -1.53$, $p = 0.125$), or naming (Mann-Whitney, $Z = -1.56$, $p = 0.119$) subtests of the WAB. (See Table 3 for language test scores for the PPA and StrAph groups.)

The two agrammatic groups, PPA-G and StrAg, did not differ on their WAB-AQs (Mann-Whitney, $Z = 0.1772$, $p = 0.081$). Similarly, there was no difference in WAB-AQ between the PPA-L and the StrAn group (Mann-Whitney, $Z = 1.103$, $p = 0.278$).

3.2. Materials and procedure

Ten two-argument (transitive) verbs were selected, including five with regular (e.g., *tickle*) and five with irregular (e.g., *eat*) past-tense morphology, with each elicited in five different forms: infinitive (e.g., *to eat*), progressive (e.g., *is eating*), present singular (e.g., *eats*), present plural (e.g., *eat*), past regular (for regular verbs, e.g., *tickled*), and past irregular (for irregular verbs, e.g., *ate*), resulting in a total of 50 experimental trials (see Table 7 for a set of sample stimuli). Note that the first two verb forms (i.e., the infinitive and progressive) are nonfinite – that is, uninflected for tense (in the progressive, tense is marked on the auxiliary verb, and the lexical verb is a participle), and the latter four are finite forms – inflected for tense. Black-and-white line drawings were prepared for all verbs, depicting an agent and a theme (e.g., a man eating a hamburger) to elicit all verb forms, except for the present plural, for which two agents and two themes were illustrated (e.g., two men eating hamburgers).

A sentence completion task, using temporal adverbs such as *everyday* (to elicit present tense singular and plural forms) and *yesterday* (to elicit past tense forms), was used to obligate production of each target verb form. Together with each stimulus picture, a sentence with a missing verb was presented and read aloud and participants were asked to complete the sentence by providing the correct verb form. To control for verb retrieval difficulties, the verb stem of each target form also was provided on each stimulus template (see Fig. 3). Responses were counted as correct if the target verb form was produced within 10 seconds of stimulus presentation. For any responses with self-corrections, the last attempt was scored.

Table 7
Verb forms assessed by the NAVI and corresponding example sentences used to elicit them in Experiment 2

Finiteness	Verb form	Example
Nonfinite (Uninflected for tense)	Infinitive	The man likes to *eat* the hamburger.
	Progressive	Now the man is *eating* the hamburger.
Finite (Inflected for tense)	Present singular	Everyday the man *eats* the hamburger.
	Present plural	Everyday the men *eat* the hamburgers.
	Past – regular	Yesterday the boy *tickled* the girl.
	Past – irregular	Yesterday the man *ate* the hamburger.

Table 8
Percent correct responses of StrAph and PPA participants for nonfinite and finite verb forms, Experiment 2

Participant	Nonfinite verb forms				Finite verb forms			
	Inf.	Prog.	Total	Pres. sin.	Pres. pl.	Past reg.	Past irreg.	Total
Primary Progressive Aphasia (PPA)								
PPA-G	92.4 (14.6)	96.2 (7.6)	94.3 (11.0)	61.0 (40.5)	59.0 (28.3)	80.0 (28.3)	71.4 (25.4)	66.7 (21.5)
PPA-L	99.0 (3.20)	99.0 (3.2)	99.0 (3.20)	92.3 (8.0)	75.3 (29.4)	95.0 (12.7)	84.0 (24.6)	87.6 (10.4)
Stroke-induced aphasia (StrAph)								
StrAg	87.3 (26.2)	90.8 (14.7)	89.1 (16.7)	67.8 (35.7)	41.9 (30.8)	55.0 (41.0)	48.0 (38.6)	53.2 (27.5)
StrAn	100 (0.0)	97.0 (4.6)	98.5 (2.3)	80.3 (12.0)	65.6 (28.3)	76.7 (22.4)	76.7 (22.4)	74.8 (18.9)

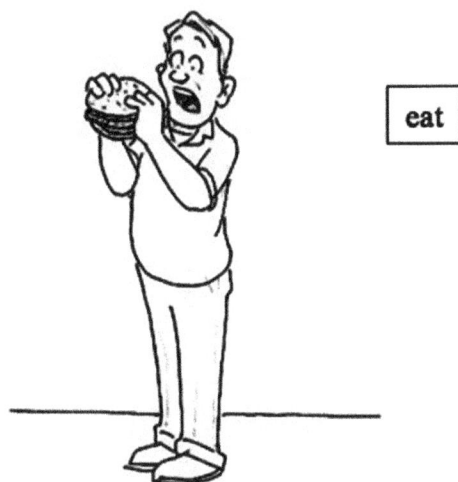

Yesterday, the man _____ the hamburger.

Fig. 4. Sample stimulus for the NAVI test, Experiment 2, to elicit the irregular past tense form, *ate*.

3.3. Results

Table 8 presents percent correct responses in each of the nonfinite and finite conditions for the PPA and StrAph participant groups, with these data presented in graphic form in Fig. 4. Analysis of the PPA data using a 2 (group) x 2 (tensed/nontensed) ANOVA revealed a main effect of group ($F(1,15) = 6.68, p = 0.021$), with PPA-G more impaired than PPA-L, and a main effect of tense ($F(1,15) = 30.8, p < 0.001$), with tensed verbs more difficult than nontensed ones. There was also an interaction between group and tense ($F(1,15) = 5.28, p = 0.036$), with the tense effect greater for the PPA-G group than for the PPA-L group. Post-hoc

comparisons showed significantly greater impairment for the PPA-G compared to the PPA-L participants on finite (Mann-Whitney, $Z = -2.01, p = 0.044$), but not on nonfinite (Mann-Whitney, $Z = -1.44, p = 0.149$), verb forms.

Similar analyses of the StrAph data also revealed a significant main effect for group ($F(1, 27) = 5.56, p = 0.026$), with StrAg more impaired than StrAn, and a main effect of tense ($F(1,27) = 36.89, p < 0.001$). In addition, as in the PPA group, post-hoc comparisons revealed a significantly greater impairment for finite, but not nonfinite, forms for StrAg compared to the StrAn group (Mann-Whitney, finite: $Z = -2.05, p = 0.04$; nonfinite $Z = -1.37, p = 0.17$).

A 2 (group) x 2 (tensed/nontensed) ANOVA for the two agrammatic groups (PPA-G and StrAg) revealed a main effect of tense ($F(1, 25) = 34.0, p < 0.001$), but no main effect of aphasia type ($F(1, 25) = 1.47, p = 0.237$) or interaction between tense and aphasia type ($F(1, 25) = 0.586, p = 0.451$) (see Fig. 4).

3.4. Discussion

As in the previous experiment, these results point to interesting symmetries between StrAph and PPA. In both cases participants with agrammatism scored lower than those with anomic or logopenic impairments on finite verb form production, though not on nonfinite verb form production. In addition, as in Experiment 1, no differences were found between the two agrammatic groups (namely StrAg and PPA-G).

These findings corroborate previous research show-ing that stroke agrammatic individuals perform sig-

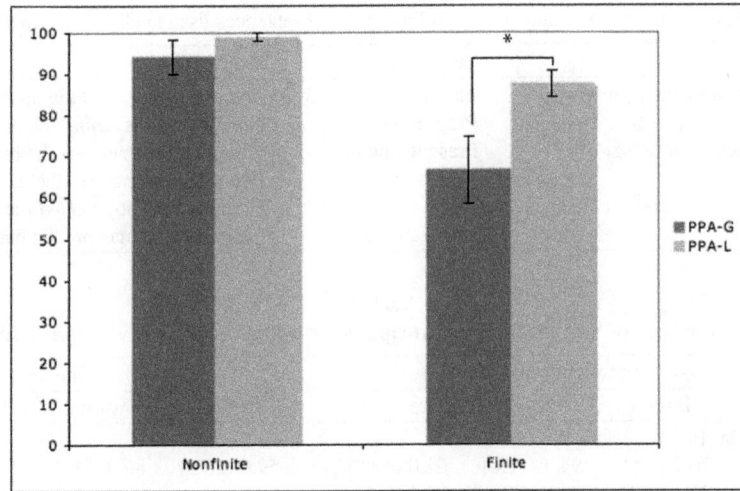

(a)

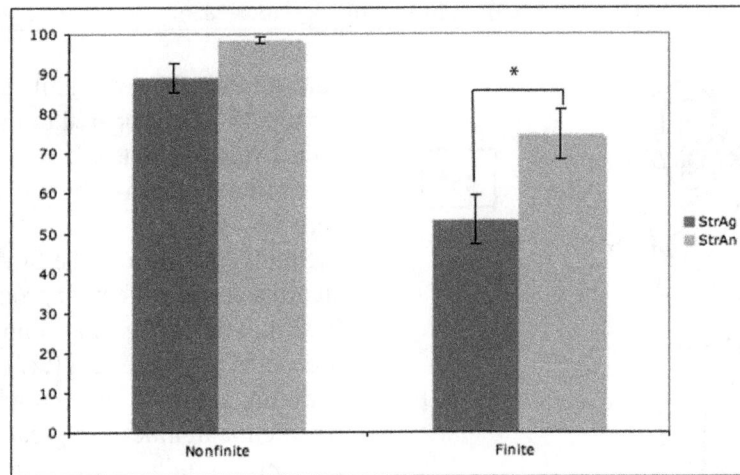

(b)

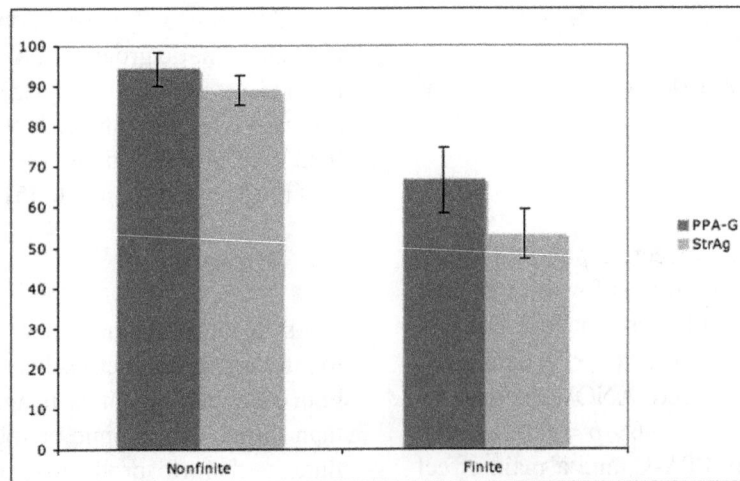

(c)

Fig. 4. Percent correct responses (with standard errors), Experiment 2: NAVI nonfinite and finite verb forms for (a) PPA and (b) stroke aphasic participants; (c) displays performance for the two agrammatic groups. $^*p < 0.05$, Mann-Whitney test, two-tailed.

nificantly more poorly than individuals with stroke-induced anomic aphasia in the production of inflected verb forms (e.g. [5]). The data also provide important new information distinguishing between agrammatic and logopenic variants of PPA. While individuals with PPA-G show impairments in production of verb tense (mirroring those seen in individuals with agrammatism resulting from stroke in this and previous studies), individuals with PPA-L do not exhibit such deficits.

4. Experiment 3. Narrative discourse analysis

Analysis of spontaneous speech enables evaluation of many different aspects of language production, and can reveal deficit patterns indicative of different linguistic impairments. For example, Saffran et al. [50] showed that individuals with stroke-induced nonfluent aphasia exhibit reduced speech rate relative to normal controls in spontaneous speech and that agrammatic individuals in particular use fewer closed-class words, either substitute or omit verb inflections, and produce fewer grammatical sentences compared to healthy control speakers (see also [8,38,49,53,62] and others).

A few studies also have examined narrative production in individuals with PPA, with several noting syntactic and morphosyntactic impairments in nonfluent PPA as compared to normal or fluent PPA speakers [3, 47,55,57,68]. Thompson et al. [55] presented the results of an in depth longitudinal analysis of four patients, then diagnosed with nonfluent PPA, and found low proportions of grammatical sentences and correct verb morphology, high ratios of open- to closed-class words, and high noun to verb ratios in the patients compared to healthy control speakers. Similarly, Gunawardena et al. [33] found fewer complex sentences; Wison et al. [68] found a greater number of syntactic errors; and Ash et al. [2] observed feature omission and incorrect use of grammatical forms in their cohorts of nonfluent PPA speakers. However, the participants with nonfluent PPA studied by Graham et al. [30] showed normal proportions of grammatical morpheme and verb productions in their narrative speech samples, suggesting that the deficit patterns in nonfluent PPA are not in line with agrammatism resulting from stroke.

Part of the lack of complete agreement across studies may relate to the diagnostic classification of nonfluent and fluent PPA, versus more precise classifications of PPA-G, PPA-L, and PPA-S. Notably, only three of the nonfluent PPA patients studied by Thompson et al. [55] showed agrammatic production patterns, which increased in severity over time, whereas one patient (Subject 2) showed a different pattern, characterized by advancing word retrieval difficulty. Notably, based on production patterns, Subject 2 would today be classified as logopenic (and he has since come to autopsy, demonstrating Alzheimer's pathology). In addition, in a more recent study, Thompson et al. [54] found that both PPA-G and PPA-L participants evinced decreased fluency (i.e., nonfluent production), measured by words per minute, compared to healthy control and PPA-S speakers. However, the PPA-G, but not the PPA-L, participants showed reductions in grammatical sentences, correct verb inflection and use of verb argument structure. Thus research examining narrative production in PPA patients is needed, comparing those presenting with PPA-G and PPA-L. Additionally, to our knowledge only two studies have compared the narrative production patterns of PPA and StrAph groups. The Thompson et al. [55] study compared PPA performance to a small group of Broca's aphasic individuals (with agrammatism), with results showing PPA production patterns (for all except Subject 2) very similar to that of the stroke-induced aphasic speakers across a range of linguistic variables. Patterson et al. [47] also examined words per minute (but no other linguistic variables) produced by progressive nonfluent aphasia (PNFA) and nonfluent aphasic (stroke-induced) participant groups. Interestingly, these authors also found no difference between the two groups.

In Experiment 3 we analyzed free narratives obtained from groups of PPA and StrAph speakers. In our analysis, we targeted the following measures: words per minute (WPM), mean length of utterance (MLU), proportion of grammatical sentences, ratio of open- to closed-class words, ratio of nouns to verbs, and proportion of correctly inflected verbs produced. Whereas the first two measures are associated with fluency, the last four are commonly taken to reflect (morpho)syntactic processing, and can be used to detect agrammatic speech.

4.1. Method

4.1.1. Participants

Nine PPA-G, 15 PPA-L, 8 StrAg and 15 healthy volunteers recruited from the subject pools of the Aphasia and Neurolinguistics Research Laboratory in Evanston, IL and the Cognitive Neurology and Alzheimer's Disease Center in Chicago, IL, participated in the study.[2] All met the same selection criteria as participants in Experiments 1 and 2. All were right-handed, except three PPA and one StrAg participants. The four groups were matched for education (Kruskal Wallis, $\chi^2(3) = 0.578, p = 0.901$). Aphasic participants ranged in age from 38 to 81 years, with a mean age of 63.0 for PPA-G, 66.5 for PPA-L, and 50.25 for StrAg, and control participants ranged in age from 50 to 74, with a mean of 62.6. Statistical analysis of age across participant groups showed significant differences (Kruskal Wallis, $\chi^2(3) = 12.09, p = 0.007$), with the PPA-G and PPA-L groups significantly older than the StrAg group (Mann-Whitney; PPA-G vs. StrAg: $Z = -2.654, p = 0.006$; PPA-L vs. StrAg: $Z = -2.908, p = 0.004$), although mean ages for the PPA and healthy control groups did not differ (Kruskal Wallis, $\chi^2(2) = 1.337, p = 0.512$) (see Table 1).

The PPA participants showed no evidence of stroke or other neurological disorder and all presented with a history of progressive language deficits with relatively spared performance in other cognitive domains. As in the previous experiments, the MMSE, WMS, Facial Recognition and Trail Making Tests were administered to rule out possible memory, visuoperceptual and attention deficits (see scores in Table 2), with all but three of the participants scoring 24 or higher on the MMSE.

As in Experiments 1 and 2, PPA variants were determined based on scores in the PPVT and the NAT. Both groups showed relatively spared word comprehension, with no significant difference between the groups (PPVT mean: PPA-G = 94.8; PPA-L – 94.0, Mann-Whitney, $Z = -0.331, p = 0.741$). On the NAT, the PPA-G group showed impaired syntactic performance, scoring significantly lower than the PPA-L group on noncanonical sentences (NAT noncanonical mean: PPA-G = 30.5; PPA-L = 78.2, Mann-Whitney, $Z = -1.411, p = 0.001$), but not on canonical ones (NAT canonical mean: PPA-G = 76.2; PPA-L = 94.5, Mann-Whitney, $Z = -3.377, p = 0.211$).

PPA participants were also administered the WAB, with mean AQs of 79.4 (range: 73.9–85.0) and 88.4 (range: 74.4–94.0) for the PPA-G and PPA-L groups, respectively, which differed significantly (Mann-Whitney, $Z = -3.369, p < 0.001$). WAB fluency scores also differed significantly (Mann-Whitney, $Z = -3.725, p < 0.001$) as did performance on the

WAB auditory comprehension (Mann-Whitney, $Z = -2.274, p = 0.023$) and repetition (Mann-Whitney, $Z = -2.158, p = 0.031$) subtests. However, there was no difference between groups on WAB naming subtest scores (Mann-Whitney, $Z = -0.627, p = 0.558$).

All of the stroke aphasic participants suffered a left-hemisphere stroke, on average 4.6 years prior to the experiment. Participants were classified as agrammatic based on performance on the WAB as well as spontaneous speech production patterns, as explained in Experiment 1. The StrAg participants in this experiment were similar in linguistic performance to those described in the former experiments, with mean WAB-AQ of 75.3 (range: 65.9–87.6), and mean WAB fluency score of 4.4 (range: 4–6) (see Table 3).

There was no significant difference between the two agrammatic groups (i.e. PPA-G and StrAg) on WAB-AQ scores (Mann-Whitney, $Z = 1.734, p = 0.093$).

4.1.2. Procedure

Narrative language samples were obtained by asking participants to tell the Cinderella story, after looking at a picture book detailing the story. The samples were recorded, transcribed, segmented into utterances, and then coded for linguistic variables using a method described by Thompson et al. [62] (also see [55, 57]). Coding involved several levels of analysis. At the utterance level, coding included identification of sentences versus non-sentential utterances and grammatical versus ungrammatical sentences (e.g. sentences where verbal tense morphology was omitted); at the bound-morpheme level, the use of inflectional morphemes (e.g., verb tense and agreement) was coded; and at the lexical level, all words were coded for open- or closed-class status and for grammatical class (e.g., noun, verb etc.).

4.2. Results

Results on the six outcome measures specified above for each participant group are shown in Table 9. A MANOVA with the six output measures as dependent variables revealed an effect of participant group on all the measures (p's < 0.001), except for noun to verb ratio ($p = 0.072$). A post-hoc Bonferroni test was further undertaken to assess between group differences. With regard to measures of fluency, for both WPM and MLU significant differences between the control group and all patient groups were found (p's < 0.01 and p's $\leqslant 0.001$, respectively). In addition, the PPA-L group produced significantly more WPM compared

---

[2] At the time the study was conducted, we were unable to recruit a large enough sample of stroke anomic participants to draw meaningful conclusions.

Table 9
Mean (standard deviation) of outcome measures in narrative analysis, Experiment 3

Participants	WPM	MLU	% Gram.	% Inflection	N:V ratio	O:C ratio
PPA-G	57.56 (25.38)	6.71 (2.08)	46.56 (18.50)	81.91 (19.54)	1.62 (0.84)	1.06 (0.20)
PPA-L	91.28 (29.61)	8.28 (1.41)	80.47 (13.88)	97.03 (4.85)	1.11 (0.68)	0.90 (0.09)
StrAg	52.62 (34.59)	4.87 (2.02)	45.13 (21.56)	82.96 (16.15)	1.71 (1.51)	1.54 (0.65)
Control	132.25 (17.43)	11.92 (3.33)	92.53 (4.41)	99.03 (2.06)	1.19 (0.22)	0.96 (0.10)

Note: WPM = words per minute, MLU = mean length of utterance, % Gram. = proportion of grammatical sentences, N:V ratio = noun to verb ratio, O:C ratio = open-class to closed-class ratio.

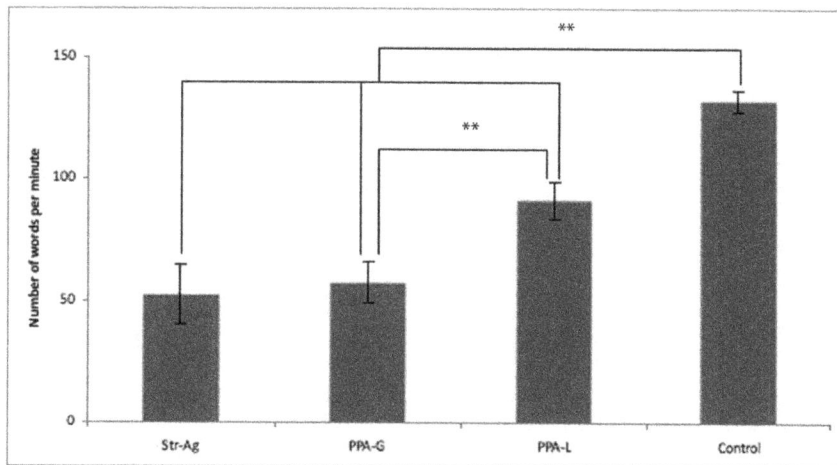

(a)

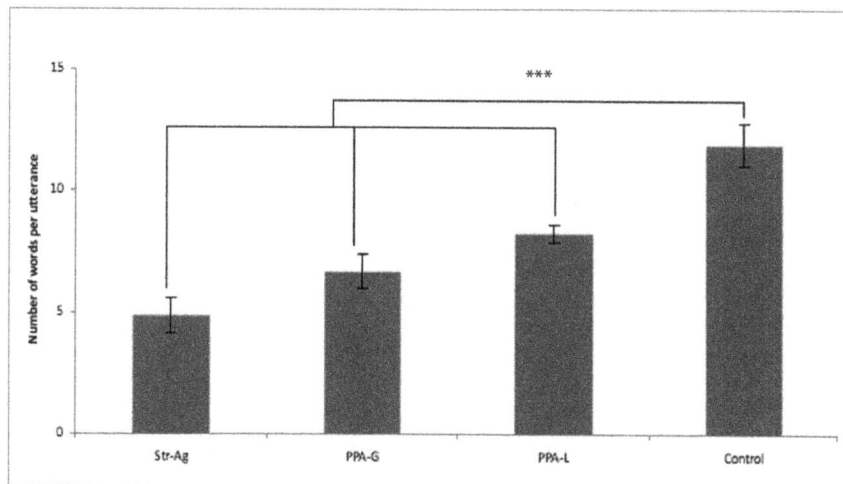

(b)

Fig. 5. (a) WPM and (b) MLU by participant group, Experiment 3. ***$p < 0.001$; **$p < 0.01$, Mann-Whitney test, two-tailed.

to the PPA-G group ($p = 0.006$), although the two groups did not differ significantly for MLU ($p = 0.827$). No significant differences were noted between the two agrammatic groups for WPM ($p = 1$) or MLU ($p = 0.758$) (see Fig. 5).

Turning next to the proportion of grammatical sentences, no significant difference was found between the control and PPA-L groups ($p = 0.309$). However, both groups differed significantly from the PPA-G group (p's

< 0.001). The StrAg group likewise displayed a lower proportion of grammatical sentence than controls ($p < 0.001$). In addition, the two agrammatic groups did not differ significantly from each other ($p = 1$). A similar pattern was noted for the proportion of correctly inflected verbs. Although significant differences were found between both agrammatic groups and the control group (PPA-G vs. control, $p = 0.005$, StrAg vs. control, $p = 0.013$), as well as between the PPA-L and PPA-G

(a)

(b)

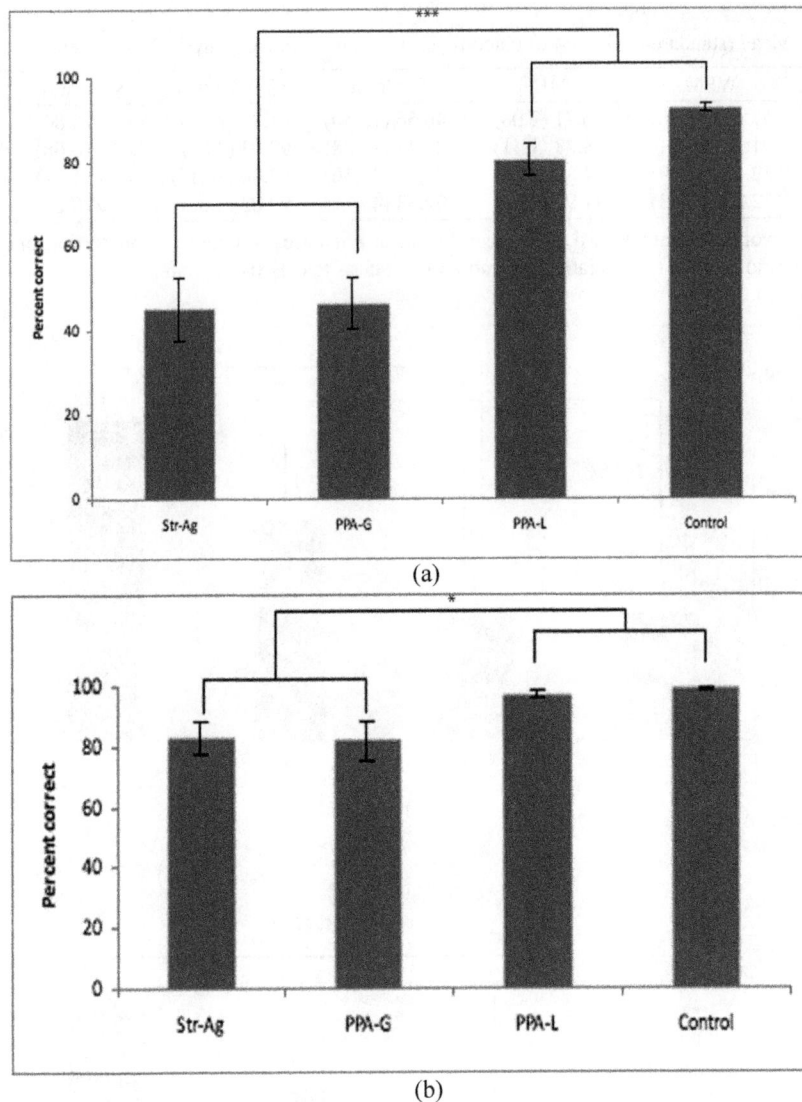

Fig. 6. Proportion of (a) grammatical sentences and (b) correctly inflected verbs by participant group, Experiment 3. $^*p < 0.05$, $^{***}p < 0.001$, Mann-Whitney test, two-tailed.

group ($p = 0.018$), the PPA-L and control groups did not differ from one another ($p = 1$). Further, no significant difference was found between the two agrammatic groups ($p = 1$). (see Fig. 6).

For noun-to-verb ratio (N:V ratio), mean ratio for the PPA-G group was higher than that for the PPA-L group, indicating that the agrammatic participants used a higher proportion of nouns in their narratives. However, this difference did not reach significance ($p = 0.245$), due to the large variability within the agrammatic group. As with previous measures, the two agrammatic groups did not differ on N:V ratio ($p = 1$). With regard to open- and closed-class word production, a significant difference was found between the StrAg group and the control group, as well as between the StrAg and PPA-G groups, for open-class to closed-class ratios

(p's < 0.01). However, PPA-G, PPA-L and control participants did not differ significantly from one another (p's $= 1$). (see Fig. 7).

4.3. Discussion

Results of the two fluency measures in the experiment, WPM and MLU, indicate that both PPA groups as well as the stroke-induced agrammatic group were less fluent than healthy controls in their narrative production. The WPM data further show that the agrammatic PPA participants were significantly less fluent than the PPA-L group, in line with previous research (e.g. [2,5, 68]). However, MLU did not differentiate the two patient groups. In support of Thompson et al. [57], these data indicate that use of the term nonfluent to classi-

(a)

(b)

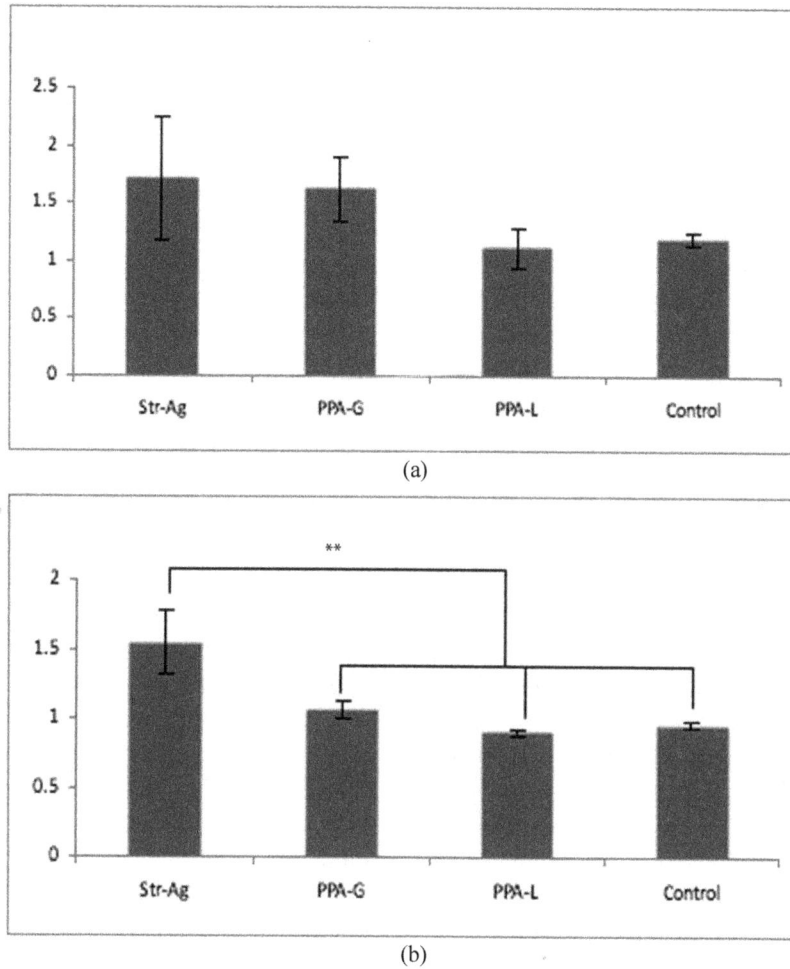

Fig. 7. (a) N:V ratio (b) O:C ratio by participant group, Experiment 3. $**p < 0.01$, Mann-Whitney test, two-tailed.

fy individuals with PPA does not differentiate between agrammatic and logopenic PPA variants. Indeed, both PPA groups demonstrate nonfluent speech compared to normal. However, the two differ in syntactic and morphosyntactic abilities. Importantly, there were no differences in fluency between the two agrammatic groups (i.e. StrAg and PPA-G).

Two of our measures, namely proportion of grammatical sentences and proportion of correctly inflected verbs, clearly indicate that the agrammatic groups are impaired with regard to (morpho)syntactic processing, showing deficits in forming syntactically correct sentences and in using grammatical morphemes to inflect verbs. These findings are consistent with previous ones, suggesting syntactic and morphosyntactic deficits in agrammatic PPA [2,55,57,68]. In contrast, performance of the logopenic PPA participants (i.e., PPA-L) was less impaired than that found in the agrammatic PPA group. These findings suggest relatively unimpaired (morpho)syntactic production ability in this patient group. However, it is worth noting that the pro-

portion of grammatical sentences produced by PPA-L individuals was smaller than that of controls, but this difference did not reach significance (i.e., 80.47% for PPA-L; 92.52% for controls). Thompson et al. [57] and Wilson et al. [68] reported similar patterns, with the PPA-L participants producing significantly fewer grammatical sentences compared to the unimpaired, control speakers, but significantly more grammatical sentences than the PPA-G group. In addition, in the present study, the PPA-L group showed very high levels of correct verb inflection (i.e., a mean of 97%), a pattern also noted in Thompson et al. [57]. Nevertheless, the mild deficit in grammatical sentence production found in PPA-L warrants further investigation to determine the robustness of this effect. For example, grammatical accuracy might be disrupted not because of syntactic processing deficits but rather because of more general word-finding difficulty, which might lead to rephrasing and resultant agrammatic output.

Results of the noun to verb ratio measure again indicate a similar deficit in the two agrammatic groups.

The agrammatic participants (both PPA-G and StrAg) showed a trend towards producing more nouns and fewer verbs, compared to healthy speakers, suggesting a grammatical deficit involving the latter category (the same trend can be seen in the PPA-G group in Thompson et al. [57]). Graham et al. [30], however, did not find evidence of verb production deficits in their nonfluent PPA patients, possibly because their patient cohort included both agrammatic and logopenic variants.

A somewhat surprising result emerged from the open-class to closed-class word production ratio measure. Whereas for StrAg participants, the ratio was higher than that of controls, suggesting, as predicted, a limited use of grammatical, closed-class morphemes, the PPA-G group patterned with the PPA-L and control groups, rather than with the StrAg group, suggesting no impairment for this variable. Notably, Graham et al. [57] likewise did not find a reduced proportion of function words in this group. Based on these results, Graham and colleagues suggested that agrammatism (or progressive nonfluent aphasia) in PPA is not akin to a true agrammatism as seen secondary to stroke aphasia. However, this conclusion is problematic in light of the other agrammatic features displayed by speakers with PPA-G, e.g. reduced proportion of grammatical sentences and correct verb inflection. Notably, Thompson et al. [57] also found significantly reduced argument structure production in their cohort of PPA-G participants, compared to other PPA groups, which also is a pervasive pattern in agrammatism resulting from stroke [5,16,37,42,62]. Indeed, Wilson et al. [68] found a significantly reduced ratio of closed class words in the agrammatic variant of PPA (albeit this was driven by only a few patients). Thompson et al. [55] also found reduced closed class word production in their three agrammatic participants. In addition, this pattern was seen in some of the PPA-G participants in Thompson et al. [57], although significant differences were not found between groups further research comparing open- to closed-class word production in primary progressive and stroke-induced aphasia is needed to determine whether this result reflects a genuine difference between PPA-G and StrAg and, if so, why.

4.4. General discussion

In the present study, we examined various measures of syntactic and morphosyntactic performance in several participant groups, including individuals with agrammatic and logopenic variants of primary progressive aphasia (PPA) and those with agrammatic and anomic aphasia resulting from stroke. We examined comprehension and production of canonical and noncanonical sentence structures using the Northwestern Assessment of Verbs and Sentences – Sentence Comprehension Test and Sentence Production Priming Test, and tested production of tensed and nontensed verb forms using the Northwestern Assessment of Verb Inflection. We further examined narrative samples, focusing on measures of speech fluency as well as properties of grammatical speech production. The results showed that agrammatic PPA and stroke-induced aphasic individuals pattern alike on several (morpho)syntactic measures. Although the two groups differed in speech of open- and closed-class words in narrative production, they showed similar deficits in production (and, to a lesser degree, comprehension) of noncanonical sentences, difficulties producing tensed verb forms, and their speech included fewer grammatical sentences and correctly inflected verbs than that of healthy speakers. Our results thus corroborate the findings of Thompson et al. [57] (as well as those of [47,55]), showing that despite the differences between PPA-G and StrAg individuals in disease etiology and mechanism, these two patient groups present with similar language deficit patterns.

In contrast, we found that logopenic PPA speakers did not display the syntactic and morphosyntactic deficits characteristic of the agrammatic groups, and performed significantly better on all tested measures, with the exception of open-to-closed class words in narratives (although other studies show closed-class word production deficits in PPA [55,68]. Notably, syntactic and morphosyntactic performance of the logopenic PPA group was comparable to that of speakers with stroke-induced anomic aphasia in Experiments 1 and 2, and to healthy speakers in Experiment 3. In general, the behavioral pattern of logopenic PPA suggests relatively intact syntactic knowledge, much like that of StrAn speakers.

It can be noted that the poorer performance of the agrammatic groups on pre-experimental language tasks may have predicted these patterns, since participants were categorized as agrammatic based on their ability to produce sentences (i.e., on the Northwestern Anagram Test for PPA participants and in spontaneous speech samples for StrAph). We note, however, that the agrammatic groups in our experiments also were significantly less fluent than the anomic/logopenic groups, based on their WAB fluency scores (the mean fluency score for PPA-G participants across the experiments was 5.52, for StrAg – 4.50, for PPA-L – 8.71, and for StrAn –

7.74). Although fluency and grammatical ability often coincide with one another in StrAg, they do not in PPA-G [57]. We also point out that the NAT only grossly addresses sentence production ability in that this test requires participants to arrange written words to form sentences and, hence, off-line strategies can be used to generate sentences. Further, the spontaneous speech samples used to classify the StrAg participants were derived from the WAB picture description task, which often results in short samples that do not adequately illustrate patient abilities (see Thompson et al. [57], for discussion of the limitations of picture description for evaluating spontaneous speech) and the samples were not thoroughly analyzed. The results for Experiments 1 and 2 were derived from constrained production tasks, and Experiment 1 also examined syntactic comprehension. In addition, Experiment 3, which tested narrative production ability, used a story-telling task and a sophisticated analysis system to quantify linguistic ability.

The systematic comparison of (morpho)syntactic impairments associated with PPA and aphasia resulting from stroke reported in this paper thus revealed symmetry between these neurolinguistic disorders, such that the deficit patterns presented by individuals with the agrammatic variant of PPA parallel, to a large degree, those of agrammatism associated with stroke, whereas the (morpho)syntactic characteristics of the logopenic variant of PPA are similar to those of anomic, stroke-induced, aphasia. These findings indicate that use of linguistically specific and sophisticated tests designed to systematically examine grammatical ability can and should be used to study the language deficit patterns seen in PPA. We further suggest that such tests be used clinically to differentiate between the different subtypes of PPA. This practice will not only contribute to our understanding of PPA and differences in deficits across PPA variants, it also will be informative with regard to how, or if, the language patterns associated with PPA differ from or are similar to those found in stroke aphasia. This latter issue, importantly, may provide insights into how language is processed in the brain. In particular, longitudinal studies examining the neural correlates of progressive (morpho)syntactic deterioration in PPA, compared to static (or improving) neurobehavioral correlates of such processing in stroke-induced aphasia may lead to important discoveries about how the brain computes syntax and morphosyntax.

References

[1] M. Arabatzi and S. Edwards, Tense and syntactic processes in agrammatic speech, *Brain and Language* **80** (2002), 314–327.

[2] S. Ash, P. Moore, S. Antani, G. McCawley, M. Work and M. Grossman, Trying to tell a tale: Discourse impairments in progressive aphasia and frontotemporal dementia, *Neurology* **66**(9) (2006), 1405–1413.

[3] S. Ash, C. McMillan, D. Gunawardena, B. Avants, B. Morgan, A. Khan, P. Moore, J. Gee and M. Grossman, Speech errors in progressive non-fluent aphasia, *Brain & Language* **113** (2010), 113–120.

[4] R. Bastiaanse, Broca's aphasia: A syntactic and/or morphological disorder? A case study, *Brain and Langauge* **36** (1995), 286–305.

[5] R. Bastiaanse and R. Jonkers, Verb retrieval in action naming and spontaneous speech in agrammatism and anomia aphasia, *Aphasiology* **12** (1998), 951–969.

[6] R. Bastiaanse and R. van Zonneveld, On the relation between verb inflection and verb position in Dutch agrammatic aphasics, *Brain and Language* **64** (1998), 165–181.

[7] A. Benton, A. Sivan, K.S. Hamsher, N. Varney and O. Spreen, *Contributions to Neuropsychological Assessment: A Clinical Manual*, (2nd edition), New York: Oxford University Press, 1995.

[8] H. Bird and S. Franklin, Cinderella revisited: A comparison of fluent and non-fluent aphasic speech, *Journal of Neurolinguistics* **9** (1995), 187–206.

[9] D. Caplan and N. Hildebrandt, *Disorders of Syntactic Comprehension*, Cambridge, MA: MIT Press, 1988.

[10] D. Caplan and G.S. Waters, Verbal working memory and sentence comprehension, *Behavioral and Brain Sciences* **22** (1999), 77–126.

[11] A. Caramazza and E. Zurif, Dissociation of algorithmic and heuristic processes in language comprehension: Evidence from aphasia, *Brain and Language* **3** (1976), 572–582.

[12] N. Chomsky, *Lectures on Government and Binding*, Mouton de Gruyter, 1981.

[13] A. Cooke, C. DeVita, J. Gee, D. Alsop, J. Detre, W. Chen et al., Neural basis for sentence comprehension deficits in frontotemporal dementia, *Brain and Language* **85**(2) (2003), 211–221.

[14] A.R. Damasio and H. Damasio, Aphasia and the neural basis of language, in: *Principles of Behavioral and Cognitive Neurology*, M. Mesulam, ed., Oxford, UK: Oxford University Press, 2000, pp. 294–315.

[15] H. Damasio, T.J. Grabowsky, D. Tranel, R.D. Hichwa and A.R. Damasio, A neural basis for lexical retrieval, *Nature* **380** (1996), 499–505.

[16] O. Dragoy and R. Bastiaanse, Verb production and word order in Russian agrammatic speakers, *Aphasiology* **24** (2010), 28–55.

[17] J. Druks, Morpho-syntactic and morpho-phonological deficits in the production or regularly and irregularly inflected verbs, *Aphasiology* **20** (2006), 993–1017.

[18] L.M. Dunn and D.M. Dunn, *Peabody Picture Vocabulary Test, fourth edition*, Minneapolis, MN: Pearson, 2007.

[19] Y. Faroqi-Shah and C.K. Thompson, Semantic, lexical, and phonological influences on the production of verb inflections in agrammatic aphasia, *Brain and Language* **89** (2004), 484–498.

[20] Y. Faroqi-Shah and C.K. Thompson, Verb inflections in agrammatic aphasia: Encoding of tense features, *Journal of Memory and Language* **56**(1) (2007), 129–151.

[21] M.F. Folstein, S.E. Folstein and P.R. McHugh, Mini-mental state. A practical method for grading the cognitive state of patients for the clinician, *Journal of Psychiatric Research* **12**(3) (1975), 189–198.

[22] N. Friedmann and Y. Grodzinsky, Tense and agreement in agrammatic production: pruning the syntactic tree, *Brain and Language* **56** (1997), 397–425.

[23] L.C. Golper, M.T. Rau, B. Erskine, J.J. Langhans and J. Houlihan, Aphasic patients' performance on a mental status examination, *Clinical Aphasiology* **17** (1987), 124–135.

[24] H. Goodglass and E. Kaplan, *Assessment of Aphasia and Related Disorders*, (3rd edition), New York: Lea and Febiger, 2001.

[25] H. Goodglass and A. Wingfield, *Anomia: Neuroanatomical and Cognitive Correlates*, San Diego: Academic Press, 1997.

[26] H. Goodglass, A. Wingfield, M.R. Hyde and J.C. Theurkauf, Category specific dissociations in naming and recognition by aphasic patients, *Cortex* **22** (1986), 87–102.

[27] M.L. Gorno-Tempini, N.F. Dronkers, K.P. Rankin, J.M. Ogar, L. Phengrasamy, H.J. Rosen et al., Cognition and anatomy in three variants of primary progressive aphasia, *Annals of Neurology* **55**(3) (2004), 335–346.

[28] M.L. Gorno-Tempini, S.M. Brambati, V. Ginex, J. Ogar, N.F. Dronkers, A. Marcone et al., The logopenic/phonological variant of primary progressive aphasia, *Neurology* **71**(16) (2008), 1227–1234.

[29] M.L. Gorno-Tempini, A.E. Hillis, S. Weintraub, A. Kertesz, M. Mendez, S.F. Cappa et al., Classification of primary progressive aphasia and its variants, *Neurology* **76** (2011), 1006–1014.

[30] N.L. Graham, K. Patterson and J.R. Hodges, When more yields less: Speaking and writing deficits in nonfluent progressive aphasia, *Neurocase* **10**(2) (2004), 141–155.

[31] Y. Grodzinsky, The neurology of syntax: Language use without Broca's area, *Behavioral and Brain Sciences* **23** (2000), 1–71.

[32] M. Grossman and P. Moore, A longitudinal study of sentence comprehension difficulty in primary progressive aphasia, *Journal of Neurology, Neurosurgery and Psychiatry* **76** (2005), 644–649.

[33] D. Gunawardena, S. Ash, C. McMillan, B. Avants, J. Gee and M. Grossman, Why are patients with progressive nonfluent aphasia nonfluent? *Neurology* **75**(7) (2010), 588–594.

[34] A. Hillis, E. Tuffiash and A. Caramazza, Modality-specific deterioration in naming verbs in nonfluent primary progressive aphasia, *Journal of Cognitive Neuroscience* **14**(7) (2002), 1099–1108.

[35] J. Hodges and K. Patterson, Semantic dementia: a unique clinicopathological syndrome, *The Lancet Neurology* **6**(11) (2007), 1004–1014.

[36] A. Kertesz, Isotope localization of infarcts in Aphasia, *Archives of Neurology* **34**(10) (1977), 590–601.

[37] M. Lee, Dissociations among functional categories in Korean agrammatism, *Brain and Language* **84** (2003), 170–188.

[38] L. Menn and L. Obler, *Agrammatic aphasia: A cross-language narrative sourcebook*, John Benjamins, 1990.

[39] M.-M. Mesulam, Slowly progressive aphasia without generalized dementia, *Annals of Neurology* **11**(6) (1982), 592–598.

[40] M.-M. Mesulam, Primary progressive aphasia: A 25-year retrospective, *Alzheimer Disease and Associated Disorders* **21**(4) (2007), S8–S11.

[41] M.-M. Mesulam, E. Rogalsi, C. Wieneke, D. Cobia, A. Rademaker, C.K. Thompson and S. Weintraub, Neurology of anomia in the semantic variant of primary progressive aphasia, *Brain* **132**(9) (2009), 2553–2565.

[42] M.-M. Mesulam, C. Wieneke, E. Rogalski, D. Cobia, C.K. Thompson and S. Weintraub, Quantitative template for sub-typing primary progressive aphasia, *Archives of Neurology* **66**(12) (2009), 1545–1551.

[43] L. Meteyard and K. Patterson, The relation between content and structure in language production: An analysis of speech errors in semantic dementia, *Brain and Language* **110**(3) (2009), 121–134.

[44] G. Miceli, M.C. Silveri, G. Villi and A. Caramazza, On the basis for the agrammatic's difficulty in producing main verbs, *Cortex* **20** (1984), 207–220.

[45] J.E. Osher, A.H. Wicklund, A. Rademaker, N. Johnson and S. Weintraub, The mini-mental state examination in behavioral variant frontotemporal dementia and primary progressive aphasia, *American Journal of Alzheimer's Disease and other Dementias* **122**(6) (2008), 468–473.

[46] J.E. Partington and R.G. Leiter, Partington's Pathway Test, *The Psychological Service Center Bulletin* **1** (1949), 9–20.

[47] K. Patterson, N.L. Graham, M.A. Lambon Ralph and J.R. Hodges, Progressive non-fluent aphasia is not a progressive form of non-fluent (post-stroke) aphasia, *Aphasiology* **20** (2006), 1018–1034.

[48] J. Rhee, P. Antiquena and M. Grossman, Verb comprehension in frontotemporal degeneration: the role of grammatical, semantic and executive components, *Neurocase* **7** (2001), 173–184.

[49] E. Rochon, E.M. Saffran, R.S. Berndt and M.F. Schwartz, Quantitative analysis of aphasic sentence production: Further development and new data, *Brain and Language* **72** (2000), 193–218.

[50] E.M. Saffran, R.S. Berndt and M.F. Schwartz, The quantitative analysis of agrammatic production: Procedure and data, *Brain and Language* **37** (1989), 440–479.

[51] A. Santi and Y. Grodzinsky, Working memory and syntax interact in Broca's area, *Neuroimage* **37** (2007), 8–17.

[52] S. Sonty, M.-M. Mesulam, C.K. Thompson, S. Weintraub, N. Johnson, T. Parrish and D. Gitelman, Primary Progressive Aphasia: Anatomical and functional analysis of the language network, *Annals of Neurology* **53**(1) (2003), 35–49.

[53] J.A. Stark, Content analysis of the fairy tale *Cinderella* – A longitudinal single-case study of narrative production: "From rags to riches", *Aphasiology* **24** (2010), 709–724.

[54] C.K. Thompson, *Northwestern Assessment of Verbs in Sentences*. Northwestern University (available at www.flintbox.com), 2011.

[55] C.K. Thompson, K.J. Ballard, M.E. Tait, S. Weintraub and M.-M. Mesulam, Patterns of language decline in nonfluent primary progressive aphasia, *Aphasiology* **11** (1997), 297–321.

[56] C.K. Thompson, B. Bonakdarpour and S. Fix, Neural mechanisms of verb argument structure processing in agrammatic aphasic and healthy age-matched listeners, *Journal of Cognitive Neuroscience* **22**(9) (2010), 1993–2011.

[57] C.K. Thompson, S. Cho, C. Ju-Hsu, C. Wieneke, A. Rademaker, B. Weitner, M.-M. Mesulam and S. Weintraub, Dissociations between fluency and agrammatism in primary progressive aphasia, *Aphasiology*, 2011.

[58] C.K. Thompson, S. Fix and D. Gitelman, Selective impairment of morphosyntactic production in a neurological patient, *Journal of Neurolinguistics* **15** (2002), 189–207.

[59] C.K. Thompson, A. Kielar and S. Fix, Morphological aspects of agrammatic aphasia, in: *Perspectives on Agrammatism*, R. Bastiaanse and C.K. Thompson, eds, Psychology Press, in press.

[60] C.K. Thompson, S. Lukic, M.C. King and S. Weintraub, Noun and verb production and comprehension in stroke-induced and

primary progressive aphasia: an introduction to the Northwestern Naming Battery Performance, *Aphasiology*, in press.

[61] C.K. Thompson, K. Lange, S. Schneider and L. Shapiro, Agrammatic and non-brain-damaged subjects' verb and verb argument structure production, *Aphasiology* **11** (1997), 473–490.

[62] C.K. Thompson, L.P. Shapiro, L. Li and L. Schendel, Analysis of verbs and verb- argument structure: A method for quantification of aphasic language production, *Clinical Aphasiology* **23** (1995), 121–140.

[63] C.K. Thompson, S. Weintraub and M.M. Mesulam, The Northwestern Anagram Test. Northwestern University (available at www.flintbox.com), 2009.

[64] R.S. Turner, L.C. Kenyon, J.Q. Trojanowski, N. Gonatas and M. Grossman, Clinical, neuroimaging, and pathologic features of progressive nonfluent aphasia, *Annals of Neurology* **39** (1996), 166–173.

[65] M. Vanier and D. Caplan, CT-scan correlates of agrammatism, in: *Agrammatic Aphasia: A Cross-Language Narrative Sourcebook,* L. Menn and L.K. Obler, eds, John Benjamins, 1990, pp. 37-114.

[66] D. Wechsler, *Wechsler Memory Scale*, (3rd edition), San Antonio, Texas: The Psychological Corporation, 1997.

[67] S. Weintraub, M.-M. Mesulam, C. Wieneke, A. Rademaker, E.J. Rogalski and C.K. Thompson, The Northwestern Anagram Test: measuring sentence production in primary progressive aphasia, *American Journal of Alzheimer's Disease and Other Dementias* **24**(5) (2009), 408–416.

[68] S.M. Wilson, M.L. Henry, M. Besbris, J.M. Ogar, N.F. Dronkers, W. Jarrold, B.L. Miller and M.L. Gorno-Tempini, Connected speech production in three variants of primary progressive aphasia, *Brain*, doi: 10.1093/brain/awq129, 2010.

[69] L.B. Zingeser and R.S. Berndt, Retrieval of nouns and verbs in agrammatism and anomia, *Brain and Language* **39**(1) (1990), 14–32.

17

Therapy efficacy in chronic aphasia

Anna Basso[a],* and Margherita Macis[b]
[a]*Department of Neurological Sciences, Milan University, Milan, Italy*
[b]*Faculty of Psychology, University of Milano-Bicocca, Milan, Italy*

Abstract. There is good evidence that aphasia therapy is effective if sufficiently prolonged or intensive and that chronic aphasic individuals can also benefit from therapy, but data on chronic aphasia are scanty.
The aim of this retrospective study was to investigate whether chronic aphasia benefits from a very intensive therapeutic regimen. We revised the files (January 2000 to December 2008) of the chronic subjects whom we suggested have periodic sessions in our Unit (generally once a week) and 2–3 hours daily of homework with the help of a family member, supervised and controlled by the speech-therapist. Treatment would go on as long as amelioration is evident. Results for 23 chronic aphasic subjects are reported. All subjects had undergone previous therapy and 10 had been dismissed because no further recovery was expected. Recovery was significant in oral and written nouns and actions naming, oral and written sentence production and Token Test scores. Only 4 subjects did not improve. Severity of the disorder did not predict success or failure. We conclude that recovery was due to the intense work done. Further, we believe such a regimen could be successful in a number of patients for whom a less intensive regimen would not be effective.

Keywords: Chronic aphasia, intensive/prolonged treatment, recovery

1. Introduction

Not everyone would agree that aphasia therapy is effective. Schoonen, for instance, wrote "How can we explain the "significant" improvement in so many studies? One of the "explanations" is that these researchers were just lucky [33]." Experimental evidence, though not definitive, is clearly in favor of aphasia therapy efficacy. Four meta-analyses [30–32,37] and two evidence-based reviews [9–12] concluded that treated aphasic subjects improve more than untreated subjects. Recently, the Cochrane review [16] came to a positive but more doubtful conclusion: "Significant differences between the groups' scores were few but there was some indication of a consistency in the direction of results which favoured the provision of SLT".

Not all studies that compared treated and untreated subjects came to the same positive conclusion; Pickersgill and Lincoln [26], for example, found no differences between treated and untreated subjects, and David et al. [13] and Lincoln et al. [18] found no significant difference in amount of recovery between subjects treated by therapists and subjects treated by volunteers. These negative results only appear to contradict the statement that aphasia therapy is effective. Bhogal et al. [7] compared intensity and quantity of therapy in positive and negative studies whose target outcome measures were the Token Test [14], the Porch Index of Communicative Abilities [27], and the Functional Communication Profile [15]. Eight studies (four positive and four negative) provided sufficient data to allow determination of the relationship between results and intensity/quantity of treatment. The total number of treatment hours in the positive studies was 98.4 and in the negative studies 43.6; the difference was significant. In effect, an insufficient amount of treatment is not efficacious. Confirmation of the importance of treatment quantity comes from a meta-analysis [31]. Intensity of treatment has also been proved to be an important factor in recovery and groups of chronic aphasic individuals who underwent intensive training based on communicative language games (CIAT) showed positive results [21,22, 28].

A thorny question for the study of aphasia therapy efficacy is spontaneous recovery, which is present in

*Corresponding author: Anna Basso, Department of Neurological Sciences, Milan University, Via F. Sforza 35, Milano, 20122 Italy. E-mail: anna.basso@gmail.com.

almost all aphasic individuals in the first months post-stroke, even if it may be very limited. Some authors [1, 8,19] report some positive results in group of chronic subjects who started treatment after the period of spontaneous recovery but more interesting are the results of a research by Moss and Nicholas [25]. They re-analyzed data from 23 studies for a total of 57 subjects, subdivided in 6 groups according to time-post-onset (TPO) – 1 to 6 years – and compared the effect of TPO on recovery. No significant difference in amount of recovery among the 6 groups was found.

The potential effect of other therapeutic strategies has recently been explored. Current research on biological approaches, such as pharmacotherapy and non-invasive cortical stimulation methods provides encouraging data [6,35]. Glutamatergic, monoaminergic, and cholinergic drugs [29] and Transcranial Magnetic Stimulation and Direct Current Stimulation [e.g. [23]] have been shown to have a positive effect on either acute or chronic aphasic individuals' performance in language tasks

In summary, there is good evidence that aphasia therapy is effective if sufficiently prolonged or intensive and that chronic aphasic individuals can also benefit from therapy. Moreover, the combined use of biological and behavioral treatment approaches seems an interesting prospective to enhance recovery [5,20].

The amount of therapy suggested to aphasic subjects at the Aphasia Unit of Milan University has increased steadily during the years. In the last years it has reached very high standards, requiring great efforts on the part of the aphasic subjects and their families. The regimen we suggest consists of periodic sessions in our Unit (generally once a week for aphasic individuals living in Milan or nearby and once or twice per month for those living far from Milan) and intensive homework (2–3 hours per day) supervised by the speech therapist; treatment is considered to be concluded when no recovery is observable between two control evaluations, 3 to 6 months apart. This regimen in not easy to implement; we must persuade aphasic individuals and their family that their convinced commitment is necessary for treatment to be efficacious, and find a way to implement the necessary homework with the help of a relative, a friend or a volunteer.

In 2001, Basso and Caporali [4] checked whether this regimen was effectively better than a more standard regimen of 5 sessions per week. Results of 3 pairs of vascular aphasic subjects comparable for sex, age, education, TPO, site and size of lesion and type of aphasia were compared. Control subjects had been treated 1-hour daily and the experimental subjects, besides daily sessions, had underwent 2–3 hours daily treatment at home with the aid of a family member. All subjects were treated for as long as some recovery was evident. All patients improved but experimental subjects improved more and, more importantly and contrary to the control subjects, used their recovered language in daily living.

Those were only 3 subjects but we were interested in knowing whether the results of such a regimen are really worth the effort and we decided that a more comprehensive study was necessary. In this paper we consider all the chronic subjects seen between January 2000 (when we regularly started to propose an intensive treatment) and December 2008 whom we suggested a similar regimen.

2. Subjects

In the period January 2000 – December 2008, 443 vascular subjects were evaluated at the Aphasia Unit of Milan University. Intensive/prolonged treatment was not suggested to 337 subjects for the following reasons: over 75 of age (56), with an incomplete evaluation (31), not or only mildly aphasic (148), in rehabilitation elsewhere (45), for other reasons (57).

Of the remaining 106 individuals to whom an intensive/prolonged treatment was suggested, 62 were acute or sub-acute (less than 6 MPO) and do not concern us here. All 44 chronic subjects (range 7-106 MPO) had undergone aphasia therapy (range 2–71 months) in different hospitals before being evaluated at the Aphasia Unit and the option to resume treatment was proposed to them. When resumption of treatment with an intensive regimen was proposed, 12 potential subjects (Group 1) refused, and an additional 9 (Group 2) abandoned treatment. Thus, the treatment group comprised 23 chronic subjects (Group 3). These persons were treated for at least 6 months.

Table 1 reports demographical and clinical data for these 23 subjects who completed at least 6 months of intensive therapy (range: 6–60). Nine had global aphasia, 3 mixed non-fluent, 6 Broca and 5 severe Wernicke aphasia. It will be remembered that all had already been treated (range 2–50 months) and 10 had been dismissed because no further recovery was expected.

Table 1
Demographic and clinical data of the 23 subjects treated for at least 6 months (Group 3)

Subject	Sex	Age	Education (years)	MPO	Previous therapy (months)	Token Test (0–36)	Aphasia type
5141	F	32	17	31	24	8	G
5170	M	54	16	7	6#	2	W
5203	M	75	17	9	8	9	W
5204	M	74	17	8	7	13	G
5223	F	41	8	64	50#	19	B
5237	F	26	13	63	36#	26	B
5250	F	67	13	7	6	9	G
5253	M	38	13	7	3	8	G
5298	M	59	12	9	8#	18	MNF
5302	M	51	11	9	8#	0	G
5334	M	66	13	16	13#	13	G
5348	M	44	13	17	7#	°	G
5406	M	42	8	25	2	20	B
5432	F	52	13	18	14	13	W
5452	M	48	13	11	9	1	W
5469	F	50	17	30	10#	18	B
5475	F	66	8	12	6	2	G
5504	F	49	8	45	17	16	B
5508	M	66	5	11	5#	6	G
5527	F	54	17	10	7	25	B
5599	M	43	8	13	3#	17	MNF
5600	M	65	13	10	6	17	MNF
5602	M	68	17	12	5	2	W

Legend: F = Female, M = Male, G = Global, W = Wernicke, B = Broca, MNF = Mixed Non Fluent, ° = Colour blind subject, # = Dismissed because it was considered that treatment was no longer effective.

3. Treatment

Except the 6 Broca aphasic individuals, all subjects were severely aphasic and aim of the treatment was to rebuild the aphasic individuals' capacity to sustain a simple conversation in daily living. The initial treatment goals were: a) improve understanding of conversational roles, b) improve comprehension of the message in "ecological" situations, including comprehension of the speaker's intention (whether it is a request of information, a communication, or a request to do something), and c) have the subjects produce more correct and longer responses.

To improve understanding of conversational roles, the clinician must make clear that she and the aphasic individual are supposed to do something in turn. Initially, this can be achieved by having the aphasic partner act in any way independently of the clinician's request, as long as this sets up a continuous exchange with the clinician. When role-switching is restored, the next step is for the clinician to make herself understood. To facilitate the hearer's job she must use some expedients: a) keep eye contact, b) make clear which speech act (ask a question, state something, or solicit the patient to do something) she is going to do

by making it explicit, c) help the aphasic patient recognize what the question is about by placing the topic of the sentence at the beginning ("London, have you ever been there?" rather than "Have you ever been in London?"), d) use all communication channels (verbal, gestural, writing, drawing, mimic), and e) verbalise the message in the simplest possible way. Questions must obviously require only short and easy responses and any response given by the aphasic subject, independently of whether it is wrong or apparently unrelated to the question posed, must be accepted and reacted to as if it were correct and related to the question. When the aphasic individual is totally unable to give a response, the clinician must offer the response for which she presumes the subject is aiming and, if he agrees, have the patient repeat it. After presenting the same question again, she poses different questions that involve the same response because it is presumable that producing a word in conversation repeatedly would facilitate its future retrieval [3]. Besides these common goals, for each patient specific goals – such as reduction of apraxia of speech, prevention of agrammatism, recovery of word finding abilities, reading aloud – were also identified.

Table 2

Comparison of mean age, education, MPO, previous therapy (months) and Token Test scores of Group 1 ($n = 12$) and Group 2 ($n = 9$) subjects

	Group 1		Group 2		T test
	Mean	SD	Mean	SD	p value
Age	56.3	12.9	58.2	15	0.760
Education (years)	10.8	3.7	12.1	3.2	0.391
MPO	33.7	22.4	29.9	32.3	0.754
Previous therapy (months)	18.3	18.2	11.8	5.3	0.311
Token Test (0–36)	11.8	8.8	8.8	8.7	0.452

Table 3

Comparison of demographic data and Token Test scores of Groups 1+2 ($n = 21$) and Group 3 ($n = 23$)

	Group 1+2		Group 3		T test
	Mean	SD	Mean	SD	p value
Age	57.1	13.5	53.5	13.4	0.371
Education (years)	11.3	3.5	12.6	3.7	0.245
MPO	32	26.4	19.3	16.8	0.061
Previous therapy (months)	15.5	14.3	11.3	11.3	0.282
Token Test scores (0–36)	10.5	8.7	11.9	7.8	0.571

The therapeutic program was more heterogeneous for the 6 Broca aphasic subjects. Four, with reduced speech and agrammatism, were asked to identify action verbs in a vocabulary, read its definition, write it down and repeat it aloud; look up in the dictionary for another action verb, repeat the whole procedure and then try to retrieve the previously rehearsed verbs. The family "therapist" had to explain the patient the structure of the verb (to kill, for instance, requires two arguments, both animate, the killer and the one killed) and ask the patient to produce a sentence with the verb and all the obligatory complements. In short, the family "therapist" were required to deliver a simplified mapping therapy [2,24]. For the two Broca aphasic that did not present agrammatism, therapy was approximately the same without, however, any particular attention on the structure of action verbs.

Tasks that could easily be explained and transferred to a naïve person or could be performed independently by the aphasic individuals were chosen and explained to the aphasic subjects and their family "therapist" and their therapeutic behavior were regularly supervised. When the therapeutic relationship between the aphasic person and their care-givers was well established, they were asked to spend 3–4 consecutive days at the Aphasia Unit and treatment of conversation was explained and shown to the care-givers; their behavior in this task was supervised.

Subjects were asked to work regularly 2–3 hours per day (partly on their own and partly with the family member) and records of their home-work was reported in our files. The frequency of their visits to the Aphasia Unit (from once a week to once a month, each time for 2–3 hours) depended on two main factors: how far they lived from Milan and the complexity of their disorders.

4. Results

Groups 1 and 2 did not differ significantly for age, education, MPO, length of therapy underwent prior to our examination or severity of aphasia as evaluated by the Token Test (Table 2).

We pooled together Groups 1 and 2 subjects and compared these variables to those of Group 3. None of the difference was significant (Table 3).

Table 4 reports percentage of correct responses in oral and written noun and action naming and picture description, and Token Test's scores at first and last evaluation of the 23 treated subjects.

Mean scores at first and last evaluation were compared by t test for paired samples. All differences were significant (Table 5 and Fig. 1).

All subjects were chronic and all had been previously treated in other hospitals and it is very unlikely that their gains could be explained by spontaneous recovery or other unspecified factors. The most obvious explanation is that amelioration was the result of treatment. However, we compared recovery in oral and written tasks because improvement in oral tasks is likely to be more sensitive to unspecific use of language in daily living but written language is not frequently used in daily living, especially by aphasic subjects and amelio-

Table 4

Percentage of correct responses in oral and written noun and action naming, sentence production, and Token Test's scores at first and last evaluation of treated subjects

| Subject | Noun naming (0–40) | | | | Action naming (0–20) | | | | Sentence production (0–20) | | | | Token Test (0–36) | |
| | Oral | | Written | | Oral | | Written | | Oral | | Written | | | |
	First	Last	First	Last	First	Last	First	Last	First	Last	First	Last	First	Last
5141	60	80	7.5	75	50	60	0	50	10	30	0	25	8	12
5170	0	32.5	0	25	0	40	0	0	0	30	0	0	2	13
5203	85	87.5	97.5	95	100	80	100	85	60	70	90	85	9	18
5204	0	15	0	10	0	35	0	0	0	5	0	0	13	23
5223	80	87.5	50	60	80	70	55	45	40	60	na	na	19	20
5237	97.5	97.5	87.5	87.5	90	95	70	85	90	90	90	100	26	27
5250	0	62.5	0	40	0	35	0	10	0	10	0	0	9	25
5253	32.5	55	0	5	15	30	0	5	0	30	0	0	8	20
5298	0	40	0	30	0	20	0	0	0	5	0	0	18	18
5302	0	15	0	0	0	5	0	0	0	0	0	0	0	3
5334	50	92.5	10	75	30	95	0	50	10	60	0	65	13	20
5348	0	7.5	22.5	55	0	0	10	15	0	0	0	25	°	°
5406	75	75	35	35	40	95	0	10	30	20	0	45	20	26
5432	2.5	82.5	5	82.5	30	80	0	80	20	60	0	80	13	19
5452	37.5	85	0	40	65	90	0	35	10	60	na	na	1	14
5469	37.5	87.5	30	90	35	70	20	80	0	90	0	90	18	25
5475	0	37.5	0	12.5	0	0	0	0	0	0	0	0	2	10
5504	70	87.5	55	90	60	85	25	85	50	90	35	70	16	29
5508	0	0	0	5	0	0	0	0	0	0	0	0	6	10
5527	52.5	82.5	62.5	95	45	85	45	90	80	100	85	100	25	28
5599	10	50	5	15	0	40	0	5	0	15	0	5	17	27
5600	20	70	7.5	65	50	75	0	80	0	70	0	50	17	23
5602	32.5	70	0	50	50	60	0	60	0	70	0	25	2	6

Legend: na = Not administered, ° = Colour blind subject.

Table 5

Comparison of oral and written noun and action naming, sentence production, and Token Test mean scores at first and last evaluation

| Task | Modality | First evaluation | | Last evaluation | | T test |
		Mean	SD	Mean	SD	(p value)
Noun naming	Oral	12.9	13.2	24.3	12.1	< 0.0001
	Written	8.3	12	19.8	13.1	< 0.0001
Action naming	Oral	6.4	6.5	10.8	6.7	< 0.0001
	Written	2.8	5.5	7.6	7.2	0.001
Sentence production	Oral	3.5	5.5	8.4	6.9	0.0002
	Written ($n = 21$)	2.9	6.4	7.3	7.7	0.002
Token Test ($n = 22$)		11.9	7.8	18.9	7.4	< 0.0001

ration in written tasks is most probably due to therapy. None of the differences was significant (Table 6).

We also considered severity of aphasia as a possible prognostic factor of recovery. We divided treated subjects in two subgroups (with Token Test's scores under or above the mean of the group) and compared their gains in the Token Test (Table 7). Token Test's scores of the "severe" subgroup were significantly lower at first and last examination but the difference between the 2 scores was not significantly different in the "severe" and "moderate" subgroups.

Particularly interesting appears to be recovery in picture description because of the use of sentences. We re-

port two examples. Subject 5602, a 68 year-old, lawyer who suffered a CVA in the left hemisphere 12 months before being evaluated at the Aphasia Unit had undergone 5 months therapy in Florence and had been dismissed because no further recovery was expected. His spontaneous speech consisted in a sort of mixed jargon (verbal paraphasias and neologisms), totally incomprehensible. Seven months later he described a picture of a living room in which a woman is knitting, a man sits in an armchair reading a newspaper, a young girl is watching television, a boy is playing with cubes, and a cat is playing with a ball of wool, as follows:

"The small cat with the small ball to play; they play

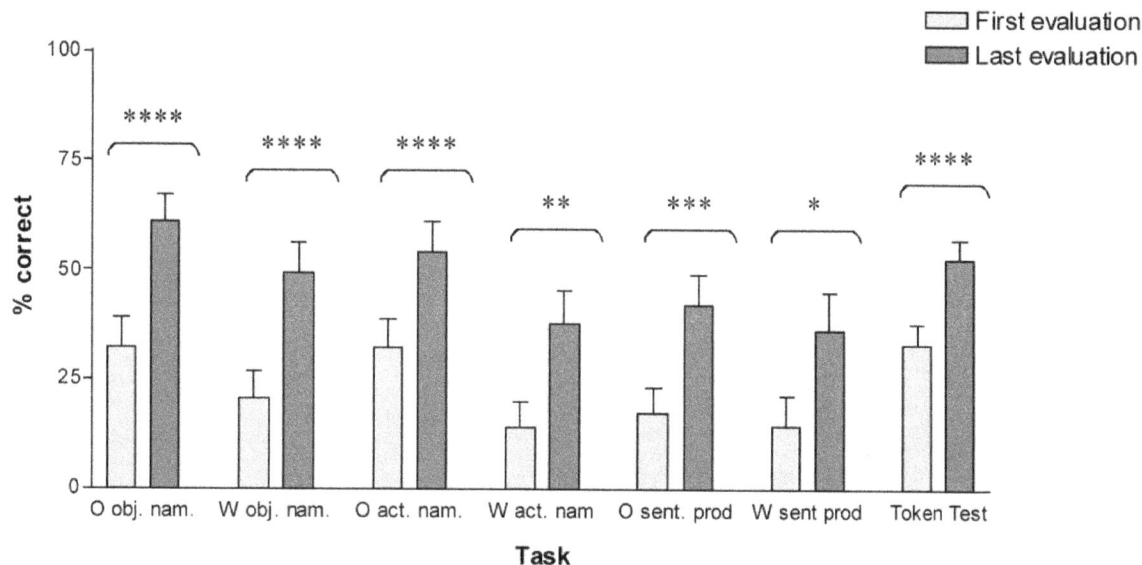

Fig. 1. Comparison of mean scores (%) in oral noun naming, written noun naming, oral action naming, written action naming, oral sentence production, written sentence production and Token Test scores at first and last evaluation of the 23 treated subjects. Error bars are SEM (standard error of the mean). Legend: O = Oral, W = Written, obj. nam = Noun naming, act. nam. = Action naming, sent. prod. = Sentence production, *$p = 0.002$, **$p = 0.001$, ***$p = 0.0002$, ****$p < 0.0001$.

with this ball with the mother to knit sweater. The girl 4–5 years old looks TV; she is the only one to look at it. The grandfather who reads the newspaper and doesn't see TV but the boy who plays with different pieces, short, long pieces."

Subject 5170 was 7 MPO when he arrived at Milan Aphasia Unit. He was 54-years-old and had become aphasic following rupture of an aneurysm. He had already been treated but after 6 months he had been dismissed because no further recovery was expected. His speech was fluent, characterized by phonemic jargon interspersed with existing words but deprived of any communicative value. Comprehension was very severely impaired. Both he and his wife were highly motivated and immediately accepted our proposal. Therapy went on for 5 years with slow but constant improvement. When they finally terminated therapy, subject 5170 described his day as follows:

"Then I eat... and then I don't know, it depends. I wanted to go with the ... with the ... (mimes cycling) with the bicycle, but now it hurts (points at his leg). Generally I go cycling and look around. I look around something here, something there, it's not like Milan. I also went along, but it was a bit painful... and then I turned and arrived to the Po. Then I come home and eat. Afterwards I look at the newspaper, what is in there, and then I go out again, not cycling I walk. I walk a little but now it hurts (points at his leg again). After I go... I look

Table 6
Comparison of recovery in oral and written tasks

	Oral task		Written task		T test
	Mean	SD	Mean	SD	(p value)
Noun naming	11.4	8.7	11.5	10	0.953
Action naming	4.4	4.3	4.7	6	0.770
Sentence production	4.9	5.4	4.4	5.7	0.776

Table 7
Comparison of Token Test scores at first and last evaluation of severe ($n = 10$) and moderate subjects ($n = 12$)

	Severe		Moderate		T test
	Mean	SD	Mean	SD	(p value)
First	4.7	3.6	17.9	4.3	< 0.0001
Last	13.1	6.6	23.8	3.8	0.0001
Difference	8.4	4.6	5.9	4	0.175

what is around... When I am at home I listen to the ... (mimes earphones), to that, do you understand? In the evening I eat and then I look (mimes TV), what's on, a bit of everything, and then I go to bed. Then everything starts again... as before."

Table 8 reports reasons why treatment was suspended, regularity of home-treatment, and the degree of improvement.

The most frequent reasons for suspension of treatment were either that subjects had reached a plateau and further recovery was not expected or that they were weary. Degree of recovery appears to be independent from suspension reasons. Regularity of home-treatment appears to be an important factor in recovery.

Table 8
Therapy length, suspension reasons, regularity of home-treatment and level of improvement

	Subject	Therapy length (months)	Reason for suspension	Regularity	Level of improvement (0–3)
Dismissed	5141	19	Plateau	Irregular	1
	5223	28	Plateau	Irregular	1
	5253	29	Plateau	Regular	3
	5334	29	Plateau	Regular	3
	5475	25	Plateau	Regular	1
	5432	18	Too dependent on therapist	Irregular	3
	5504	13	Too dependent on therapist	Irregular	3
	5298	11	Don't work	Irregular	1
	5348	36	Don't work	Irregular	0
	5527	7	Don't work	Irregular	3
Self-dismissed	5170	60	Too weary	Regular	3
	5237	10	Too weary	Irregular	0
	5302	24	Too weary	Regular	0
	5406	7	Too weary	Irregular	2
	5599	9	Too weary	Regular	2
	5600	6	Too weary	Regular	3
	5204	12	Health	Regular	1
	5250	20	Health	Regular	3
	5452	22	Health	Irregular	2
	5508	12	Health	Irregular	0
	5203	6	Moved	Regular	2
Still in treatment	5469	17		Regular	3
	5602	7		Regular	3

Legend: 0 = no improvement, 1 = little improvement, 2 = good improvement, and 3 = very good improvement.

5. Discussion

In summary the conclusions that can be drawn from our study are the following: 1) 50% of the subjects, even after a previous treatment, agreed to start an intensive and supposedly very long period of treatment with the help of a family member; 2) no difference was found between subjects who agreed to treatment and those who refused it in type and severity of aphasia, MPO, age, education and previous treatment; 3) as a group, treated subjects recovered significantly in all behaviors studied and severity of aphasia was not a negative prognostic factor; 4) recovery appears to be due to treatment, particularly because it was not different in oral and written tasks and it is difficult to imagine that writing ameliorate spontaneously in chronic severe aphasic individuals; 5) in all cases it was reported that they were more communicative in their daily living. Finally, although no definitive conclusion is possible, inspection of Table 8 seems to indicate a convincing relationship between regularity of home-treatment and recovery.

This is a retrospective study and its aim was clinical. The question was: do chronic aphasic individuals still benefit from therapy and do we have enough evidence that the therapeutic regimen we suggest is worth while the effort it requires? The answer can only be given by the aphasic subjects and their family but the very fact that in many cases treatment lasted more than a year can be read as a positive answer. Sometimes we had to insist to put an end to it; the aphasic subjects and their "family therapists" appear very much motivated and are prepared to go on forever as was the case with subject 5170 and his wife who went on for 5 years regularly working 2–3 hours per day, showing some improvement at each control evaluation. From our point of view the response is an unequivocal "yes", even for subjects that are considered to represent the most unlikely examples of likely recovery: subjects were chronic, most were very severely impaired, all had already been treated, and 10 had been dismissed because no further recovery was expected. Only 4 subjects did not show any improvement and as many as 10 showed a substantial improvement.

Probably the question of aphasia therapy efficacy could have been settled satisfactorily, if it were recognized that treatment regimen is an important determinant of recovery and that the main reason why therapy was not found to be efficacious in some studies that compared treated and untreated subjects [17,18,34,36] is that it was not sufficiently intensive and/or prolonged.

In efficacy studies the content of therapy has rarely been taken into account but it goes without saying that results depends on what is done and not only for how long or with what frequency it is done. Treatment was specifically devised and different for each of the 23 treated subjects but due to the severity of the disorder the goal was the same for most of them: sustain a simple conversation in daily living, conversation being the fundamental and primary type of language use. Moreover, the involvement of naïve "therapists" reduced the choices of possible tasks. It is possible that with different and more varied therapeutic interventions better results would have been achieved. What we do want to stress, however, is that recovery never showed up suddenly after a short period of treatment; amelioration was slow and continuous. Recovery, and particularly their use of language for communication purposes, was the result of the intense work done and we argue that such a regimen could be successful in a number of patients for whom a less intensive regimen would be ineffective.

Therapy cannot be delivered with such an intensity and for such a long time by speech therapists alone; it must be a mutual endeavor which sees the aphasic subjects, their families, and the speech therapists as active collaborators. Meinzer et al. [22] trained a group of family members to deliver CIAT to 10 chronic aphasic individuals and compared their results to those of 10 chronic aphasic subjects treated by experienced therapists. Both groups improved and there was no significant difference between the 2 groups.

In this perspective, speech therapists' tasks are more varied and more demanding. They have to locate the damage, decide what is the best treatment, establish which tasks aphasic subjects can carry out on their own and which with the help of a family member, show them how to perform the required tasks, regularly check what is going on between the subject and the lay person delivering therapy, perform the control evaluations, and adapt the intervention to the subject's recovery. Put differently, they are no longer the first violinists but conductors of a harmonious orchestra.

References

[1] J.L. Aten, M.P. Caligiuri and A.L. Holland, The efficacy of functional communication therapy for chronic aphasic patients, *The Journal of Speech and Hearing Disorders* **47** (1982), 93–96.

[2] A. Basso, *Aphasia and Its Therapy*, Oxford University Press, 2003.

[3] A. Basso, Natural conversation: A treatment for severe aphasia, *Aphasiology* **24** (2010), 466–479.

[4] A. Basso and A. Caporali, Aphasia therapy or the importance of being earnest, *Aphasiology* **15** (2001), 307–332.

[5] M.L. Berthier, C. Green, J.P. Lara, C. Higueras, M.A. Barbancho, G. Dávila and F. Pulvermüller, Memantine and constraint-induced aphasia therapy in chronic poststroke aphasia, *Annals of Neurology* **65** (2009), 577–585.

[6] M.L. Berthier and F. Pulvermüller, Neuroscience insights improve neurorehabilitation of poststroke aphasia, *Nature reviews Neurology* **7** (2011), 86–97.

[7] S.K. Bhogal, R. Teasell and M. Speechley, Intensity of aphasia therapy, impact on recovery, *Stroke; a journal of cerebral circulation* **34** (2003), 987–993.

[8] H. Broida, Language therapy effects in long term aphasia, *Archives of Physical Medicine and Rehabilitation* **58** (1977), 248–253.

[9] S.F. Cappa, T. Benke, S. Clarke, B. Rossi, B. Stemmer and C.M. van Heugten, EFNS guidelines on cognitive rehabilitation: report of an EFNS task force, *European Journal of Neurology* **10** (2003), 11–23.

[10] S.F. Cappa, T. Benke, S. Clarke, B. Rossi, B. Stemmer and C.M. van Heugten, EFNS guidelines on cognitive rehabilitation: report of an EFNS task force, *European Journal of Neurology* **12** (2005), 665–680.

[11] K.D. Cicerone, C. Dahlberg, K. Kalmar, D.M. Langenbahn, J.F. Malec, T.F. Bergquist, T. Felicetti, J.T. Giacino, J.P. Harley, D.E. Harrington, J. Herzog, S. Kneipp, L. Laatsch and P.A. Morse, Evidence-based cognitive rehabilitation: recommendations for clinical practice, *Archives of Physical Medicine and Rehabilitation* **81** (2000), 1596–1615.

[12] K.D. Cicerone, C. Dahlberg, J.F. Malec, D.M. Langenbahn, T. Felicetti, S. Kneipp, W. Elmo, K. Kalmar, J.T. Giacino, J.P. Harley, L. Laatsch, P.A. Morse and J. Catanese, Evidence-based cognitive rehabilitation: updated review of the literature from 1998 through 2002, *Archives of Physical Medicine and Rehabilitation* **86** (2005), 1681–1692.

[13] R. David, P. Enderby and D. Bainton, Treatment of acquired aphasia: speech therapists and volunteers compared, *Journal of Neurology, Neurosurgery, and Psychiatry* **45** (1982), 957–961.

[14] E. De Renzi and P. Faglioni, Normative data and screening power of a shortened version of the Token Test, *Cortex* **14** (1978), 41–49.

[15] A.L. Holland, *Communicative Abilities in Daily Living*, Baltimore: University Park Press, 1980.

[16] H. Kelly, M.C. Brady and P. Enderby, Speech and language therapy for aphasia following stroke, *Cochrane Database of Systematic Reviews Online* **5** (2010), CD000425.

[17] E. Levita, Effects of speech therapy on aphasics' responses to Functional Communication Profile, *Perceptual and Motor Skills* **47** (1978), 151–154.

[18] N.B. Lincoln, E. McGuirk, G.P. Mulley, W. Lendrem, A.C. Jones and J.R. Mitchell, Effectiveness of speech therapy for aphasic stroke patients. A randomised controlled trial, *Lancet* **1** (1984), 1197–1200.

[19] C. Mackenzie, An aphasia group intensive efficacy study, *The British Journal of Disorders of Communication* **26** (1991), 275–291.

[20] P.I. Martin, M.A. Naeser, M. Ho, E. Treglia, E. Kaplan, E.H. Baker and A. Pascual-Leone, Research with transcranial magnetic stimulation in the treatment of aphasia, *Current Neurology and Neuroscience Reports* **9** (2009), 451–458.

[21] M. Meinzer, D. Djundja, G. Barthel, T. Elbert and B. Rockstroh, Long-term stability of improved language functions
in chronic aphasia after constraint-induced aphasia therapy,
Stroke: A Journal of Cerebral Circulation **36** (2005), 1462–
1466.

[22] M. Meinzer, S. Streiftau and B. Rockstroh, Intensive language
training in the rehabilitation of chronic aphasia: efficient training by laypersons,*Journal of the International Neuropsychological Society JINS* **13** (2007), 846–853.

[23] C. Miniussi, S.F. Cappa, L.G. Cohen, A. Flöel, F. Fregni, M.A.
Nitsche, M. Oliveri, A. Pascual-Leone, W. Paulus, A. Priori and V. Walsh, Efficacy of repetitive transcranial magnetic
stimulation/transcranial direct current stimulation in cognitive
neurorehabilitation, *Brain Stimulation* **1** (2008), 326–336.

[24] C.C. Mitchum, M.L. Greenwald and R.S. Berndt, Cognitive
treatments of sentence processing disorders: what have we
learned? *Neuropsychological Rehabilitation* **10** (2000), 311–
336.

[25] A. Moss and M. Nicholas, Language rehabilitation in chronic
aphasia and time postonset: a review of single-subject data,
Stroke; a journal of cerebral circulation **37** (2006), 3043–
3051.

[26] M.J. Pickersgill and N.B. Lincoln, Prognostic indicators and
the pattern of recovery of communication in aphasic stroke
patients, *Journal of Neurology, neurosurgery, and psychiatry*
46 (1983), 130–139.

[27] B.E. Porch, *Porch Index of Communicative Abilities: Therapy
and development* **1**, Palo Alto, CA: Psychologists Press, 1967.

[28] F. Pulvermüller, B. Neininger, T. Elbert, B. Mohr, B. Rockstroh, P. Koebbel and E. Taub, Constraint-induced therapy of
chronic aphasia after stroke, *Stroke: A Journal of Cerebral
Circulation* **32** (2001), 1621–1626.

[29] F. Pulvermüller and M.L. Berthier, Aphasia therapy on a neuroscience basis,*Aphasiology* **22** (2008), 563–599.

[30] R.R. Robey, The efficacy of treatment for aphasic persons: a
meta-analysis, *Brain and Language* **47** (1994), 582–608.

[31] R.R. Robey, A meta-analysis of clinical outcomes in the treatment of aphasia, *Journal of Speech, Language, and Hearing
Research* **41** (1998), 172–187.

[32] M.L. Rohling, M.E. Faust, B. Beverly and G. Demakis, Effectiveness of cognitive rehabilitation following acquired brain
injury: a meta-analytic re-examination of Cicerone et al.'s
(2000, 2005) systematic reviews, *Neuropsychology* **23** (2009),
20–39.

[33] R. Schoonen, The internal validity of efficacy studies: design and statistical power in studies of language therapy for
aphasics, *Brain and Language* **41** (1991), 446–464.

[34] C.M. Shewan and A. Kertesz, Effects of speech and language
treatment on recovery from aphasia, *Brain and Language* **23**
(1984), 272–299.

[35] S.L. Small and D.A. Llano, Biological approaches to aphasia
treatment, *Current Neurology and Neuroscience Reports* **9**
(2009), 443–450.

[36] L.A. Vignolo, Evolution of aphasia and language rehabilitation: a retrospective exploratory study, *Cortex* **1** (1964), 344–
367.

[37] R. Whurr, M.P. Lorch and C. Nye, A meta-analysis of studies
carried out between 1946 and 1988 concerned with the efficacy
of speech and language therapy treatment for aphasic patients,
European Journal of Disorders of Communication **27** (1992),
1–17.

18

Decision making cognition in primary progressive aphasia

Ezequiel Gleichgerrcht[a,b,*], Teresa Torralva[a,b], María Roca[a,b], Daniela Szenkman[a],
Agustin Ibanez[a,b,c,d], Pablo Richly[a], Mariángeles Pose[a] and Facundo Manes[a,b,*]

[a]*Institute of Cognitive Neurology (INECO), Buenos Aires, Argentina*
[b]*Institute of Neurosciences, Favaloro University, Buenos Aires, Argentina*
[c]*Universidad Diego Portales, Santiago, Chile*
[d]*National Scientific and Technical Research Council (CONICET), Buenos Aires, Argentina*

Abstract. We sought to investigate the decision making profile of Primary Progressive Aphasia (PPA) by assessing patients diagnosed with this disease ($n = 10$), patients diagnosed with behavioral variant frontotemporal dementia (bvFTD, $n = 35$), and matched controls ($n = 14$) using the Iowa Gambling Task, a widely used test that mimics real-life decision making. Participants were also evaluated with a complete neuropsychological battery. Patients with PPA were unable to adopt an advantageous strategy on the IGT, which resulted in a flat performance, different to that exhibited by both controls (who showed advantageous decision making) and bvFTD patients (who showed risk-appetitive behavior). The decision making profile of PPA patients was not associated with performance on language tasks and did not differ between sub-variants of the disease (namely, semantic dementia and progressive nonfluent aphasia). Investigating decision making in PPA is crucial both from a theoretical perspective, as it can shed light about the way in which language interacts with other cognitive functions, as well as a clinical standpoint, as it could lead to a more objective detection of impairments of decision making deficits in this condition.

1. Introduction

Decision-making is a complex process requiring the interaction of many cortical and subcortical regions. It is widely accepted that the ventral prefrontal cortex (PFC) plays a pivotal role in social and emotional decision-making [1–3]. Additionally, converging evidence indicates the importance of other brain regions, including the dorsal prefrontal cortex and the amygdala, and highlights the relevance of lesion laterality and lesion etiology across regions [4]. The cognitive demands prompted by this complex processes can be difficult to capture with neuropsychological batteries, but in the last decade, the assessment of decision making has prompted the development of new tasks, and it is now a cognitive process that lends itself to laboratory measurement.

We have recently reviewed the way in which decision making is affected in neurodegenerative disease [4]. For instance, patients with Alzheimer disease (AD) seem to engage in random choice-making, leading to non-advantageous outcomes. Basal ganglia degeneration in patients with Parkinson disease (PD) and Huntington disease (HD) deteriorates their efficient decision-making abilities, in part, because the disruption of cortico-subcortical cognitive loops affect their executive performance and their reward-associated learning. In turn, patients with behavioral variant frontotemporal dementia (bvFTD) show a real risk-appetitive behavior characterized by their consistent choice of options presenting immediate reward but long term punishments, which is most likely associated with the degeneration of the prefrontal cortex.

In the current study, we investigated decision making in patients with Primary Progressive Aphasia (PPA). Mesulam originally described PPA as "a slowly pro-

*Corresponding author: Ezequiel Gleichgerrcht or Facundo Manes, Pacheco de Melo 1854, Buenos Aires, Argentina (1126). E-mail: egleich@ineco.org.ar; fmanes@ineco.org.ar.

gressing aphasic disorder without the additional intellectual and behavioral disturbances of dementia. Memory, judgment, and executive function should be intact at least in the two first years of the disease". Although there have been some studies of cognitive performance beyond language functions in PPA [5–7], to the best of our knowledge, however, no research has been conducted on the decision making cognition of patients with this pathology.

PPA is most frequently associated with frontotemporal pathology and three clinical types of aphasia have been described: nonfluent aphasia (PNFA), semantic dementia (SD), and logopenic aphasia. Patients with PNFA exhibit effortful, halting speech characterized by a loss of grammatical complexity and a high frequency of errors. In turn, SD patients show a more fluent speech with a loss semantic knowledge, thus affecting the content of their discourse, which is also reflected in their poor performance on confrontation naming tasks. Because of its relatively recent description, some of the core characteristics of the logopenic subtype are still matter of debate [8,9], but it is generally accepted that these PPA patients present with low speech rates and impaired complex syntactic comprehension and difficulties in naming [10]. The differences between PPA patients are thought to result from distinct patterns of cortical atrophy and their underlying pathological changes. While patients with PNFA tend to show left posterior frontoinsular atrophy [11] and, more typically, FTD-tau pathology [12], SD patients tend to exhibit anterior temporal lobe atrophy [11] and FTLD-TDP pathology [12].

The importance of understanding decision making in PPA is at least twofold. On the one hand, it can further our knowledge about the way in which cortical degenerations leading to prominent language deficits can impact on other higher cognitive functions. Secondly, it bears a fundamental clinical relevance for legal reasons, because as we will argue later in this article, it can contribute to the way we judge faulty decisions made by patients with PPA. For these reasons, the present study sought to investigate the decision making profile of patients diagnosed with PPA and its relationship with language impairment.

2. Methods

2.1. Participants

Patients with diagnosis of PPA ($n = 10$; 5 PNFA and 5 SD) and bvFTD ($n = 35$), as well as healthy controls

($n = 14$), were consecutively recruited from our clinic. Diagnosis was initially made independently by two experts in the FTD complex (FM and MP) and confirmed in the context of a multidisciplinary meeting (comprising cognitive neurologists, psychiatrists, neuropsychologists and speech pathologists) during which each patient's case is reviewed individually. Inter-reliability diagnosis was excellent (Cohen's kappa = 0.92). BvFTD and PPA diagnosis was made on the basis of published criteria [13] and on the new classification of PPA [10], as one of the authors was involved in said classification. All patients in the former group presented with prominent changes in social behavior and personality as verified by a close relative as well as frontal atrophy on MRI and/or frontal hypoperfusion on SPECT, when available. Classification of PPA patients into PNFA and SD was confirmed by an experienced speech pathologist and linguist expert in neurodegenerative pathologies (DS). Patients included in the present study did not meet criteria for specific psychiatric disorders, as determined by exhaustive psychiatric examination. They were in the mild stages of the disease, as determined by a score of 0.5 or 1 on the Clinical Dementia Severity Rating Scale (CDR) [14]. Healthy controls were matched for age, gender, and years of education, and they reported no history of traumatic brain injury, psychiatric disorders, or substance abuse. All participants gave their informed consent prior to inclusion in this study.

2.2. Procedure

The study was initially approved by the ethics committee at the Institute of Cognitive Neurology (Buenos Aires, Argentina) following the ethical standards established by the 1964 Declaration of Helsinki. Participants completed a series of interviews, including neurological and psychiatric assessment, and standard neuropsychological assessment. All participants were administered the Iowa Gambling Task (IGT).

2.2.1. Neuropsychological assessment

Participants in all groups were assessed with an extensive neuropsychological battery assessing (a) general cognitive status, with the Mini Mental State Examination (MMSE) [15], and the Addenbrooke's Cognitive Examination – Revised (ACE-R) [16]; (b) verbal memory through the Rey auditory verbal learning test (RAVLT) [17] and the logical memory subtest of the WAIS-R [18], as well as non-verbal memory with the Rey Complex Figure (RCF) test [17]; (c) attention with the forward digits span task of the WAIS-III [18] and the Trail Making Test Part A (TMT-A) [19]; (4) executive function using the backward digits span test [18], Part B of the Trail Making Test (TMT-B) [19], and the modified version of the Wisconsin Card Sorting Test (WCST) [20]; and (e) language with the Boston Naming Test [21] for naming, the Token Test [22] for comprehension, phonological (letter "P") and semantic (animals) fluency, and the Pyramid and Palm trees test [23] for semantic knowledge.

2.2.2. The Iowa Gambling Task

Bechara et al. [24] developed the Iowa Gambling Task (IGT) in order to provide a more realistic scenario for the assessment of decision-making. Participants are asked to choose between four decks of cards A–D and are instructed that the goal of the task is to maximize their profit with an initial loan of $2000. After picking a card, participants always earn a certain amount of money. However, repeatedly throughout the trails, certain cards may also subtract money (e.g. participant picks a card and is awarded $200 yet loses $50). Participants are unaware that two of the decks are 'advantageous' – cards selected from these decks are associated with either small monetary rewards or, in comparison to the rewards, smaller losses – whereas the other two decks are 'disadvantageous' – cards selected from these decks are associated with either large monetary rewards or even larger losses. As such, an advantageous deck may award the participant with $60 and the deduct $50 (i.e., net gain), while a disadvantageous deck may award $300, but subtract $1200 (i.e., net loss). For this reason, repeatedly selecting cards from the 'advantageous' decks will result in overall profit, whereas repeatedly selecting cards from the 'disadvantageous' decks will result in a net loss over time. Participants are also unaware that they must choose 100 cards before the task is over. For the purposes of performance analysis on the IGT, five blocks of 20 consecutive cards are defined (i.e., cards 1 through 20, cards 21 through 40, and so on), and a net score is calculated for each block as the number of cards chosen from the advantageous decks (C + D) minus the number of cards chosen from the disadvantageous decks (A + B). A total net score is also obtained by adding the individual net scores for each of the five blocks. The IGT is thought to measure decision making beyond the basic executive function capabilities measured by classic laboratory tests. This is supported by the fact that correlations between such executive tasks and IGT performance have not been found consistently throughout the literature, thus suggesting

that IGT measures an ability to make decisions that mimics more closely the demands of real-life scenarios (for further discussion on this issue, please see [4]).

2.3. Statistical analysis

Demographic and neuropsychological data were compared between the three groups using a one-way ANOVA design followed by Bonferroni post hoc tests when appropriate. When analyzing categorical variables (e.g. gender, recognition), the Freeman-Halton extension of the Fisher exact probability test for 2×3 contingency tables was used. Performance on the IGT was analyzed using a 3 (group) $\times$ 5 (IGT blocks) ANOVA. For comparisons of test performance between subtypes of PPA (SD and PNFA), U Mann-Whitney comparisons were used because of the nonparametric nature of the variables in this sample. The relationship between different variables was calculated using Spearman's correlation coefficient. The α value was set at 0.05, two-tailed for all analyses.

3. Results

3.1. Demographic and neuropsychological performance

As seen in Table 1, groups were successfully matched for age ($F_{2,54} = 0.72$, $p = 0.49$), gender ($\chi^2 = 0.25$, df $= 2$, $p = 0.98$) and years of education ($F_{2,54} = 2.23$, $p = 0.17$). Performance on neuropsychological tests was as expected for each patient group. Naming as measured by the BNT ($F_{2,54} = 38.9$, $p < 0.001$) and semantic fluency differed significantly between PPA and bvFTD patients ($p < 0.001$ and 0.018, respectively). PPA patients also showed a significantly lower performance ($p < 0.01$) on the ACE-R ($F_{2,54} = 17.2$, $p < 0.001$) but not ($p = 0.89$) on the MMSE ($F_{2,54} = 5.15$, $p < 0.01$) since the former test includes a more comprehensive and extensive section on language.

3.2. Iowa Gambling Task

As Fig. 1 shows, a 3 (group) $\times$ 5 (IGT blocks) repeated ANOVA design revealed no significant main effect of block ($F_{4,204} = 1.41$, $p = 0.23$) but both a significant main effect of group ($F_{2,51} = 14.9$, $p < 0.001$) and a significant group $\times$ block interaction ($F_{8,204} = 2.51$, $p = 0.01$). Indeed, a significant difference was found between the groups particularly on block 2 ($F_{2,51} =$

Table 1
Demographic information and neuropsychological test performance. Values are shown as Mean (SD)

			PPA (n = 10)	bvFTD (n = 35)	CTR (n = 14)	Group Comparison	P	CTR vs. PPA	CTR vs. bvFTD	PPA vs. bvFTD
Demographics	Age (years)		69.6 (8.9)	68.5 (7.3)	65.5 (6.5)	$F = 0.72$	0.49	n.s.	n.s.	n.s.
	Gender (M: F)		5:5	18: 17	7: 7	$\chi^2 = 0.25$	0.98	n.s.	n.s.	n.s.
	Education (years)		16.6 (2.4)	13.6 (4.5)	13.9 (3.0)	$F = 2.23$	0.17	n.s.	n.s.	n.s.
Cognitive status	ACE-R		69.7 (12.6)	81.9 (10)	94.5 (5.3)	$F = 17.2$	< 0.001	< 0.001	0.001	< 0.01
	MMSE		25.9 (2.7)	26.8 (2.9)	29.2 (1.0)	$F = 5.15$	< 0.01	0.02	0.03	n.s.
Memory	Logical Memory	Immediate	14.3 (11.7)	16.9 (7.6)	24.1 (8.3)	$F = 4.39$	0.02	n.s.	0.03	n.s.
		Delayed	9.33 (9.4)	9.71 (8.6)	18.9 (7.9)	$F = 5.74$	< 0.01	n.s.	< 0.01	n.s.
		Recognition	12.8 (4.0)	12.9 (4.9)	16.9 (2.9)	$F = 3.90$	0.027	n.s.	0.012	n.s.
	RAVLT	Immediate	22.4 (9.4)	28.1 (10)	25.1 (8.9)	$F = 12.3$	< 0.001	< 0.001	< 0.001	n.s.
		Delayed	3.63 (3.8)	3.77 (2.9)	20.1 (8.9)	$F = 13.2$	< 0.001	< 0.01	< 0.001	n.s.
		Recognition	8.13 (4.2)	9.63 (3.5)	17.1 (2.9)	$F = 5.51$	< 0.01	0.022	0.012	n.s.
	RCF	Delayed	18.2 (8.6)	6.86 (7.7)	18.5 (9.1)	$F = 12.9$	< 0.001	< 0.01	< 0.001	n.s.
		Recognition	50% hit	50% hit	92% hit	$\chi^2 = 0.39$	0.04	0.04	0.04	n.s.
Attention	Digit span forward		5.44 (1.6)	5.94 (1.3)	5.0 (1.1)	$F = 8.69$	0.001	< 0.01	< 0.01	n.s.
	TMT-A (sec)		128.4 (181)	66.4 (31)	39.4 (16.4)	$F = 3.83$	0.028	n.s.	0.026	n.s.
Executive functions	Digit span backwards		3.33 (0.9)	3.83 (1.3)	5.0 (1.1)	$F = 6.61$	< 0.01	< 0.01	< 0.01	n.s.
	Phonologic fluency		7.67 (4.1)	12.4 (7.1)	17.5 (5.7)	$F = 7.00$	< 0.01	< 0.001	0.033	n.s.
	TMT-B (sec)		251.1 (162)	182.8 (72)	94.1 (44.3)	$F = 8.71$	0.001	< 0.001	0.012	n.s.
	WCST (total score)		3.60 (2.3)	3.29 (1.8)	5.6 (0.7)	$F = 7.22$	< 0.01	n.s.	0.001	n.s.
Language	BNT (/20)		6.43 (7.1)	17.8 (2.9)	19.8 (0.4)	$F = 38.9$	< 0.001	< 0.001	n.s.	< 0.001
	Token test (/32)		25.8 (5.1)	22.7 (4.6)	25.2 (1.1)	$F = 2.82$	0.39	n.s.	n.s.	n.s.
	Semantic fluency		7.44 (5.3)	13.5 (6.0)	20.7 (5.2)	$F = 13.9$	< 0.001	< 0.001	< 0.01	0.018
	Pyramid and Palm Trees		44.7 (8.6)	49.6 (3.5)	51.9 (0.3)	$F = 6.90$	0.001	< 0.01	0.018	n.s.

PPA = Primary Progressive Aphasia; bvFTD = behavioral variant Frontotemporal Dementia; CTR = Control; ACE-R = Addenbrooke's Cognitive Examination – Revised; MMSE = Mini-Mental State Examination; RAVLT = Rey Auditory Verbal Learning Test; RCF = Rey Complex Figure; TMT = Trail Making Test (-A and -B parts); WCST = Wisconsin Card Sorting Test; BNT = Boston Naming Test; n.s. = not significant.

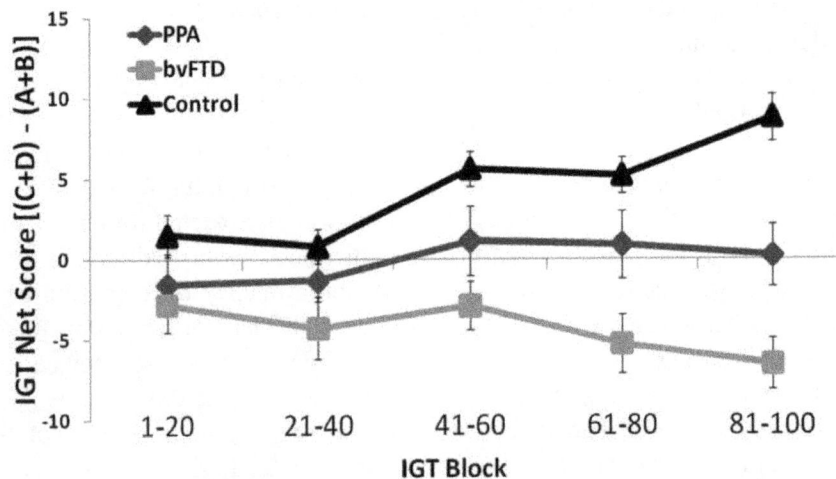

Fig. 1. *Mean (SEM)* group performance on the IGT, as measured by the net score ("good decks" minus "bad decks") on each 20-card block.

4.05, $p = 0.023$), block 3 ($F_{2,51} = 5.31$, $p < 0.01$), block 4 ($F_{2,51} = 8.14$, $p = 0.001$), and block 5 ($F_{2,51} = 15.3$, $p < 0.001$). In all of these cases, bvFTD patients were outperformed by controls (block 2: $p = 0.021$; blocks 3 and 4: $p < 0.01$; block 5: $p < 0.001$). Controls showed significant differences from PPA patients exclusively on block 5 ($p = 0.027$). PPA patients showed a significantly better performance than bvFTD

patients particularly on blocks 4 ($p = 0.05$) and block 5 ($p = 0.024$).

Total net score on the IGT (i.e., the sum of the five block net scores) significantly differed between the groups ($F_{2,51} = 15.35$, $p < 0.001$), with PPA patients differing significantly from bvFTD patients ($p = 0.036$) but not from controls ($p = 0.076$), although the bvFTD and control groups differed significantly ($p < 0.001$)

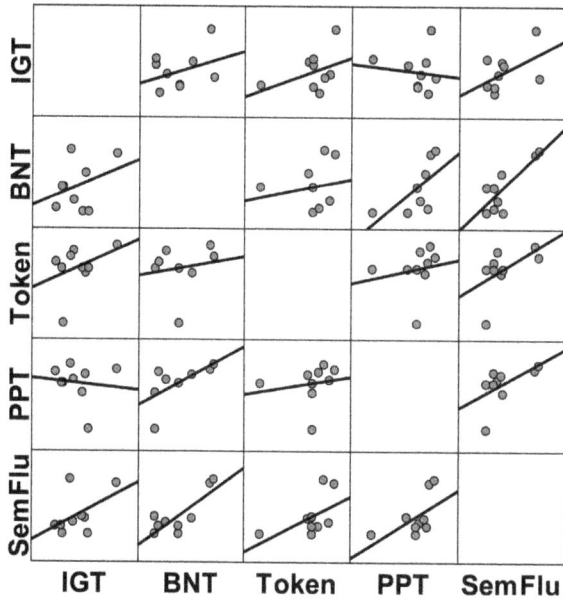

Fig. 2. Correlation matrix for language variables and total net score on the IGT (Iowa Gambling Task). No significant correlations were found. BNT = Boston Naming Test; Token = Token Test; PPT = Pyramid and Palm Trees; SemFlu = Semantic Fluency.

between each other.

3.3. Correlation analyses (Fig. 2)

No significant correlations were found within PPA patients between the total net score on the IGT and the BNT ($r = 0.08$, $p = 0.83$), Token test ($r = 0.16$, $p = 0.65$), PPT ($r = -0.04$, $p = 0.91$), or semantic fluency ($r = 0.36$, $p = 0.31$). Yet, when looking at correlations between language tasks, performance on the PPT was significantly associated with BNT scores ($r = 0.74$, $p = 0.015$) and the number of words produced on the semantic fluency task ($r = 0.64$, $p = 0.04$). Correlations sought between other scores derived from the IGT (e.g. block 5 score) and language tasks were also non-significant.

3.4. PNFA vs. SD

No significant differences were found between PN-FA and SD patients on the IGT for any of the blocks (1: $U = 6.0$, $p = 0.26$; 2: $U = 7.0$, $p = 0.35$; 3: $U = 9.5$, $p = 0.61$; 4: $U = 11.0$, $p = 0.91$; and 5: $U = 10.5$, $p = 0.76$). The groups did not differ on the total IGT net score either ($U = 11.0$, $p = 0.91$). Correlations between IGT performance and language variables remained non-significant within each PPA subgroup analyzed independently.

3.5. Positive vs. negative total net score

In order to further explore the possibility of differential decision making profiles within the PPA population, patients were divided into two groups based on whether they obtained a positive (i.e., greater than zero; $n = 4$) or negative (i.e., lower than zero; $n = 6$) total net score on the IGT. No significant differences were found on any of the demographic variables (age: $U = 6.0$, $p = 0.67$, gender: $\chi^2 = 0.74$, $p = 0.39$, education: $U = 7.5$, $p = 0.71$, and age at onset: $U = 6.50$, $p = 0.26$). Similarly, positive and negative IGT net score PPA patients had comparable cognitive status (ACE-R: $U = 10.0$, $p = 0.76$, MMSE: $U = 9.0$, $p = 0.91$). No significant differences were found on the BNT ($U = 4.0$, $p = 0.63$), the Token test ($U = 3.0$, $p = 0.51$), semantic fluency ($U = 7.50$, $p = 0.71$), and the PPT ($U = 3.0$, $p = 0.51$). Similarly, the groups had comparable performance on tasks of memory, attention, and executive functions (all $p > 0.24$).

4. Discussion

Decision making cognition, as assessed using the Iowa Gambling Test, was impaired in patients with PPA. In the present study, patients with PPA showed a decision making profile characterized by lack of adoption of an advantageous strategy, which led to a "flat performance" on the Iowa Gambling Task. Said flat performance is characterized by a net score (i.e. advantageous – disadvantageous choices) that is close to null throughout the task, reflecting the fact that card choices favored neither advantageous nor disadvantageous decks. This profile differed significantly from that of healthy control subjects, who showed more frequent choice-making from the "good" decks, resulting in an overall gain. Importantly, the decision making profile of PPA patients also differed significantly from that of patients with bvFTD, since the latter group showed risk-appetitive behaviors by which long term losses were masked by immediate rewards, a decision making pattern which has been consistently reported in the literature for this population [25,26]. It must be noted that because of this proximity to a "zero" net score, PPA patients could be perceived as being more risk-appetitive than controls. In this sense, it is important to consider that PPA patients showed a significantly less risky decision making profile than the bvFTD group, a truly risk-appetitive population. This suggests that risk taking among PPA patients is most likely unrelated to an inability to foresee the negative outcome of risky choices, as it occurs in bvFTD.

PPA performance on the IGT seemed neither to be related to their language deficits nor to differ between subtypes of PPA. Several hypotheses could potentially explain the flat IGT performance exhibited by PPA patients in our study. First, it could be the case that language deficits affected patients' understanding of the task. This seems unlikely, however, as no significant differences were found between the groups on the Token test, which is widely used to measure comprehension of verbal instructions. Moreover, while one would expect a positive significant correlation between IGT scores and the Token test (i.e., the worse comprehension is, the poorer the performance on decision making), no such correlation was found. Second, deficits on other language functions other than comprehension could be influencing performance on the IGT directly. But again, no significant correlations were found between the IGT and other language variables, including semantic fluency, confrontation naming, and semantic knowledge. Furthermore, when correlation analyses were conducted for each variant (i.e. SD and PNFA) independently, correlations remained non-significant. As well, when PPA patients were classified based on whether they had an overall positive or negative net score on the IGT, no significant differences emerged on any of the language variables. Thus, given that performance on the IGT appears to be unrelated to language abilities, it is likely that the non-advantageous, non-risky (i.e. "flat") decision making profile of PPA patients is not the *direct* result of language deficits typical of this condition.

Perhaps a more promising explanation, given the complex neural networks underlying the decision making process, is that language deficits may have an *indirect* influence on IGT performance. For instance, Rogalski et al. [27] have shown that aphasia in PPA patients contributes to the difficulty they experience in choosing items within the same semantic class. One can thus hypothesize that PPA patients may have been unable to distinguish the potential differences between several decks of cards; perhaps, these were all interpreted as part of the same semantic category (i.e., they were unable to process the differences between the "safe" and the "risky" decks on the IGT). Furthermore, it has been recently reported that PPA patients have difficulties in the representation of quantities in real-life scenarios [28], which could have also contributed to the decision making profile found in this study. On top of the direct and indirect influences of language deficits

on decision making, it is also plausible that a shared underlying mechanism affects both decision making and language simultaneously. After all, there are some major common features between both cognitive processes. One such feature, for instance, is the need to access mental representations, which are essential both for language content and for the evaluation of distinct choices (in this case, advantageous vs. disadvantageous) when making a decision. If shared mechanisms are indeed affected in PPA patients, then language and decision making, as well as any other processes feeding on such mechanisms, are prone to being impaired.

These preliminary reflections on the influence of language impairment on IGT performance must of course be interpreted with caution given the small sample size of PPA patients in this study. Of special interest is the prediction that semantic deficits may diminish performance by means of an inability to properly and differentially categorize "safe" vs. "bad" decks, which must be tested in future studies using a larger PPA population of SD patients, whose performance – but not that of PNFA patients – should be affected by impairments in their semantic ability.

The potential role of cognitive deficits typical of PPA patients in decision making performance need not be limited to language problems alone. For example, Banks and Weintraub [29] found a loss of self-awareness in PPA patients, which could also affect performance on the IGT, especially if patients feel their cognitive assessment is useless or a waste of time. In fact, the "flat" profile exhibited by PPA patients in this study resembles that of patients with psychiatric disorders - such as euthymic bipolar patients – who tend to choose randomly between good and bad decks [30, 31]. In this regard, future studies should attempt to compare the performance on the IGT of patients with PPA and with psychiatric disorders in order to determine whether there is a potential common denominator between these conditions that could explain such flat performance. Naturally, it is likely that the performance exhibited by PPA patients on the IGT is the combined result of multiple factors rather than one in particular, including those detailed above, as well as other underlying mechanisms that are yet to be identified.

The findings of the present study must be considered in the context of certain caveats, of which the small sample size of our PPA group is a major limitation. However, this is the first empirical study to examine decision making cognition in PPA. The results hereby presented are supported by the fact that the groups were accurately paired with healthy controls, as well as the fact that we did find robust significant effects in terms of performance on the IGT. Importantly, the groups in this study are similar in size to those employed in the other relevant reports on the neuropsychological aspects of PPA (ten patients in ref. [7], five patients in ref. [32]; etc.). Future studies should try to replicate these findings in larger populations, paying particular attention to potential differences between subtypes of PPA. While the diagnosis of patients with PPA in our study was based solely on clinical assessment and not on pathological analyses, it is important to note that patients were longitudinally studied as part of our FTD program, and all of them went on to exhibit the typical clinical syndrome of PPA.

In this seminal study on the decision making profile of patients with PPA, we have found a very distinct performance pattern compared to that exhibited by healthy controls and to patients with another variant under the umbrella of frontotemporal dementias. Identifying the way in which patients with this condition make decisions in real life has relevant implications from many angles. Theoretically, it provides information about the potential relationship between patterns of cortical degeneration, language deficit profiles, and impairments in decision making. By the same token, it can provide evidence for a possible dissociation between performance on language and decision making tasks, which can further help us dissect the complexity of the frontal and temporal circuitry involved in these higher cognitive processes. From a clinical perspective, our findings stress the need to include measures such as the IGT as part of neuropsychological assessment batteries for PPA patients. Among other measures aimed at detecting executive and social cognition deficits [33], the IGT has been shown especially capable of detecting cognitive and behavioral impairments otherwise missed by classical laboratory tests [34]. Understanding the decision making profile of PPA patients is also fundamental in the development of evidence-based policies regarding behavioral problems in this population. If patients affected by this condition fail to make advantageous choices, to what extent can they be considered responsible for their actions? Can they be found guilty for committing a crime? Should the medical decisions considering their own health be left to the patients' own criteria? How should we proceed should the relatives of a patient argue that he/she can no longer take care of the family's financial matters? The answers to these and other similar important questions are not without controversy, but by furthering our understanding of decision making in patients with PPA,

we will be able to provide more solid and consistent arguments to contribute towards policy making that will eventually affect the everyday living of these patients and their beloved ones.

Acknowledgements

The present study was supported by a FINECO grant.

References

[1] S.W. Anderson, J. Barrash, A. Bechara and D. Tranel, Impairments of emotion and real-world complex behavior following childhood- or adult-onset damage to ventromedial prefrontal cortex, *Journal of the International Neuropsychological Society* **12**(2) (2006), 224–235, JINS. [10.1017/S1355617706060346].

[2] A. Bechara and M. Van Der Linden, Decision-making and impulse control after frontal lobe injuries, *Curr Opin Neurol* **18**(6) (Dec 2005), 734–739.

[3] F. Manes, B. Sahakian, L. Clark, R. Rogers, N. Antoun, M. Aitken et al., Decision-making processes following damage to the prefrontal cortex, *Brain: A Journal of Neurology* **125**(Pt 3) (2002), 624–639.

[4] E. Gleichgerrcht, A. Ibanez, M. Roca, T. Torralva and F. Manes, Decision-making cognition in neurodegenerative diseases, *Nat Rev Neurol* **6**(11) (Nov 2010), 611–623.

[5] J. Rhee, P. Antiquena and M. Grossman, Verb comprehension in frontotemporal degeneration: the role of grammatical, semantic and executive components, *Neurocase* **7**(2) (2001), 173–184.

[6] C.E. Leyton, M. Hornberger, E. Mioshi and J.R. Hodges, Application of Addenbrooke's cognitive examination to diagnosis and monitoring of progressive primary aphasia, *Dement Geriatr Cogn Disord* **29**(6) (Jul 2010), 504–509.

[7] S. Bozeat, M.A. Lambon Ralph, K. Patterson, P. Garrard and J.R. Hodges, Non-verbal semantic impairment in semantic dementia, *Neuropsychologia* **38**(9) (2000), 1207–1215.

[8] M.L. Henry and M.L. Gorno-Tempini, The logopenic variant of primary progressive aphasia, *Curr Opin Neurol* (2010 Sep 16).

[9] M.F. Bonner, S. Ash and M. Grossman, The new classification of primary progressive aphasia into semantic, logopenic, or nonfluent/agrammatic variants, *Curr Neurol Neurosci Rep* **10**(6) (Nov 2010), 484–490.

[10] M.L. Gorno-Tempini, A.E. Hillis, S. Weintraub, A. Kertesz, M. Mendez, S.F. Cappa et al., Classification of primary progressive aphasia and its variants, *Neurology* (2011 Feb 16).

[11] M.L. Gorno-Tempini, N.F. Dronkers, K.P. Rankin, J.M. Ogar, L. Phengrasamy, H.J. Rosen et al., Cognition and anatomy in three variants of primary progressive aphasia, *Ann Neurol* **55**(3) (Mar 2004), 335–346.

[12] M. Grossman, Primary progressive aphasia: clinicopathological correlations, *Nat Rev Neurol* **6**(2) (Feb 2010), 88–97.

[13] D. Neary, J.S. Snowden, L. Gustafson, U. Passant, D. Stuss, S. Black et al., Frontotemporal lobar degeneration: a consensus on clinical diagnostic criteria, *Neurology* **51**(6) (Dec 1998), 1546–1554.

[14]   C.P. Hughes, L. Berg, W.L. Danziger, L.A. Coben and R.L. Martin, A new clinical scale for the staging of dementia, *Br J Psychiatry* **140** (Jun 1982), 566–572.

[15]   M.F. Folstein, S.E. Folstein and P.R. McHugh, "Mini-mental state", A practical method for grading the cognitive state of patients for the clinician, *J Psychiatr Res* **12**(3) (Nov 1975), 189–198.

[16]   E. Mioshi, K. Dawson, J. Mitchell, R. Arnold and J.R. Hodges, The Addenbrooke's Cognitive Examination Revised (ACE-R): a brief cognitive test battery for dementia screening, *Int J Geriatr Psychiatry* **21**(11) (Nov 2006), 1078–1085.

[17]   A. Rey, L'examen physiologique dans le cas d'encephalopathie traumatique, *Archives de Psychologie* **28** (1941), 286–340.

[18]   D. Wechsler, WAIS-R: Manual: Wechsler adult intelligence scale-revised: Harcourt Brace Jovanovich [for] Psychological Corp; 1981.

[19]   J.E. Partington and R.G. Leiter, Partington's Pathway Test, *The Psychological Service Center Bulletin* **1** (1949), 9–20.

[20]   H.E. Nelson, A modified card sorting test sensitive to frontal lobe defects, *Cortex; a Journal Devoted to the Study of the Nervous System and Behavior* **12**(4) (1976), 313–324.

[21]   E. Kaplan, H. Goodglass and S. Weintraub, The Boston Naming Test Philadelphia: Lea and Febiger: Inc; 1983.

[22]   O. Spreen and A.L. Benton, Neurosensory Center Comprehensive Examination for Aphasia (1977 revision). Victoria, BC: Neuropsychology Laboratory, Univ of Victoria, 1977.

[23]   D. Howard and K. Patterson, The Pyramids and Palm Trees Test: Thames Valley Test Company, 1992.

[24]   A. Bechara, A.R. Damasio, H. Damasio and S.W. Anderson, Insensitivity to future consequences following damage to human prefrontal cortex, *Cognition* **50**(1–3) (Apr–Jun 1994), 7–15.

[25]   E. Gleichgerrcht, A. Ibáñez, M. Roca, T. Torralva and F. Manes, Decision-making cognition in neurodegenerative diseases, *Nature Reviews Neurology* **6**(11) (2010), 611–623.

[26]   T. Torralva, C.M. Kipps, J.R. Hodges, L. Clark, T. Bekinschtein, M. Roca et al., The relationship between affective decision-making and theory of mind in the frontal variant of fronto-temporal dementia, *Neuropsychologia* **45**(2) (2007), 342–349, [10.1016/j.neuropsychologia.2006.05.031].

[27]   E. Rogalski, D. Blum, A. Rademaker and S. Weintraub, False recognition of incidentally learned pictures and words in primary progressive aphasia, *Neuropsychologia* **45**(2) (28 Jan 2007), 368–377.

[28]   C.L. Julien, J.C. Thompson, D. Neary and J.S. Snowden, Understanding quantity in semantic dementia, *Cogn Neuropsychol* **27**(1) (Feb 2010), 3–29.

[29]   S. Banks and S. Weintraub, Self-awareness and self-monitoring of cognitive and behavioral deficits in behavioral variant frontotemporal dementia, primary progressive aphasia and probable Alzheimer's disease, *Brain Cogn* **67**(1) (Jun 2008), 58–68.

[30]   S. Rahman, B.J. Sahakian, R. Cardinal, R. Rogers and T. Robbins, Decision making and neuropsychiatry, *Trends Cogn Sci* **5**(6) (1 Jun 2001), 271–277.

[31]   B.D. Dunn, T. Dalgleish and A.D. Lawrence, The somatic marker hypothesis: A critical evaluation, *Neuroscience and Biobehavioral Reviews* **30**(2) (2006), 239.

[32]   J.R. Hodges and K.S. Graham, A reversal of the temporal gradient for famous person knowledge in semantic dementia: implications for the neural organisation of long-term memory, *Neuropsychologia* **36**(8) (Aug 1998), 803–825.

[33]   T. Torralva, M. Roca, E. Gleichgerrcht, T. Bekinschtein and F. Manes, A neuropsychological battery to detect specific executive and social cognitive impairments in early frontotemporal dementia, *Brain* **132**(Pt 5) (May 2009), 1299–1309.

[34]   E. Gleichgerrcht, T. Torralva, M.A. Roca and F. Manes, Utility of an Abbreviated Version of the Executive and Social Cognition Battery in the Detection of Executive Deficits in Early Behavioral Variant Frontotemporal Dementia Patients, *Journal of the International Neuropsychological Society* (2010), First View:1-8, [10.1017/S1355617710000482].

Permissions

List of Contributors

Hiroo Ichikawa, Nobuyoshi Takahashi, Soutaro Hieda, Hideki Ohno and Mitsuru Kawamura
Department of Neurology, Showa University School of Medicine, Shinagawa-ku, Tokyo, Japan

Lieve De Witte
Department of Linguistics, Vrije Universtiteit Brussel, Brussel, Belgium

Jo Verhoeven
Department of Communication Sciences, City University, London, UK
Institute of Behavioural Neuroscience, Antwerp, Belgium

Sebastiaan Engelborghs and Peter P. De Deyn
Department of Neurology and Memory Clinic, Middelheim General Hospital (ZNA), Antwerp, Belgium
Laboratory of Neurochemistry and Behavior, Institute Born-Bunge Foundation, University of Antwerp, Antwerp, Belgium
Department of Health Care Sciences, University College Antwerp, Antwerp, Belgium
Department of Nursing Sciences, Faculty of Medicine, University of Antwerp, Antwerp, Belgium

Peter Mariën
Department of Linguistics, Vrije Universtiteit Brussel, Brussel, Belgium
Institute of Behavioural Neuroscience, Antwerp, Belgium
Department of Neurology and Memory Clinic, Middelheim General Hospital (ZNA), Antwerp, Belgium
Laboratory of Neurochemistry and Behavior, Institute Born-Bunge Foundation, University of Antwerp, Antwerp, Belgium

Serena Amici
Memory and Aging Center, Department of Neurology, University of California, San Francisco, USA
Department of Neurosciences, University of Perugia, Perugia, Italy

Maria Luisa Gorno-Tempini
Memory and Aging Center, Department of Neurology, University of California, San Francisco, USA

Jennifer M. Ogar
Memory and Aging Center, Department of Neurology, University of California, San Francisco, USA
VA Northern California Health Care System, Martinez, CA, USA

Nina F. Dronkers
Memory and Aging Center, Department of Neurology, University of California, San Francisco, USA
VA Northern California Health Care System, Martinez, CA, USA
University of California, Davis, Davis, CA, USA

Bruce L. Miller
Memory and Aging Center, Department of Neurology, University of California, San Francisco, USA

Davide Crepaldi and Claudio Luzzatti
Department of Psychology, University of Milano-Bicocca, Milan, Italy

Wei-Chun Che
Otorhinolaryngology Department, Taichung Veterans General Hospital, Taichung, Taiwan

I.-Fan Su
Division of Speech and Hearing Sciences, University of Hong-Kong, Hong-Kong, China

Kyrana Tsapkini
Department of Neurology, Johns Hopkins Medical Institutions, Baltimore, MD, USA
Department of Psychology, Aristotle University of Thessaloniki, Thessaloniki, Greece

Christina Helen Vlahou
Department of Psychology, Aristotle University of Thessaloniki, Thessaloniki, Greece

Costantin Potagas
Department of Neurology, University of Athens, Eginition Hospital, Athens, Greece

Jacquie Kurland and Margaret A. Naeser
Harold Goodglass Boston University Aphasia Research Center, Department of Neurology, Boston University School of Medicine and the Veterans Affairs Boston Healthcare System, USA
University of Colorado at Boulder, Departments of Speech, Language and Hearing Sciences and Neuroscience, USA

Errol H. Bakera, Karl Doron, Paula I. Martin, Heidi E. Seekins and Andrew Bogdan
Harold Goodglass Boston University Aphasia Research Center, Department of Neurology, Boston University School of Medicine and the Veterans Affairs Boston Healthcare System, USA

Perry Renshaw and Deborah Yurgelun-Todd
Brain Imaging Center, McLean Hospital, Belmont, MA and Harvard Medical School, USA

Maria Kambanaros
Cyprus Acquisition Team, Department of English Studies, University of Cyprus, Nicosia, Cyprus

Lambros Messinis
Department of Neurology, Neuropsychology Section, University of Patras Medical School, Patras, Greece

Emmanouil Anyfantis
Department of Speech and Language Therapy, Technological Educational Institute Patras, Patras, Greece

Claudia Repetto, Maria Cotelli and Orazio Zanetti
IRCCS S. Giovanni di Dio Fatebenefratelli, Brescia, Italy

Rosa Manenti
Department of Neuroscience, Vita Salute University and San Raffaele Scientific Institute, Milan, Italy

Marco Calabria
Department of General Psychology, University of Padua, Italy

Barbara Borroni and Alessandro Padovani
Department of Neurology, University of Brescia, Italy

Carlo Miniussi
IRCCS S. Giovanni di Dio Fatebenefratelli, Brescia, Italy
Department of Biomedical Sciences and Biotechnologies, University of Brescia, Italy

Argye E. Hillis
Department of Cognitive Science, Johns Hopkins University, Baltimore, MD, USA
Department of Neurology, Johns Hopkins University School of Medicine, Baltimore, MD, USA
Department of Physical Medicine and Rehabilitation, Johns Hopkins University School of Medicine, Baltimore, MD, USA

Paolo Caffarra
Department of Neuroscience, University of Parma, Parma, Italy

Outpatient Clinic for the Diagnosis and Therapy of Cognitive Disorders, AUSL, Parma, Italy

Simona Gardini, Letizia Concari and Federica Barocco
Department of Neuroscience, University of Parma, Parma, Italy

Francesca Dieci
Outpatient Clinic for the Diagnosis and Therapy of Cognitive Disorders, AUSL, Parma, Italy

Stefano Cappa
Department of Clinical Neuroscience, Vita-Salute San Raffaele Hospital, Milan, Italy

Caterina Ghetti
Medical Physic Department, Azienda Ospedaliero-Universitaria, Parma, Italy

Livia Ruffini
Department of Nuclear Medicine, Azienda Ospedaliero-Universitaria, Parma, Italy

Guido Dalla Rosa Prati
Poliambulatorio Dalla Rosa Prati, Centro Diagnostico Europeo, Parma, Italy

Andreia V. Faria and Susumu Mori
Department of Radiology, Johns Hopkins University School of Medicine, Baltimore, MD, USA

Melissa Newhart and Cameron Davis
Department of Neurology, Johns Hopkins University School of Medicine, Baltimore, MD, USA

Jenny Crinion
University College London, London, UK

Shannon Cooley
Johns Hopkins University, Baltimore, MD, USA

Krist A. Noonan, Sheeba Eshan and Matthew A. Lambon Ralph
School of Psychological Sciences, University of Manchester, Manchester, UK

Elizabeth Jefferies
Department of Psychology, University of York, York, UK

Peter Garrard
Stroke and Dementia Research Centre, St George's University of London, London, UK

Emily Rogalski, Emily Shaw, Sabrina Sawlani and Christina Wieneke
Cognitive Neurology and Alzheimer's Disease Center, Northwestern University Feinberg School of Medicine, Chicago, IL, USA

Sandra Weintraub
Cognitive Neurology and Alzheimer's Disease Center, Northwestern University Feinberg School of Medicine, Chicago, IL, USA
Department of Psychiatry and Behavioral Sciences, Northwestern University Feinberg School of Medicine, Chicago, IL, USA

Alfred Rademaker
Department of Preventive Medicine, Northwestern University Feinberg School of Medicine, Chicago, IL, USA

M.-Marsel Mesulam
Cognitive Neurology and Alzheimer's Disease Center, Northwestern University Feinberg School of Medicine, Chicago, IL, USA
Ken and Ruth Davee Department of Neurology, Northwestern University Feinberg School of Medicine, Chicago, IL, USA

M.L. Henry, M.C. Babiak, B.L. Miller and M.L. Gorno-Tempini
Memory and Aging Center, Department of Neurology, University of California, San Francisco, CA, USA

M.V. Meese
Alta Bates Medical Center, El Cerrito, CA, USA

S. Truong
San Francisco State University, San Francisco, CA, USA

Susy Paolini, Lucia Paciaroni and Osvaldo Scarpino
Unit of Neurology, Italian National Research Center on Aging, Via della Montagnola, Ancona, Italy

Antonio Manca, Roberto Rossi and Daniela Fornarelli
Unit of Radiology, Italian National Research Center on Aging, Ancona, Italy

Stefano F. Cappa
Vita-Salute University and Division of Neuroscience, San Raffaele Scientific Institute, Milan, Italy

Angela M. Abbatecola
Scientific Direction, Italian National Research Center on Aging, Ancona, Italy

Cynthia K. Thompson
Department of Communication Sciences and Disorders, Northwestern University, Evanston, IL, USA

Department of Neurology, Northwestern University, Evanston, IL, USA
Cognitive Neurology and Alzheimer's Disease Center, Northwestern University, Evanston, IL, USA

Aya Meltzer-Asscher and Jiyeon Lee
Department of Communication Sciences and Disorders, Northwestern University, Evanston, IL, USA

Soojin Cho
Department of Communication Sciences and Disorders, Northwestern University, Evanston, IL, USA
Cognitive Neurology and Alzheimer's Disease Center, Northwestern University, Evanston, IL, USA

Sandra Weintraub
Department of Neurology, Northwestern University, Evanston, IL, USA
Cognitive Neurology and Alzheimer's Disease Center, Northwestern University, Evanston, IL, USA
Department of Psychiatry and Behavioral Sciences, Northwestern University, Evanston, IL, USA

Anna Basso
Department of Neurological Sciences, Milan University, Milan, Italy

Margherita Macis
Faculty of Psychology, University of Milano-Bicocca, Milan, Italy

Ezequiel Gleichgerrcht, Teresa Torralva, María Roca and Facundo Manes
Institute of Cognitive Neurology (INECO), Buenos Aires, Argentina
Institute of Neurosciences, Favaloro University, Buenos Aires, Argentina

Daniela Szenkman, Pablo Richly and Mariángeles Pose
Institute of Cognitive Neurology (INECO), Buenos Aires, Argentina

Agustin Ibanez
Institute of Cognitive Neurology (INECO), Buenos Aires, Argentina
Institute of Neurosciences, Favaloro University, Buenos Aires, Argentina
Universidad Diego Portales, Santiago, Chile
National Scientific and Technical Research Council (CONICET), Buenos Aires, Argentina

Index